Death in old age

Death in old age

How a pandemic makes us rethink mortality

Barbara A. Misztal

PETER LANG
Oxford • Bern • Berlin • Bruxelles • New York • Wien

Bibliographic information published by Die Deutsche Nationalbibliothek. Die Deutsche Nationalbibliothek lists this publication in the Deutsche Nationalbibliografie; detailed bibliographic data is available on the Internet at http://dnb.d-nb.de.

A catalogue record for this book is available from the British Library.

Library of Congress Cataloging-in-Publication Data
Names: Misztal, Barbara A., author.
Title: Death in old age : how a pandemic makes us rethink mortality / Barbara A. Misztal.
Description: Oxford ; New York : Peter Lang, [2023] | Includes bibliographical references.
Identifiers: LCCN 2022046290 (print) | LCCN 2022046291 (ebook) | ISBN 9781800790025 (paperback) | ISBN 9781800790032 (ebook) | ISBN 9781800790049 (epub)
Subjects: LCSH: Death. | Mortality. | Old age.
Classification: LCC HQ1073 .M576 2023 (print) | LCC HQ1073 (ebook) | DDC 306.9--dc23/eng/20220930
LC record available at https://lccn.loc.gov/2022046290
LC ebook record available at https://lccn.loc.gov/2022046291

Cover design by Brian Melville for Peter Lang Ltd.

ISBN 978-1-80079-002-5 (print)
ISBN 978-1-80079-003-2 (ePDF)
ISBN 978-1-80079-004-9 (ePub)

Published by Peter Lang Ltd, International Academic Publishers,
Oxford, United Kingdom
oxford@peterlang.com, www.peterlang.com

This publication has been peer reviewed.

For those who are in our memories and for a new bright star, Alfie.

It has come to seem
there is no perfect ending.
Indeed, there are infinite endings.
Or perhaps, once one begins,
there are only endings

Louise Gluck, Faithful and Virtuous Night

Contents

INTRODUCTION:

A special time to talk about death in old age

Why is the topic of death in old age so important and timely?

The main theme of this book is death in old age, with a focus on contemporary Western societies prior to COVID-19 and during the recent pandemic. Such a concern with a singular type of death in these specific contexts means that, while recognizing mortality as a universal human condition, the book does not meditate on death in general or abstract terms. Without delving into discussions of the timeless aspects of mortality in philosophy, theology, art history, psychology, medicine, anthropology, law and education, it views death as one of the most difficult, complex and diverse events in human life. While acknowledging that the awareness of mortality has played a different role in different societies through history, it explores the place and narratives of death in old age in 'greying' Western societies. By placing the discussion of death in old age in the context of the period of 'the normality of our previous normal' (Zizek 2020) and the very abnormal times of the COVID-19 pandemic, this book aims to prompt rethinking of societal obligations to the aged and to reflect on possible ways to handle death in old age. It looks at death in old age in normal times, when broader cultural and moral tales would 'try to inoculate us against fear of death by banalizing and de-toxicating the sight of dying' (Bauman 2011: 392), and compares this with death from COVID-19, which has been unpredictable, statistical, depersonalized and lonely. While accepting that attitudes towards dying and death prevalent in the present are 'neither unalterable nor accidental' (Elias 1985: 84) and without assuming that the impact of COVID-19 will result in a total or permanent alteration of standards, the book discusses which values and orientations towards death in old age have been reinforced and which have been challenged by the pandemic. Thus, the book offers a platform to debate society's responsibility to old people and to explore the legacy of the pandemic in order to reflect on the quality of end-of-life care.

The topic of death in old age is very timely and important for several reasons, including that by talking about death in old age we can create a much-needed space for debates about death. In Western societies until recently, the topic of death generally was perceived to be something of a taboo. Until the beginning of this century, the sociological literature on death and dying built its theoretical paradigms upon Philippe Aries's (1981) assumption of the taboo of death in modern society. However, from the 1970s onwards, the topic of death has gradually become less unmentionable as the 'thanatological revolution' animated death studies across Western Europe and the United States. Since then, the number and quality of studies dedicated to death have been growing (Broom 2015; Hockey 1990; Holloway 2007; Lawton, Julia 2000; Kellehear 2009; Neimeyer 1995; Walter 2020). Moreover, the popularity of self-help manuals about how to secure a 'good death or 'death with dignity' – works ranging from Jane Feinman's (2006) *How to Have a Good Death* to Lyons and Winter's (2021) *We All Know How This Ends)* has increased, while images of death – especially of sudden and heroic death – have frequently been presented on TV screens and other media. With these trends making death more visible, today's culture can no longer be described as a culture of 'death denial' or the 'death taboo' (Walter 2020). Yet, even though death is no longer always invisible, death in old age still remains a topic that is removed from the everyday experience of many people and is not explored (Gawande 2014; Zimmermann 2012). In our society, death in old age – which is often a medicalized, prolonged, lengthy and complex process – is hidden from public view (Carr and Luth 2019; Lloyd 2015).We avoid planning for it and feel awkward around old people who are grieving. However, precisely because death is now most likely to occur at the end of a long life, it is important to know how to ensure the quality of the end-of-life care for the elderly as well as to understand their views and values in relation to 'the greatest event' in life, as death is portrayed in Rilke's poem 'The Song of the Life and Death'.

Death is 'not the problem of the dead, but of the living, and that means us' (Oz 1972: 240). Hence, by confronting mortality and by broadening our understanding of the role of death in old age in modern society, we can throw light on the cultural values that influence how we understand mortality in the West. Coming face to face with mortality not only makes life seem vulnerable and fragile; it also enhances our receptiveness to morality because the awareness of mortality can make one a more moral person (Genna 2020). The sense of mortality is the essential part of why our lives matter, why we care, why we take on responsibilities and why we value freedom, justice and dignity (Hägglund 2021). Although we need to admit that it would be disparaging to live with the continual awareness of our mortality, there is a need to acknowledge that now is a unique time to talk about death in later life. We have been led to rethink mortality in contemporary times because people who live under the protections of modern medicine, and who will be kept alive for longer than would have been conceivable even a century ago, now perceive death as not their problem, as something very distant that they know little about, and have no desire to consider (Engelhart 2022). In other words, the engagement with the issue of death in old aged has never been so important as now, when new moral dilemmas are triggered by the deferral of dying to old age and, at the same time, there is an absence of ethical attention to death in old age (Davis 2020). Because of the absence of conceptualizations of death in old age in today's cultural narratives, and because people no longer expect to die before their old age, they feel immune from death and see it as a very distant topic. Hence the issue of death in the elderly – which is often death from disabling, chronic and degenerative diseases, which may take many months or years – tends to be kept well hidden in the background. Yet the marginalization of death in old age can impact the quality of the end-of-life care, and this means this issue requires urgent rethinking in our ageing societies.

Above all, the topic of death in old age is connected to the fact that death now increasingly occurs at the end of a long life. As the large post-war baby boomer generation is ageing, all developed nations can expect a big increase in death rates until around 2050. In the United Kingdom, as a result of the significant decline in mortality from 2001 to 2020, 18%

of the population is now above 65 years of age (Spiegelhalter and Masters 2021: 136), while over the last thirty years, the number of people aged 90 years or more has increased by more than two and a half times, reaching recently 609,503 (Office of National Statistics 2020). The same trends are visible in other Western countries. For instance, 23% of the Italian population is now above 65 years old, while in Japan, the country with the highest life expectancy, 29% of people were over 65 years old in 2020 (Spiegelhalter and Masters 2021: 136). Now, with the average length of life in the developed world being above 80 years, death in old age is the most common modern type of death (Lloyd 2015). For example, in the United Kingdom between 1990 and 2017, the share of deaths in the over-seventies age cohort has increased from one-third to half of all deaths (Richie and Roser 2019), while in 2021 two-thirds of 585,412 deaths registered in England and Wales were among people aged over 75 years (Scobie and Hutchings 2022). Presently in Britain, most people die when they are over the age of eighty, with approximately 90% of deaths being of people aged over 65 years (Age UK 2015). In the United States in 2015, 2.7 million deaths – that is, 32% of all deaths – were of persons aged 85 years and older, 24% were of persons aged between 75 and 84 years and 19% were of persons aged between 65 and 74 years (Carr and Luth 2019: 517). In other words, in 'greying' Western societies, social and political concerns about death in old age are becoming more pressing.

Finally, the subject of death in old age is timely because the recent COVID-19 pandemic has not only made death more visible; it has also disproportionately affected the elderly. This has raised questions about how modern societies can best protect the aged. The World Health Organization (WHO 2022) has estimated that the global actual excess deaths – that is, the number of deaths that occurred beyond those expected without the pandemic – reached almost 15 million. The WHO report, released in May 2022, also found that age mattered, with 82% of the deaths occurring among people above the age of 60 (Balloux 2022: 49). The WHO figure points out that older people, especially if they suffer from chronic illnesses, have been at higher risk of death from COVID-19 than younger age groups. Already in the first year of the COVID-19 pandemic, the international data showed that once infected with the virus, the chance of death was one in 100 at age sixty-five, one in twenty-five at age 75, and one in seven at age 85, while for the youngest age groups, the risk from COVID-19 was 'broadly comparable to those [from] everyday activities' (Levin, Cochran and Walsh 2020: 24). The United Kingdom was also hit hard by COVID-19, with the country recording over 170,000 deaths linked to the disease and seeing the biggest rise in age-standardized mortality rates for seventy years since the major flu epidemic of 1951 (Spiegelhalter and Masters 2021). In Britain in 2020, people aged over 90 years had 35,000 times the risk of dying of COVID-19 as young children. Hence, it can be observed that 'this virus, just, like normal life, persecutes older people' (Spiegelhalter and Masters 2021: 125).

Because of COVID-19's age-specific pattern of mortality – namely, that each ten-year increase in age more than doubles the risk of death for the virus (Webb 2020), since the beginning of the pandemic, there has been a need for government to take on social and public health responsibilities to protect older people from the COVID-19 risk in hospitals, homes and care settings. Yet, despite the high level of deaths in the elderly population and despite the Office of National Statistics (2021) data showing the high proportion (25.7%) of deaths of care home residents involving COVID-19, the problem of the threat posed to older people by the virus has not been addressed adequately. Fortunately, the rates of hospitalization and death for the aged have been reduced as a result of the successful vaccination programme, which in the United Kingdom began on 8 December 2020. In the following months, apart from vaccines and antiviral drugs, better treatments and greater knowledge of how the disease progresses have contributed to lowering the rates of hospitalization and to saving the lives of many elderly people. Yet through the whole pandemic, even though the vaccine uptake among the aged has been above 90%, the risk for aged people has continued because the effectiveness of the vaccines declines more quickly in older people and new variants of the virus have emerged. Moreover, with the growing public weariness and with the United Kingdom, in April 2022, passing the responsibility for everyday protective behaviour on to individuals, elderly people – especially those with underlying health conditions – and any other people with a compromised immune system have continued to face the risk in public places. Despite the evidence that the overall mortality rate has varied hugely by age through the whole pandemic, the particular risk posed by the coronavirus to the elderly did not become a key focus of British policy during the health crisis.

As many studies show, despite COVID-19's age-specific mortality pattern, several governments – including Britain's – have shown total disregard for social and public health responsibilities towards elderly people by not prioritizing the protection of the aged (Calasanti 2020; Calvert and Arbuthnott 2021; Clarke 2021; Dodsworth 2021; Martin and de Saille 2022). In other words, together with the pandemic, there has been 'a parallel outbreak of ageism' (Ayalon et al. 2020) or discrimination against older adults rooted in the acceptance of the difference between old and young as justifying the exclusion of the aged (Calasanti 2020). By neglecting its obligations to increase efforts to protect the elderly who have been at the greatest risk from the COVID-19 pandemic, and by employing the ageist rhetoric and accepting 'the brutal fact' that losing people in old age 'does not cause as much economic or social disruption as losing children or people of working and childbearing age' (MacKenzie 2020: xxv), the UK government has been relaying on and reinforcing ageist prejudices and stereotypes. The UK policy of managing the health crisis, rooted in viewing the pandemic as affecting 'just some elderly in care homes', and comments that people dying from COVID-19 are 'just essentially all over 80' have scapegoated the elderly. According to Caroline Abrahams, director of the charity Age UK, it is ageism not to be concerned about the elderly dying of COVID-19. Tedros Adhanom Ghebreyesus, director-general of the WHO goes further, describing this policy as 'moral bankruptcy at its highest'.

The COVID-19 crisis has revealed that ageism is still embedded in British society and has exposed its application in the UK government's handling of the recent pandemic. Because of the ageism inherent in the British government's COVID-19 policy, the United Kingdom's elderly people have faced a double risk. Apart from their low adaptive immunity, which puts them at risk of both catching and dying from the virus, and the waning effects of the vaccine, the aged have also faced additional risks as a result of government policy failures. For instance, aged people have been faced with the risk of being transferred from hospitals to care homes without testing for COVID-19, and have been denied access to hospitals and/or ventilators so this equipment might be reassigned to younger people who are more likely to survive (Calvert and Arbuthnott 2021; Clarke 2021; Cooper and Szreter 2021; Francis 2020, 2021; Horton 2020). The underlying ageism of the governmental policies of handling the recent pandemic has also had a negative impact on older people's feelings of security, been detrimental to their mental health and affected their physical condition. In addition to the use of the narrative of ageism, the 'fear-based' policy narrative has been applied to manipulate the general public's deep-rooted fears of contagion and death (Dodsworth 2021).

Moreover, the pandemic has revealed the faultlines in British society in terms of poverty, lower incomes and higher-risk jobs and ethnicity, as well as regional disparities in healthcare resources and access to health and care services. The COVID-19 crisis has not only exposed and supplemented the existing discrimination against older adults and fuelled many injustices, but has also revealed the structural problems that exist in the UK medical and care systems, both seen as struggling to provide palliative and hospice care. Hence, it is important to question how we should proceed in terms of the quality of end-of-life care after the current crisis has abated. To learn lessons from the COVID-19 pandemic about how older people should be protected and how the quality of the end-of-life care should be ensured, we should acknowledge that although the pandemic has disrupted daily routines, and brought tragedy and disorder to concrete human lives, the coronarius crisis, like other collective threats, has also created an opportunity to review and revise people's priorities and to mobilize for change. A new value of solidarity, together with the inequalities connected with age, ethnicity, race, and class revealed by the pandemic, might mean that COVID-19 can contribute to enlarging the scope for social change and for much-needed reforms of the health and care systems.

While looking at government attempts to balance obligations towards the aged with other values, such as economic growth and the needs of the younger generations, this book discusses the impact of governmental policies of 'prioritising the young over the old' on quality of the older population's end-of-life care (Reisz 2020: 3). By exposing the underlying tensions in handling old people's care at the end of life both before and during the health crisis, the volume aims to reflect on the ethical dimensions revealed by the pandemic. While showing the increased visibility of death of older people during the pandemic, the book argues that the death of the old cannot be regarded simply as an untimely problem or inconvenient cost because all deaths count: with every death, an entire and irreplaceable world is lost (Derrida 1992).

The content of the book

The structure of the book reflects its two main topics: death in old age and the impact of the pandemic on the quality of elderly people's end-of-life care, with all chapters dealing with the issues connected with death in old age in both pre-COVID and COVID times. While not dealing with death in spiritual and physical terms, this book aims to show death as the ultimate diverse and hard-to-predict event, as for 'all the death, we die unrehearsed', as Les Murray (2013) states in his poem 'Corniche'. Writing about death in old age in two different contexts and writing mainly about the United Kingdom – one of the world's less religious societies – do not just limit our possibility of tackling the universality of the mortal condition, but do not leave a space for in a detailed consideration of the role of religion in death. While recognizing the impact of secularization on attitudes towards death in modern societies, the book also acknowledges that even within multicultural contexts where secularism is a significant mode of belief and personal practice, death and dying are embedded within forms of religiosity (Broom 2015; McManus 2013). The volume does not analyse changes in the social construction and experiences of death in old age from any religious perspective, and it is not concerned with the ideas of afterlife and immortality offered by world religions. Yet, as older people are much more likely than younger people to declare that they have a religion (Woodhead 2016), and as religion still often plays a part in people's engagement with death, the book pays attention to the role of religion and other cultural resources in negotiating death practices and following death rituals. For example, as many death ceremonies still take place in formal religious institutions, when describing funeral rituals or other death-related practices, the significance of religion cannot be overlooked.

To explore death in old age under two different health and structural conditions, we will focus on older people when they are approaching death as a consequence of an inevitable and irreversible deterioration of their ageing organisms. Although British official accounts assume that old people are generally those of pensionable age – that is, over 65 years of age – here, as the main theme of the volume confines our attention to old people in the last stage of their lives – we are interested in the distinct chronological period associated with 'the oldest old, typically after the age of 80' (Carr and Luth 2019: 515). The impact of the recent COVID-19 pandemic on death in old age will be approached through a sociological lense. Even though many books have been published about COVID-19 (e.g. Clarke 2021; Hennessy 2022; Horton 2020; Sridhar 2022; Spiegelhalter and Masters 2021); however, they are mainly written from the medical, biological, statistical or journalistic perspectives and their contents are dominated by issues of the pandemic's origin, treatments, tests, vaccine and policies. As I am a sociologist, I am not interested in the COVID-19 pandemic as a biomedical occurrence, but rather as the sociological phenomenon shaped by social variables, values, fears and anxieties. The social construction of the coronavirus pandemic involves its social costs and a recognition of the significance of the social processes shaping it. Such a perspective also leads to viewing pandemics as times of loss and grief, alterations in people's social relationships, routines, livelihoods and ways of dying and being interred. Although much of the book's discussion of death in old age will apply to modern Western societies generally, debates about COVID-19 narratives and policies will be placed explicitly in the British context. As the COVID crisis has increased risks and introduced new challenges for the elderly, we look at what has happened to care and circumstances of death in old age during the pandemic in the United Kingdom, and at the implications of these new threats and changes in conditions of dying for our sense of mortality and our responsibility for old people who are in their final stage of life.

While acknowledging that the pandemic has exacerbated the deep-seated economic and social inequalities that exist in the United Kingdom, and revealed the country's ethnic and regional divisions, this book focuses only on older people and the policies that applied to them during COVID-19. It recognizes that the pandemic highlighted the scale of health inequalities regarding the risks faced by those living with chronic diseases and disabilities, including individuals with immunocompromised systems. For example, 35% more lives were lost in the 20% most deprived areas in the United Kingdom than in the least, with 45% more years of life lost in total (Health Foundation 2022). Moreover, there was disproportionality in the deaths from COVID among Black, Asian and minority ethnic healthcare staff, as 21% of all staff are Black, Asian or minority ethnic but 63% of healthcare workers who died were Black, Asian or minority ethnic (Marsh and McIntyre 2020). The book also concedes that the COVID-19 pandemic brought suffering not only to older people but also to younger people who, while being at low risk from the virus, have forgone education, friends and work. Yet, because of its subject matter, it is only concerned with the pandemic and the impact of relevant policies on older people.

To achieve its aims – that is, to compare death in old age under two different health and structural conditions – this book brings together various approaches, perspectives, materials and disciplines. Contrasting death in old age under two different circumstances requires a rich collection of research across disciplines and genres, from gerontology and death studies to statistics and literature. In order to fully account for people's experiences of the COVID-19 emergency, it is also essential to incorporate relatively recent and various types of works, from journalistic reports and freshly published political and medical studies of the pandemic, through people's recollections and memories of COVID-19 (such as diaries and memories preserved on various digital platforms), to reviews of government policies by two select committees on the early response of the British government to the coronavirus pandemic. Only such a 'trespassing' (to use Albert Hirschman's 1993 phrase), which brings together various genres and disciplines, can offer us the possibility to bridge fragmentations and gaps between various approaches in debates on death about the end of life and discussions about the legacy of COVID-19 and its impact on our ways of thinking about death in old age.

The book is divided into three parts, each consisting of three chapters, with each chapter exploring a given topic in both contexts: the pre-COVID period and during the pandemic. Part I, while questioning common assumptions that old people 'know how to die', that old age 'makes dying easier' and that death of the elderly is 'natural' (Lloyd 2004: 237), discusses the tendency of modern Western societies to keep the deaths of old people hidden and in the background. It argues that despite the recent extension of life, which has made death in old age the dominant type of death in developed nations, contemporary societies still lack a language to help people to understand and talk about death in old age. The analyses in the last segments of each chapter in the first part of the book demonstrate that the COVID-19 pandemic has increased the visibility of death in old age and has brought to the surface modern ageism, which is one of the last socially sanctioned biases to be embedded in social institutions and interactions (Holstein 2015). This part of the book concludes that, by exposing ageist prejudices and revealing intergenerational tensions, the recent health crisis raises questions about background assumptions of societal perceptions of older people and about society's responsibilities towards the aged.

Part II illustrates how death implicitly inhibits older people's everyday experiences and practices. It argues that older adults increasingly live in the shadow of death, not only because they often suffer from multiple chronic conditions but also due to their numerous encounters with the deaths of their friends and family members, and because of their confrontation with the problem of death in the public sphere. When the risk and visibility of death in the public sphere increase rapidly, as they did during the pandemic, the scope for a profound reckoning with life and death shrinks and older adults reflect on death and dying in the light of new fears about their own vulnerability, worries about their loss of control over the end of life and anxiety about a lack of contact with loved ones in their final moments. During the COVID-19 crisis, the higher frequency of encounters with death and new rules for burial services meant the traditional role of cemeteries as places where one could communicate with the whole family and friends was compromised. With the pandemic imposing restrictions on intimacy in death, these new circumstances were very unsettling for many older people.

Part III explores the variety of conditions, places and ways of dying that are found in later life and their alteration in the context of COVID-19.

It starts by debating what is happening in the context of the *memento mori* (the remembrance of death) and goes on to show the implications of the awareness of mortality in the process of the transformation associated with ageing. After acknowledging that experiences and perspectives on death differ within and among cultures, and presenting a short review of arguments and studies of the fear and acceptance of death in older age, this part focuses on two extreme ways of dying. The first refers to a situation where the old person is aware of the impending death and still has the chance to maintain some control and choice at the end of life. The second type of death denotes death in 'the fourth age' – that is, the experience of dying where the process of deterioration in physical and mental capacities means that the dying person is unable to manage and control the end of life (Gilleard and Higgs 2010). Both kinds of dying have been affected by the COVID-19 pandemic, which has added new layers of vulnerability, enforced loneliness and confusion to the lives of frail older people, who were already feeling abandoned.

The Epilogue, while assuming that the worst of the pandemic is behind us, calls for the continuation of debating what COVID-19 has left behind, and what lessons are to be learnt from it. It makes a case for the importance of talking about death in later life and for a recognition of the significance of choice regarding how we want to die and the quality of end-of-life care.

PART I

The only normal death-age

CHAPTER 1

Too old to die young: *The perception and visibility of death in old age*

Part I of this book, while questioning the assumption that death in old age is 'natural' and 'on schedule' (Lloyd 2004: 237), proposes a rethink of whether 'the old is dreaded because it has become the only normal death-age' (Blythe 1979: 96). All three chapters dispute the factors behind the invisibility of death in old age, including the role of language in stereotyping the old, the dominant conceptualizations of ageing process and viewing the ageing population as a burden and a threat. They also explore the COVID-19 pandemic's impact on longevity and on the profile of death in old age, and discuss how the recent health crisis has exposed ageism and generational tensions.

This chapter argues that the marginalization of death of older persons is still upheld by the perception of death in old age as timely, expected, appropriate, distant and normal – in other words, as not 'our' problem. It further critically reviews the assumption that death in old age is natural by exploring the historical trends in longevity and changes in ways of dying, including the medicalization of death. The chapter also indicates that characterizing death in old age as a normal and natural implies acceptance or resignation on the part of elderly people while in reality older people are often actively engaged in controlling and remaking the dying process. The final section of the chapter explores how the coronavirus pandemic, by the inclusion of death in the normal fields of everyday life and by exacerbating anxieties about the futility of life, has not only impacted the visibility of death in old age but also led us to rethink how older people are cared for at the end of their lives.

The theme of death has been engaging philosophers, religious communities and civic cultures for centuries. While the awareness of mortality has always been seen as the defining truth of human existence, the persistence of varieties of understandings of this tragic and inconsolable event reflects the notion of death's complexity, difficulty and ambiguity. These features of death are revealed in an enormous body of literature on this topic, ranging from philosophy, theology, psychology and sociological theories of death, to studies of narratives of death in literature and poems, to images of death in photographs and theatre, and research into the relationship of the dead body with technology. All these approaches represent the diversity of understandings and conceptualizations of the notion of death; moreover, these disciplines do not speak in one voice. Even philosophy, which tends to concern itself very much with death and adopts death as the muse of its craft, is full of contradictory thoughts on death. For example, while some philosophers – from ancient to contemporary examples – idealize death (Plato), others glorify it (Schelling); some portray death as terrifying fate (Aristotle), while still others see death as a liberation from an unbearable existence (Nietzsche). Moreover, in contrast to thinkers such as Epicurus who appreciate death's moralizing effect and value death for giving rise to reflections on life, other philosophers, such as Sartre, view death as depriving life of all sense and making our existence meaningless (Choron 1965). Symbolic presentations of death have always varied widely, from an 'inevitable evil' to the Grim Reaper, the Great Leveller, the Dark Angle, the Pale Rider with a deadly scythe and 'an unwelcome and devilish adversary' (Black 2018: 3), to metaphors of death as a benign occurrence, such as a 'deep sleep', 'a fine and quiet place' and 'the Welcome Visitor' (Stark 2016:197).

The human experience of death has changed over the course of history. In the past, when the common symbols, traditions, religions and ceremonies of society were giving meaning to people's experience of death, the ambiguities and difficulties in understandings of death were constrained by the main cultural and religious narratives. In such societies, death was less ambiguous and less subjective as people were prepared for death by the ordering rituals and normative guidance that existed (Aries 1981). However, in our modern Western nations, this is no longer the case. In contemporary cultures, as common symbols and shared traditions have faded or disappeared altogether, the meaning of death has become more private and more ambiguous. Today's lack of rules, directions and shared expectations about how to care for and cope with challenges of the end of life means that the majority of us are puzzled by the complex relationship between life and death. As our knowledge about death and dying is has expanded little, and as ambivalence and difficulties in our understanding of death are not confined by cultural practices and narratives, we tend to cope with these problems by covering them with great social salience (Davis 2020).

Hence, even though the total taboo or denial of death is no longer the underlying feature of modern culture (Aries 1981; Kellehear 2007; Walter 2020), we deal with the ambivalence of our attitudes to death by keeping a distance from death in our daily lives. Nothing is more indicative of such attempts to distance ourselves from death than the silence about death in old age that characterizes today's modern culture. In advanced Western societies, there is not only a tendency to marginalize the elderly and keeping the death of old hidden in the background, but also 'a profound tendency to prevent or deny the changes and declines of age' (Lamb 2015: 42). In today's developed nations, where the gains in life expectancy have displaced death into old age, most people assume they will live into older age, even consider death in old age as their right, and designate old age as the appropriate time to die. Hence, seen as being too far away in the future to constitute a central component of people's lives, death in old age tends to be framed as a problem that does not need to be dealt with by society. Moreover, this type of thinking is assisted by viewing older people's acceptance of life coming to an end as 'natural' (Blythe 2005: 133). The roots of this idea can be traced back to the ancient thought that old age is preparing us for death. From Stoics, through Montaigne, to modern times, old age has been seen as making death more desirable than life, showing courage in the face of death and as opting for death as a way of escaping the disabilities, boredom, decline and miseries of old age. According to this perspective, older people's death makes more sense than continuing to live forever. Since death frees them from pain and suffering, and since they have already had a long life, old people 'ought not to be repining at the approach of death' (Socrates, quoted in Choron 1965: 45).

The perception of death of elderly people as a normal occurrence can be found in today's everyday expressions, which stress how timely, expected, appropriate and normal the death of older people should be. Daily phrases also suggest that old people have died because they 'have worn out' or 'got tired' (Humphrys and Jarvis 2010: 44), 'were getting on a bit' or 'lived to a ripe grand age' (Hockey 1990: 37). Typical comments after the death of older persons, while conveying grief, also emphasize that as the older elderly have 'lived long enough' and 'had a good life', one 'shouldn't feel so full of grief' (Terkel 2002: xxiii). In other words, if the person who died 'was an old man' who 'had a good life', one should 'try not to let it get to you so much' (O'Hagan 1999: 231). Moreover, when somebody old dies, it is 'unsurprising', as 'what could be more ordinary?' (Terkel 2002: 227). And, after all, such a death is not threating as it is only 'the old [who] died' (Enright 2020: 321). In contrast to death in old age, which does not increase our fear of the end and is seen as timely, death prior to old age is perceived as threatening, tragic, premature and wasteful. For example, the cancer-related death of a younger person is commonly associated with the terms 'untimely' and 'tragic', while the death of an older person, regardless of the causes, is viewed as 'normal' and 'expected' (Lawton 2000; Lloyd 2004).

Such everyday expressions and talking about older people's death as a 'natural', while reducing our own fear of death, also help to hide the death of old people. By viewing death in old age as 'a normal', we tend to keep death in a distance, reduce the sense of futility of life and therefore uphold a sense of normality. In other words, we make death not relevant to us, or neutralize death's sting, by considering older people's death as a 'natural'. In short, by viewing death in old age as a distant and normal, we tend to keep death in old age a private, and hidden issue. This type of approach, together with the institutionalization of death in old age (which will be discussed in Part III), while perhaps not necessarily diffusing our fear of death, reduces social concern about responsibility for older people and for the quality of the end-of-life care by contributing to the invisibility of the death of old people.

This invisibility of death of old people in Western society today is also sustained by the media's language and images, which tend to protect viewers' enjoyment and reflect the celebration of youth in popular culture. Even though there has been an increasing presence of actual deaths in news bulleting and a growing number of portrayals of fictional death in films and television series since the last decade of the twentieth century, these references are very rarely portrayed as death in old age. Thus, despite the fact the different generations are defined by their different media habits, the majority of us still get a similarly evasive message about death that comes with ageing,. Since nothing sells like fear, the media are populated with the presentation of death as violent, tragic, dramatic, unexpected, heroic or involving a famous person. News programmes or documentaries tend to try to avoid images of death in old age as this type of death is seen being 'too close home' and 'not selling' well (McManus 2013: 226). Although representations of death in old age cannot totally be eliminated – especially from soap operas, which is the genre most associated with representations of everyday issues – even in this genre, the deaths of older people are infrequently represented, as deaths in soap operas are 'almost three time more likely to be from violent causes than would be expected from a character's age and sex' (Crayford et al. 1997: 16). In many new fictional presentations of death – for example, in such television series as *Six Foot Under* or *The Big C*, ordinary death mainly means the death of young people, such as a suburban young mother diagnosed with terminal cancer (McManus 2013: 212). Thus, both fictional and actual accounts of extraordinary death and ordinary death tend to overlook death in old age. Journalists, bloggers and reality TV producers all adhere to the lack of concern in popular culture with the real issues connected to mortality, while focusing on forensics, dissection, decay and crime, with corpses at centre stage. News, documentaries, soap operas, video games and internet memorial and grief sites all convey messages about how death is to be seen as distant and not frightening – as not yet part of one's life's journey (Haunch 2010). In short, the media play a vital part in the process of hiding death in old age.

It can therefore be argued that the knowledge about death that comes from the media is lacking on two accounts. First, although death is becoming more present in the media, we are still not very familiar with death of old people hidden away in care homes or hospitals. Despite the fact that 'the mediated sharing of the stories of strangers' deaths maybe the most common death experience in modern culture' (Kitch and Hume 2008: xvii), this experience has never – until recently – included stories about death in old age, particularly elderly people residing in nursing homes or hidden away in hospitals, as this type of death was seen as not newsworthy. For the whole of history, people have experienced dying at close range, at home;

people were therefore familiar with it, and death was not alien to young or older people (Kellehear 2007). Furthermore, although mediated experiences of death are important for our understanding of death in the modern age (Hanusch 2010), these provide only a partial knowledge of death; this is not only because the media rarely offer encounters with deaths of older people, but also because media-relayed knowledge is not first-hand experience. Moreover, this secondary – or mediated – experience of death not only limits the scope of our understanding the death in old age, but also plays role in defusing our fear of death with the help of neutralizing metaphors and the viewing of death in old age as 'natural' or 'normal' death.

Apart from making older people's deaths invisible and reducing our own fear of death, such representations and also views that the death of an older person is a 'natural progression' can be seen as a part of society's negative stereotyping associated with ageing. Our attitudes to the death of elderly people, as exposed by our daily narratives, are based on the assumption that elderly people are 'not us'; they are strangers as 'they have one foot in the grave' (Blythe 2005: 21). By introducing distance from older people's fate, and ultimately between life and death, younger generations in contemporary society set the deaths of older people apart from themselves and stigmatize the aged as 'others'. Moreover, the assumption that an elderly person sees death as a natural event marking the completion of their life, and the expectation that they will embrace their finitude without fear, can facilitate ageism and is not necessarily helpful for elderly people themselves. The vocabulary of this viewpoint draws on such notions as 'living well, dying well' and stresses the importance of a proper 'timing' of death, while painting a picture of 'a gross mistimed' death – that is, death that is not easy and natural, but rather a social embarrassment and a burden to society and its resources (Kellehear 2007: 248). The rhetoric of elderly people's acceptance of and responsibility for death as an inevitable and normal event implies not only resignation on the part of elderly people but, by characterizing death in old age as easy and natural, also assumes that everyone dies at the right time and without too much pain, suffering and dependency.

The assumption that death loses its frightening character as the individual becomes older overlooks the fact that the older people are not an homogenous group, but rather differ not only in terms of their social, ethnic and economic characteristics, but also in terms of their past experiences and their levels of suffering and incapacity of body and/or mind (Lloyd 2000). This group is shaped by larger social and cultural factors, gender differences, and health and age differences – for example, those aged over 85 years compared with a group of those aged between 70 and 85 years accepted dependency more easily and gave up control over some aspects of their lives (Cruikshank 2003: 21). The diversity of older people's life-courses, attitudes and experiences means that some of them would like to have total control of over the process of dying, while others would wish for help and support through the process of dying. Furthermore, many studies of attitudes to death and dying focused on people over the age of 75 revealed that death in old age is not always an easy and welcome experience (Howarth 2007). With today's dying being characterized by making choices among medical procedures and ways of dying – including assisted dying – the language that constructs old age as a natural timing of death is no longer appropriate for such a debate. The notion of natural death in old age as an abstract cultural ideal and as 'a somehow ethically neutral event that is unhampered by technological interference' (Kaufman 2005: 323) overlooks the fact that older people can have different resources and opinions on the use of medical interventions at the end of life.

In what follows, we will discuss two main reasons for not seeing the death of the elderly as a part of the natural order: the historical relationships between old age and death; and the advances in medical science and technology that have occurred, which have put decisions about prolongation of life and the timing of death into human hands.

Changes to life expectancy and ways of dying

Every society has ideas about the 'right' time to die, and in contemporary Western nations this is usually believed to be in old age (Howarth 2007: 52). To realize just how modern this relationship between old age and death is, it is enough to remember that in the 1660s, when people firstly became interested in the idea of calculating life expectancies, the average British person lived to just over thirty years, while a child born in the United Kingdom today can expect to live more than fifty years longer than that (Johnson 2021). Another good illustration of the past idea about death in old age is Montaigne's (1533–92) belief that it was total foolishness to expect to die from 'draining away of one's strength caused by extreme old age'. In his day, dying in old age was a 'rare death', unique and outside the normal order, a 'singular and extraordinary death', so 'less natural than others' (Montaigne 1987: 101, 103). Montaigne retired from active life at the age of 39 and died at the age of 59, which was above his own prediction and above the average life expectancy at birth for Europeans at that time, which was just under 40 years.

In pre-industrial Europe, death rates were high at all ages but a small numbers of people survived to old age, thus the age structure of these societies was characterized by the small proportion of the older population, the high volume of death and the low life expectancy at birth. For example, English society between 1574 and 1821 had a higher proportion of very young children and a lower proportion of older people (Laslett 1969: 217), while there was a very high rate of infant and child mortality – over 12% of all children would die in their first year of life in in the late sixteenth and early seventeenth centuries, which contributed to the low life expectancy (Marshall 1980: 23). Although death visited the young more frequently than the old, all lives were threatened by outbreaks of plagues, epidemics and famines, as well as poverty. Since the second half of the eighteenth century, the historical changes in mortality as a result of the decline in infant mortality and the control of infectious diseases have been lowering the death rate and increasing life expectancy in Europe. The Industrial Revolution brought about an accelerated improvement in mortality rates and consequently, since 1840 in most European countries, there has been an increase in life expectancy of three years every year (Grant and Scott 2016: 17). The increased life expectancy at birth in the industrialized countries from 40 years in 1840 to 45 years by 1880 and to over 50 years by the end of century was a result of the decline in infant and child mortality rates (Marshall 1980: 13). During the latter part of the nineteenth century in England, the infant mortality rate was 150 per 1,000 (Marshall 1980: 13), while in 1900 in England and Wales, 25% of deaths were of infants under 12 months of age and by the end of the century, this had fallen to only 1% of deaths (Walter 2017: 7).

In Western countries during the transition from pre-industrial to today's post-industrial societies, death has largely been postponed into old age (Walter 2020). In 1900, 12% of deaths were among those aged over 75 years, despite the age structure of European societies at that time still including a low proportion of older people (Walter 2017: 7). For example, the 1900 figure of the percentage of population over the age of 65 for England and Wales was 4.7, while for Germany the figure was 4.9 (Marshall 1980: 13). The significant increases in the proportion of the aged population occurred only in the twentieth century, when all Western societies witnessed a decline in child mortality, and a subsequent improvement in longevity. Since the mid-nineteenth century, people in the United States have also been living longer, but in 1900, the life expectancy of an average American at birth was still only 47 years (Emanuel 2014). In the twentieth century, life expectancy at birth in developed countries was almost double what it had been in 1841. This doubling of life expectancy happened not only because of medical advances, such a as vaccines, antibiotics and better medical care that saved more children from premature death and effectively treated infections, but also as a result of developments in public health and improvement in living standards, artificial fertilizers, hygienic plumbing, fewer famines and the introduction of safety technology and regulations (Johnson 2021).

In the United Kingdom, the population steadily grew older through the latter half of the twentieth century: in 1990 there were 9.1 million UK residents aged 65 years and over, representing 15.8% of the total population, while in 2016 there were 11.8 million, accounting for 18% of the total population (ONS 2018). The probability of death for an 80-year-old man in England in 1950 was 14%; this has now fallen to 8%. For a 90-year-old, the probability has fallen from 30% to 20% over the same period (Grant and Scott 2016: 18). At the end of the twentieth century, the age at which people died had changed significantly, as deaths among the over-75s had increased to 59% of all deaths; thus death has moved from 'the province of infancy and childhood to that old age' (Walter 2017: 7). In the United

States by 1930, the life expectancy of an average American at birth was approximately 59.7 years; by 1960, it was 69.7 years; by 1990, it had increased to 75.4 years and in the last several decades increases in longevity have been achieved mainly by extending the lives of people over 60 years as the infant mortality rate has stabilized (Emanuel 2014). In the United Kingdom in the first two decades of the twenty-first century, mortality rates continued to improve: the proportions of all deaths in the younger age groups are small, while two-thirds of deaths occur in people over 75 years of age (Wolpert 2011: 222). All age groups have benefited from an improvement in mortality rates as the proportions of all deaths in the younger age groups are small, while people are living longer and 80% of all deaths are among people aged 65 and over (Wolpert 2011: 222). In the United Kingdom, deaths under 60 years of age accounted for just 9% of all male deaths and around 6% of all female deaths in the period 2012–14 (ONS 2015).

Although the global average life expectancy has more than doubled since 1900, and is now above 70 years, and although it can be claimed that this the global doubling of life expectancy is one of the greatest achievement in human history (Johnson 2021), the story of this human progress is not totally unproblematic. First, there has never been equality in the expansion of longevity between developed and less-developed nations. The high global inequality in life expectancy, although declining, is still very large both across and within countries. In the twentieth century, when life expectancy at birth in developed countries doubled, for a very long it stayed low in the rest of the world. Even though developing countries' death rates have recently dropped considerably and rapidly, and in Africa the average life expectancy in 2016 had increased to 61.2 years, overall increased life expectancy has benefited mainly richer countries (World Life Expectancy 2016). In other words, despite global life expectancy increasing dramatically over the last few decades, being born into an affluent, developed nation is still the biggest contributor to longevity.

However, although economic development is strongly associated with greater longevity, it is not the only factor shaping rates of mortality as, even in affluent countries, social and economic inequalities undermine longevity. For example, the United States has the highest infant mortality rate and the lowest life expectancy among industrialized nations (Case and Deaton

2020). Hence, how one experiences of dying has always been influenced by one's social location, gender, ethnicity and region. In many nations, the class-based differences within mortality statistics began to be documented only from the beginning of the twentieth century; nonetheless, there is much evidence of 'the influence of wealth and culture on mortality and morbidity' for the previous centuries as well (Townsend 1979: 369). The inequality in life expectancy continued through the course of the twentieth century, even in countries with well-developed national health systems and welfare states, in which the level of socio-economic division was reduced. Since the beginning of the second decade of the twenty-first century, some deterioration in mortality rates has also been exhibited in several European countries (Netherlands, France, Germany, Belgium) and in the United States. Yet it is the United Kingdom, which already had lower life expectancy than many comparable nations, that stands out as the country where there has been the greatest deterioration in mortality improvements and where the benefits from an increase in longevity were most unequally distributed.

In the United Kingdom there was a decline in life expectancy in the first couple of years of the 2020s, accompanied by a larger gap in life expectancy between the poor and the wealthy. Calling this process a stalling of mortality, Murphy et al. (2019) show how the deterioration in mortality improvements trends appeared to be particularly marked among older persons and among those living in the most deprived areas of the United Kingdom. Moreover, since the beginning of the second decade of the twenty-first century, the gap between life expectancy in the best-off and worst-off areas has been widening, a growing disparity accompanied by a larger gap between male and female life expectancies. This latter gap has continued to widen since the late eighteenth and early nineteenth centuries, mainly as a result of men's working conditions and because of the decline in tuberculosis, which affected women more than men. This gap increased further in the first part of the twentieth century in developed countries, with more women surviving childbirth and having fewer children, thus reducing the risk of dying in labour. However, in the United Kingdom, after it peaked at 6.3 in 1971, the difference between male and female life expectancies has been decreasing, with mortality falling faster in males than females because of decreases in smoking and less mortality from cardiovascular diseases among men. In 2016–18 in England, life expectancy for women at birth was 83.2 years and for men it was 79.6 years; this disparity, due to faster improvements in mortality for men than for women, has continued to narrow (Raleigh 2019).

Looking at the UK evidence about the deterioration in mortality improvements from the beginning of the second decade of this century, Murphy et al. (2019: 2) conclude 'that there is no clear evidence for any specific explanation or combination of causes'. Yet other researchers blame the stalling of longevity on the UK Government's policies, particularly on its cuts to welfare, social care and health services (Davis 2018). Several studies have documented that since the 2008 financial collapse, and in the context of the growing financial costs of care, the policy of austerity that has been responsible for real cuts to people's incomes and the erosion of institutional support and provision for people in later life has had a negative effect on life expectancy (Fordham 2017; Hiam et al. 2018; Kingston et al. 2018). As a result of austerity measures, the British National Health Service (NHS), in the context of increasing demands – which were mainly due to the ageing of the British population and a greater burden caused by rising levels of chronic conditions – was unable to fully protect the nation's health, contributing to a stalling of life expectancy (Phillipson 2015). This inability to meet the increased demand for services resulted in England's highest death rates of older patients and the highest death rates of frail and older hospitalized patients in the Western world, as well as higher mortality rates among hip fracture patients and patients with heart failure who had diabetes than in all other developed countries (Gregory 2021).

Apart from the 'greying' of modern developed nations, another factor behind changing the profile and nature of dying in old age in the twenty-first century is the new leading causes of deaths among older people. The redefinition of leading causes of death in old age and ways of dying, like the gains in longevity, has resulted from advances in medical technology, knowledge and intervention Before modern medicine modified or eliminated fatal diseases, infections were one of the main causes of death in old age. For example, in England in the late Victorian and Edwardian period, pneumonia, which was the most feared disease after tuberculosis and nearly always fatal, accounted for death of the big proportion of the elderly, while in the United States, prior to the introduction of antibiotics, pneumonia was credited with causing one-quarter of all deaths (Honigsbaum 2020:41). William Osler, the so called father of modern medicine, named pneumonia the 'Captain of the Men of Death' because it promised a quick, painless exit from life. In his classic textbook, *The Principles and Practice of Medicine*, Osler (quoted in Emanuel 2014) added: 'Pneumonia may well be called the friend of the aged. Taken off by it in an acute, short, not often painful illness, the old man escapes those "cold gradations of decay" so distressing to himself and to his friends.' Although pneumonia is no longer ranked among the top causes of death for older persons, it is still among the most serious infections in the elderly, especially those aged 85 and over (Gorina and Lentzner 2005: 11).

In Western societies today, dying in older age is unlike the more sudden deaths experienced by most humans in the past. Now dying in old age is an extended, gradual, slower, incremental and more prolonged process resulting from various chronic and degenerative diseases of ageing (Lloyd 2015). In the context of more old people dying in this way and the growing difficulties involved in determining the main cause or causes of death, to facilitate the unified classification of leading causes of death in old age, the International Classification of Diseases (ICD 2020) recommends that old age is not classified as 'a disease or a cause of death'. For example, in the United States since 1955, nobody has died of old age (Wolpert 2011: 225). Although in the United Kingdom a death certificate can list the cause of death as old age, this cause is only used in very limited circumstances, such as 'a gradual decline in patients' general health and functioning'. Moreover, as the UK Guidance for doctors certifying cause of death does not clarify just how old 'old age' is, further sorting was required. After much discussion, the Death Certification Advisory Group recommended that 'deaths certified as due to old age or senility alone should be referred to the coroner unless the deceased was aged 80 or older, the conditions listed above are all fulfilled and there is no other reason that the death should be referred' (GP Notebook 2022). Now old age tends not to be listed as the main cause of death, although it is still assumed that 'ageing does lead to the inability to deal with disease that may be partly due to the ageing process itself' (Wolpert 2011: 226).

Today, death in later life is the result of varieties of prolonged diseases that in the past caused immediate death but can now be managed for many additional years of life. Older people are dying as a result of heart disease, vascular disease including strokes, respiratory disease and cancer. For example, in the United Kingdom the main causes of death of over 65 are heart disease and cancer (Wolpert 2011: 226). In the United States between 2000 and 2010, the number of deaths from stroke declined by more than 20% (Emanuel 2014), thus strokes and accidents have been replaced as the top killers by cancer, heart disease and Alzheimer's disease (Erickson 2013: 8). Many more people are living long enough to experience many debilitating conditions, such as Alzheimer's disease and other forms of dementia, which strip people of their autonomy and agency, and exclude them from decision-making when life is drawing to an end, while rendering them more vulnerable to dying. For example, Alzheimer's disease has gained importance as a cause of death among older persons in the United States over the past two decades (Gorina and Lentzner 2005: 4), while in the United Kingdom from 2015, dementia has become one of the main cause of death (Mannix 2018). Living with such conditions, which decrease functioning and dramatically lower quality of life, illustrates one of the costs of medicine's success in expanding longevity.

The dying process has been made a more complex, often more lonely and more ambiguous phenomenon by the increasing medicalization of death – that is, the expansion of intensive treatments for older people and the increased room for explicit decisions about death in terms of control and quality at the end of life puts decisions about the prolongation of life and the timing of the end into older people's hands and those of their loved ones. Through the ability of preventive medicine to diagnose and treat (e.g. medications to lower blood pressure and regulate cholesterol) and through life-extending medical and surgical technologies (such as coronary artery bypass, graft surgery, medications to lower blood pressure and regulate cholesterol, cardiac procedures, cancer treatments, organ transplantation), more older people are living for longer and dying of different diseases than their ancestors. By confronting older people with a challenge to seek medical treatment and intervention, the medicalization of death has also raised new ethical dilemmas and brought some new problems and anxieties. Although it has reshaped death in older age into a more private issue, it has also made the dying process more demanding and more expensive, and has not always taken older people's preferences and abilities to cope, understand and accept dependence and vulnerability into account.

With the medicalization of death, today death in old age has entered the domain of choice and has moved from rare occurrence to 'right' for most people, making it the central issue in ethical debates. Dying in old age has thus been remade into a less traditional process (Broom 201; Erickson 2015; Kaufman 2005; Walter 2017). Moreover, when both ageing and death are treated medically, medical interventions and medical technologies can create a zone of indistinction between dying and living, and add to the ambiguity of what is natural about dying in older age, including 'the mistaken perception that death itself can be controlled' (Erickson 2015: 9). The vision of natural death, 'understood to be a somehow ethically neutral event that is unhampered by technological interference', becomes increasingly difficult to sustain in 'a society with insatiable demands for medical intervention' (Kaufman 2005: 323). In other words, we do not know 'what dying as a natural phenomenon in later life looks like because of frailty, debility and decline are today defined and – thus constrained – by the language of medicine' (Kaufman 2005: 82).When the vision of 'old-age-as-disease' drives hospital practice, there is a risk of 'excessive medical intervention, or even medical technology can extend life beyond all sense' (Erickson 2015: 111).

Such a singular focus in medical care on living longer worries bioethical critics, who are concerned that dying is being seen as an emergent problem, the nature and timing of which can be controlled and constructed by technology. They question Western societies' recent tendency to prolong dying regardless of the impact of such efforts on the conditions and quality of a person's end-of-life experience. For example, bioethicist Daniel Callahan (1993: 40), who is critical of unlimited attempts to extend life and negatively evaluates the trend for the dying process to be shaped by 'technological brinkmanship', argues that we must learn to accept the idea of a 'natural lifespan' and remember that being mortal is 'to live a life that will be marked by illness, injury decline, and death' (Callahan 1993: 40).

In total contrast to this rejection of any form of dependency and medical intervention is the stand of the global anti-ageing industry, which promotes the view of ageing as a curable disease. Declaring a distaste for mortality, immortalists or 'scientists, dreamers and – crucially – billionaires, who want us to think of age as a curable disease and that death is something that could be indefinitely postponed', the anti-ageing industry repudiates death in old age as being so 'anti-aspirational' or as almost 'sort of an affront' to modern life (Harris 2021). In this new version of ageism, ageing without any help from the 'anti-ageing' business is viewed as a failure and death is proclaimed to be a 'disaster'. But even if scientific advances can make ageing a thing of the past, death cannot be avoided; thus we should concentrate on assisting and helping the exit rather than on delaying the inevitable at huge expense. Such a focus on easing the process of death in old age is especially important in modern societies as elderly persons live for a long time with multiplicity of ailments and face various choices of treatments, and their dying is prolonged, slower, gradual and overseen by doctors.

As the recent COVID-19 pandemic has undermined the historical trends in improvements in longevity and has weakened the view that the timing of death is a controllable event, in what follows we explore how the pandemic has strengthened the relationship between old age and death, and changed the perception and profile of the death of elderly people.

The pandemic's impact on the profile of longevity and death

The COVID-19 pandemic has shed light on many old issues, added new troubles, exacerbated some trends and altered other trajectories. Among the problems and difficulties brought to our attention by the pandemic are not only health-related issues but also society's awareness and cultural preparedness for pandemics and state–society relations – which have all been crucial in the fight against the coronavirus. The COVID-19 crisis has impacted longevity and the profile of death in old age. But above all, the pandemic has made death far more visible, and more specifically it has enhanced the public's awareness of the death of old people. This consequence of the COVID-19 crisis is connected with this pandemic's specific mortality pattern.

There are many similarities between pandemics in history; however, from the perspective of our topic here, the most essential is the difference between these traumatic events in terms of their impact on different age groups. The varied mortality patterns of different pandemics can be visualized by a range of differently shaped curves: there are pandemics with U-, L- and W-shaped curves. The most common are pandemics with a U-shaped curve, as generally two groups – small children and older persons, which are the groups with the weakest immune systems – are likely to be most vulnerable. However, these two groups are not always equally effected – for example, the Spanish flu had a W-shaped curve, as adults aged 20–40 years accounted for half the total influenza deaths (Honigsbaum 2020). This most striking aspect of the Spanish flu pandemic – the fact its victims were mainly younger people – meant that, while younger people were perishing, the life expectancy of older people barely changed (Spinney 2017). There are also epidemics with forward looking L-shaped curves, such as polio, in which there is an increased risk for the very young and a relatively low risk for others (Chrisakis 2020). COVID-19 has been the pandemic with 'a backward-looking L-shape' with 'a low risk for the young and elevated risk for the elderly' (Chrisakis 2020: 181). In contrast to the mortality patterns of other pandemics, COVID-19's very unusual pattern means that during this pandemic the most vulnerable people have been the elderly. The number of deaths from coronavirus for each thousand people has increased with age, thus the extraordinary difference in risks from COVID-19 faced by different generations is the pandemic's main feature. In age groups up to and including 60–69 years, fewer than one in 1,000 people have died from coronavirus; in the 70–79 years age group, it is two in every 1,000 people; for the age group 80–89 years, it is seven in every 1,000 people; and for those aged 90 years and over, it is 18 people in every 1000 people (Webb 2020). To explore how the pandemic has changed British older people's accommodation with mortality, their experience and management of the end of life, we will evaluate the United Kingdom's preparedness for the pandemic and outline, in a compact way, the pandemic's three waves and three lockdowns.

The first thing that the history of pandemics tell us is that they are always met with shock, disbelief and astonishment because people prefer to forget the plagues of the past and believe that pandemics have been controlled in modernity (Harari 2020). This sentiment is well illustrated by a quote from Albert Camus's novel *The Plague* (2020: 42): 'There have been as many plagues and wars; yet always plagues and wars take people equally by surprise.' Until recently, the cultural amnesia about past pandemics has been sustained by a common belief in the success of modern medicine to control viral, bacterial and other disasters, a confidence supported by the fact that infectious diseases have faded as a leading cause of death. With the absence of collective and personal memories of lethal pandemics, even alarms and wake-up calls raised by the outbreak of AIDS and by later infectious diseases, such Severe Acute Respiratory Syndrome (SARS), pandemic influenza and Ebola, did not increase the urgency and understanding of the need to prepare for future pandemics (Hardt 2017). The short-sightedness of such a stand had translated itself into a lack of funding, a lack of anticipation and inadequate preparation for next health crisis. This failure of planning is seen as being responsible for mishandling of the COVID-19 pandemic in many countries, including the United Kingdom (MacKenzie 2020).

Despite scientists and health experts' warnings, the United Kingdom lacked effective planning for the pandemic (Sridhar 2022). Although the experts' report, based on a pandemic planning exercise in 2016, alerted the British government to the need to stockpile emergency personal protective equipment (PPE) and advised about the demands any pandemic could place on hospitals and care homes, the UK government had not implemented the required actions and this lack of preparedness resulted not only in a lack of investment in required equipment but also a lack of training of medical staff in dealing with the realities of a contagious virus (Horton 2020). Furthermore, if there were any evidence of the UK Government's preparations for a pandemic, these were focused on influenza – that is, on 'the wrong type of disease' (UK Parliament 2021). Although both influenza and COVID-19 are respiratory diseases, there are several important differences between them. First, the SARS-CoV-2 virus, the COVID-19 disease-causing agent, which is part of a family of viruses that includes respiratory severe diseases such as SARS, is more infectious than seasonal flu. Second, the COVID-19 virus is more deadly as the fatality rate of standard flu is typically below 0.1%, while the proportion of all those infected by the coronavirus who died of the disease was 1.1% in the first wave of the pandemic (Spiegelhalter and Masters 2021: 147). As news about the COVID-19 threat reached the United Kingdom in December 2019, the high cost of ignoring the lessons from the last pandemic – SARS, which was the forerunner to COVID-19 – became clear. This lack of preparedness led to chronic shortages and out-of-date PPE, a lack of effectiveness of the trace-and-test system and delays in imposing restrictions to stop the spread of the virus from abroad as well as delays the introduction of lockdowns (Horton 2020).

The first lockdown in the United Kingdom, which began on 23 March 2020 and lasted until 4 July 2020, was presented as the only way to cut the lines of transmission, save lives and protect the National Health Service. The official announcement, while introducing restrictions such as closure of all non-essential high street businesses and schools, identified older chronological age as a risk factor for COVID infection, disease severity and mortality. While others were permitted to leave their homes – although only for essential purposes – older (aged 70 and over) and clinically vulnerable people were asked to shield and self-isolate themselves. This shielding group comprised of 66.2% of 18.5 million individuals aged 70 years or over, while the remining 33.8% were younger people with an underlying health conditions and therefore also at risk of severe COVID-19 (Walker et al. 2020). Although the governmental handling of the COVID-19 pandemic was initially supported by the public, with growing evidence of the state's many failures, such as too late introduction of the first lockdown, a lack of required PPE, a lack of travel restrictions for too long, too slow increases in testing for the virus, problems with the test-and-trace system and a lack of promised protection of care homes – public trust in state policies declined (Calvert and Arbuthnott 2021). With the proof of the drastic impact of the pandemic on the health and morale of older people, and with the delays and failures that occurred in the management of the health crisis, the public increasingly questioned the government's management of the pandemic (Clarke 2020; Hall 2020).

With winter 2020–21 approaching, it became clear that COVID-19 occurring at same time as an outbreak of flu could significantly increase risk of death of the most vulnerable people. At the beginning of October 2020, there were 21,915 cases of COVID-19 across the United Kingdom, more than 10,000 COVID patients in hospital and 326 deaths reported. These data, according to the chief scientific adviser Patrick Vallance, painted 'a very grim picture'. He warned that deaths over the winter could be 'twice as bad or more than the first wave' (Sage et al. 2020: 7). Hence, after the period of local restrictions, orders for all non-essential high street businesses to be closed and prohibitions of meetings with people from outside one's support bubble, on 3 October 2020, the second lockdown was implemented to protect the NHS from being overburdened with a winter surge of COVID-19. With fatalities from the coronavirus being 'hugely concentrated in a subset of 10 to 20% of the population: the elderly, frail and those with co-morbidities' (Safi 2020), the vulnerable and those over 70 years of age were advised to be especially careful and minimize their social contacts, although there was no return of a formal request that they shield themselves. The function of the second lockdown was to shelter the health system from the risk of 'a one-two punch', or the threat of growing numbers of older people becoming infected first with flu and then with COVID-19 (Kormann 2020). Its other role was to prevent the health system and its practitioners from any exposure to the ethical dilemmas connected with difficult choices and prioritizations of patients for ventilators and treatments (Weeks 2020). Hence, the second lockdown's narratives were about the necessity of 'an operational tsunami' and about the need to avert a 'moral crisis'. The first of these stressed the importance of preventing the NHS from being overwhelmed by coronavirus and flu cases; the second aimed to ensure that nurses and doctors could avoid moral decisions about who to help and who did not qualify for treatment. The government promised to do all that was required to reduce the burden faced by the NHS and to protect doctors and nurses from being forced to choose 'who would live, who would die' (Sage et al. 2020: 7).

During the second lockdown, as was the case during the first lockdown, the government operated on the basis that controlling the virus was a trade-off between the heath of the nation and the health of the economy (Calvert and Arbuthnott 2021) – hence, the government's focus on the minimalization of economic disruptions, which led to delays in lockdowns and which can best be illustrated by its catchy slogan 'eat out help out', aimed to ensure the economic recovery of the hospitality industry, while ignoring the potential risk of such actions to the health of the public. The hope for a return to normality at that time was uplifted by announcements from several companies (Pfizer/BioNTech, Moderna and Oxford University and AstraZeneca on 9, 16 and 23 November 2020 respectively) that their vaccines has been 90% successful in large-scale trials (Spiegelhalter and Masters 2021). The United Kingdom, as the first country to do so, started administering jabs on 8 December 2020. The successful start of vaccination programmes and the country's early lead in administering vaccinations, together with the end of the second lockdown – which formally finished on 2 December 2020 – buoyed hopes for an end to the pandemic. However, without a strong vaccination rate, with winter being the best season for transmitting the virus and with a rising number of coronavirus cases attributed to a new variant, 75% of the country spent the end of the year under restrictions.

From mid-December 2020, the spreading of the new Delta variant of the virus, with cases of transmission, hospitalization and deaths rising steadily, was the main concern. With new infections growing and with mortality rates ascending, together with the government's failure to manage the test-and-trace system and to handle outbreaks of the infection in care homes, it became obvious that in order to prevent the spread of the new variant there was a need for the third lockdown. On 6 January 2021, with 407 new deaths reported and with 58,784 COVID-19 cases – the highest ever daily figure – and as new COVID-19 infections passed the 50,000 mark for the seventh day in a row, England went into third national lockdown (Spiegelhalter and Masters 2021: 45). A total of 75,431 people had died since the start of the pandemic and 2,713,563 cases had been reported.

The restrictions of the third lockdown were more like the rules of the first lockdown rather than those of the second lockdown. Aiming to bring the Delta variant under control and keep vaccines rolling out, the third lockdown's rules banned leaving home for outdoor recreation and both primary and secondary schools were closed and learning was conducted online.

People were advised to stay home until mid-February 2021 and during that time were only allowed to leave home for essential work, medical reasons, exercise, shopping or providing care to the vulnerable. In the third lockdown, as in the first wave, in order to 'protect the NHS and to save lives', the nation was instructed to suspend its unnecessary activities. However, despite vaccines reducing the likelihood of serious illness and death, and the age-targeted vaccination strategies, the government's COVID-19 policy still continued to be mistrusted. This lack of confidence was exacerbated by the public's dissatisfaction with a lack of open discussion of the ethical problems raised by the state's policy to fight the spread of COVID-19. The 'invisibility of ethics', or the absence of debates of ethical issues – such as what is the limit to restrictions on freedom, whether chronological age should be an accepted criterion for the shielding and treatment, who should be prioritized for the COVID-19 vaccine and what kind of the frailty assessment should be used to decide a person's eligibility for treatment – further undermined trust in state–society relations (Seedhouse 2021).

From March 2021, England began a gradual exit out of the lockdown by lifting several restrictions, reopening schools, outdoor activities and settings. The growing levels of vaccination, which were reducing the levels of hospitalization and death from COVID-19, prompted the UK Government to announce 'Freedom Day' on 19 July 2021, when most remaining pandemic restrictions were lifted: social distancing, masks and some travel restrictions were dropped. However, although the mass vaccinations continued to keep deaths and hospitalizations at much lower levels than in previous waves, and despite the fact that for first time on 1 June 2021 daily deaths were zero, the level of infection in the United Kingdom picked again up at the end of summer 2021. The autumn saw the continuation of infections, which implied that, despite being the most important tool in fighting the virus, the coronavirus vaccine alone could not be expected to halt the country's experience of the pandemic. Moreover, the vaccine's ability to prevent infection with COVID-19 wanes over time and this decreased of effectiveness of the vaccine is related to age. This, together with the Delta variant – which was more infectious than the old strains – surging around the world, resulted in the rise of COVID-19 cases in the second part of 2021. For example, on 21 September 2021 31,564 people in the United

Kingdom tested positive for COVID-19, 861 people were admitted to hospital and 203 people had died within 28 days of a positive COVID-19 test (*The Guardian*, 22 September 2021).

The risk of another wave and waning immunity – especially in older people – have prompted a call for booster shots, or third vaccine doses, for the aged and vulnerable to prolong their protective immunity. Following the recommendation from the Joint Committee on Vaccination and Immunisation (JCVI), aged and extremely vulnerable people were offered COVID-19 booster vaccinations six months after their last dose. While the clinical benefits of booster vaccinations could not be questioned, among 51,284 people who died with COVID-19 in the period from 2 January to 2 July 2021, there were 640 people who were fully vaccinated (Vesty 2021). This showed that, regardless of vaccination status, coronavirus could still be a threat to life. Moreover, of the 640 people who died while fully vaccinated, 256 were classed as 'breakthrough deaths', as they were diagnosed with COVID-19 some fourteen days or more after their second vaccine (Vesty 2021). The statistics also showed that old people were most at risk, as the median age of 'breakthrough deaths' was 84 years in the first part of 2021, compared with 82 years for other COVID-19 deaths and for non-COVID deaths (Vesty 2021).

As England entered its second pandemic winter, the steep rise in COVID-19 cases in Europe in the last months of 2021 and the emergence of a new variant, Omicron, caused concern. On 27 November 2021 the British government announced new rules to combat the Omicron variant, including compulsory masks on public transport and in shops – but without any extra restrictions, such as social distancing, wearing masks in pubs or working from home. As delivering booster jabs was proclaimed 'our new national mission', from 1 December 2021 until the end of January 2022, the NHS offered 25 million booster jabs – all adults were eligible for boosters from three months after their last COVID-19 shot. Even though Omicron was spreading rapidly in late 2021, the UK Government – relying on studies showing that this variant, although more infectious, was less deadly than other versions of the virus – did not consider a total lockdown. Despite stronger measures in Scotland, Wales and Northern Ireland, the UK Government resisted calls to go further. Yet on 8 December 2021, in response to new concerns over the high risk of reinfection from Omicron, the UK government announced new COVID-19 restrictions for England, adding to mandatory face coverings in public, the call for people to work from home where possible and demands to show COVID status for entry into many venues.

From January 2022, as a result of high immunity levels, the milder effects of the Omicron variant and the growing effectiveness of hospital treatment, there was a steady and continuing fall in cases of hospitalizations and death. On 21 February 2022, with 63% of all adults having received their third jab, and with deaths and hospitalizations falling, the restrictions in England were lifted. The government also announced that from 1 April 2022, charges for lateral flow tests would be introduced, while people aged 75 years or over and residents in aged care homes, and anyone aged 12 or above who was immunosuppressed would be offered additional boosters (*The Guardian*, 2022). Yet as infection levels among the over-70s remained high, the additional vaccinations for over-75s and the clinically vulnerable started earlier. Even with the fourth booster being available from March 2022, the health crisis continued until mid-April 2022.

By this stage, as government figures confirmed the country was slowly returning to normality, the United Kingdom had recorded more than 21 million cases of COVID-19 and over 174,440 deaths linked to the disease. While the UK Government statistics for deaths included any deaths that had occurred within 28 days of a positive test, separate figures published by the Office for National Statistics (ONS) for the same period showed there had been more than 190,000 deaths registered in the United Kingdom where COVID-19 was mentioned on the death certificate and that more than four in five, or more than 80%, of those people were aged 70 years and over. Until the arrival of the vaccination and high vaccination coverage among elderly persons, COVID-19 presented older people with a much higher risk of death than it did younger people. Interestingly, throughout the pandemic, apart from age and underlying health conditions – including compromised immune systems – another factor increasing the risk of death was poverty. For example, people in the 20% most deprived parts of England were twice as likely to die from COVID and they died at younger ages because the existing health inequalities meant they may have had lower life expectancy (Health Foundation 2022).

COVID-19 has not only presented older people with a higher risk of death, but it may also hasten non-COVID deaths and result in an increased number of cases of untreated serious illness. While in the pre-COVID period older people spent an average of nine years in poor health before dying (Teggi 2020: 5), during the pandemic, people aged over 75 years – that is, people in the age group where three-quarters of those with the virus died from COVID – lost an average 6.5 years of life (Health Foundation 2022). During the pandemic, older people's death came sooner, was unpredictable and took place in the context of many restrictions on visitations, new difficulties and disruptions in access to a range of health services. Moreover, the pandemic also contributed to lowered life expectancy in the United Kingdom, which even before the pandemic was lower than in many other Western European countries and was already 'stalling' (Murphy et al. 2019: 2). In 2020, the life expectancy of the United Kingdom declined to its lowest level lowest since 2011 for both sexes: the 'very high level' of excess deaths caused life expectancy to fall by 1.3 years for men, to 78.7 years, and to fall by 0.9 years, to 82.7 years, for women (UK Government 2021). The difference in life expectancy between the best and worst parts of the United Kingdom was preserved, if not increased, during the pandemic – for example, that female life expectancy was reduced by 1.1 years in Derby, but it increased by 1.7 years in Kensington and Chelsea (Owen 2021). Other countries also saw falls in in life expectancy in 2020, yet while the average reduction driven by coronavirus deaths across the OECD nations was 0.6 years, Britain's drop of a year, falling from 81.4 years in 2019 to 80.4 years in 2020, was the second worst (Lay 2021).

From the beginning of the pandemic, the topic of death – and especially the death of old people – was at the core of the daily news and daily government announcements. Statistics, discussions and coverages of deaths from COVID-19 could be found on the front pages of all newspapers, in the lead stories of television news and in social media. At the height of the coronavirus outbreak, people became familiar with the government publications of the death tolls, with reports about numbers of deaths involving COVID-19 released each day. While presenting the challenges arising from the COVID-19 pandemic as being unprecedented and demanding extensive measures from everybody, the media constructed the image of the United Kingdom as a nation struck very hard by COVID-19 and trying its best to come together to handle the pandemic. The media paid special attention to the fate of elderly people and often checked whether all required measures to protect old and vulnerable people had been taken. By widely broadcasting that thousands of care residents died from confirmed or suspected COVID-19 cases, the media conveyed a dramatic portrait of the impact of the pandemic on the life and death of elderly people. In other words, by reporting on COVID-19 death rates and the fate of old people in hospitals and care homes, the British media brought the death of elderly people to the attention of their readers and viewers in an unprecedented way.

While showing the hospital wards where many elderly people, gowned and masked or on ventilators, struggled to survive, television programmes informed us that age was the biggest risk factor for dying from the coronavirus; that the risk of dying from COVID-19 in the 65–74 years age group was 90 times higher as eight out of ten COVID-19 deaths have been of people aged over 65 (BBC1 *News at 6*, 2 October 2020). From newspapers, social media and TV reports from hospitals and care homes, we learned that about 66% of critical care patients aged 80 years or over died within 28 days, compared with 12% of those aged 16–39 years, and that many elderly people in fact acquired the virus in hospital (Spiegelhalter and Masters 2021: 81, 104). Journalists, who frequently visited care homes around the United Kingdom, informed their viewers, listeners and readers that among people already diagnosed with COVID-19, people who were 80 years or older were 70 times more likely to die than those under 40 years. The tragedy of such death rates was reinforced by the media pictures of older people shielding, being taken care of in residential homes or being transported to hospital. These images of fragile and vulnerable elderly people were often accompanied by stories about the inadequacy of testing and the unavailability of protective measures in care homes, as well as about the low priority given to the plight of residents of care homes into which patients were discharged from hospital without testing (to be discussed further in Chapter 9). The media also told their audiences about the loneliness of isolated older people and their fear of 'uncertainty, of danger, of the loss of everything' (Miller 2020: 22).

CHAPTER 2

Too old not to remind us about death

Too old to 'live happily ever after'

This chapter debates whether aged people, seen as 'having one foot in the grave' and as 'not having that long' to live (Blythe 2005: 21, 22), tend to be dismissed because they are 'reminding us of death', to paraphrase the phrase from Larkin's (1977) poem 'The Old Fools'. While in the previous chapter we argued that the tendency of contemporary Western societies to keep the deaths of aged people hidden in the background is sustained by viewing death in old age as being timely and appropriate, here we will discuss the degree to which today's culture, with its myth that we can age without ageing, assists the marginalization of older people and helps to hide their deaths, and therefore does not equip society and its older population to deal adequately with death. After showing the current boom in narratives about ways of being old and the heterogeneity of today's older population, it asserts that these developments, while slowly transforming our cultural narrative of ageing, have not yet effectively challenged socially sanctioned ageism. The chapter argues that, by focusing on our desire to prevent the decline associated with the ageing process, contemporary discourses of ageing have neither changed seeing the elderly as 'a buffer zone between society and death' (Erickson 2013: 9), nor contributed to the development of a more holistic approach to old age and dying. It also asserts that, by boosting our hopes for 'growing without ageing' (Katz 2003), modern societies have prepared us badly for old age and death. After discussing conceptualizations of the ageing process and the ways in which various generations have confronted mortality, the chapter concludes by looking at both the impact of the COVID-19 pandemic on the visibility of the death of old people and ageism in UK society.

Over the last couple of decades in Europe and North America, the demographic changes, mainly brought about by the greater life expectancy, the first baby boomers reaching retirement age, the increased participation of older people at the employment, the voluntary sector, and leisure activities and travel adventures, have increased scholars and policymakers' interest in the ageing population (Misztal 2020). There are many approaches and perspectives in debates over the definition of ageing, but all these voices agree that ageing is a complex and multi-factorial process. Yet, unsurprisingly, the various attempts to identify the meaning of the concept of ageing have yet not reached a single agreed-upon definition of ageing (Armstrong 2019). Since there is no space here to map all the voices that are present in debates about the definition of ageing, we will sketch only the main perspectives within age studies and cultural gerontology. The main conclusion from the examination of the concept of ageing developed in these fields is that the proposed definitions of ageing and narratives of old age tend to overlook the special status and importance of the period of the deterioration taking place in the years leading up to death. This failure to acknowledge the significance of the end of life is a common feature. The first perspective invoked the inevitability of physical ageing, perceived it as a natural decline, and adopted a complementary view of nature and culture as distinct realms, each with its own appropriate forms of knowledge and expertise (Marshall 2015). The growing criticism of this biological-foundationalist approach, and subsequent efforts to undermine its nature–culture binary, have been inspired by attempts to turn age into a cultural phenomenon. The subsequent emergence of the constructionist perspective, which renders the body's physical aspects either negligible or as a purely medical matter, has prompted a view of ageing as a matter of thinking positively and keeping the mind active (Tulle 2015). By rejecting the metaphor of old age as decline and dependency, this approach has contributed to overcoming the stereotyping of the elderly as 'smiling old dears' and 'unbearable bores' in sensible shoes and 'old-fashioned cardigans', without their own free will and autonomy (Lively 2014: 53).

However, by excluding the body, such a perspective has not taken into account the significant aspect of older people's experience. The recognition of the materiality and lived experience of bodies has established the importance of a phenomenological perspective that enables us to understand that 'body matters are at the heart of ageing as experience but also … the target of social and cultural practices' (Tulle 2015: 127). This stance allows us to explore how older people experience the materiality of their bodies while viewing their embodied action as shaped by a cultural context, not as pre-social or somehow 'natural'. Subsequently, feminist gerontologists and cultural sociologists, who view ageing as a phenomenon mediated by external factors such as gender expectations, have oriented the study of age and ageing towards the adoption of a more explicitly cultural approach, while at the same time drawing attention to the embodied nature of age (Gilleard and Higgs 2015). Following the inclusion of not only gender, but also race, ethnicity, sexuality and disability, in re-examinations of previous assumptions about later life has led to age being seen through the lenses of 'intersectionality' – that is, 'the cross disciplinary arena that sees social phenomena through the lenses of multiple identities and positions that destabilize and render contingent dominant interpretations of later life' (Gilleard and Higgs 2015: 30).

Alongside academic works, contemporary societal discourses contribute to our understanding of ageing. The dominant cultural narratives, while overlooking the possibility of any bodily and mental decline and avoiding mention of the proximity of death as one of the symptoms of old age, propagate that 'older people should actively pursue active ageing, mostly understood as economically productive ageing, the adoption of healthy lifestyle and the prizing of ageless appearance (via fitness, clothing, cosmetic management)' (Tulle 2015: 128). The demographic changes in society, and the new cultural context, have established later life as a universal expectation associated with the advantages of 'successful' or 'good' ageing. The popular discourses about 'productive' and 'successful' ageing offer an image of old people as free and unencumbered agents, able to exercise choice and autonomy. Yet this narrative of self- sufficiency and independence is based not only on the deficient conception of the old person, but also on inadequate understanding of the nature of the last stage of life, or the 'evening of life' (Kierkegaard, quoted in Davis 2020: 8), which always denotes the period of life when we can expect death. In other words, we lack a cultural framework for old age that could provide older people with opportunities to define ageing on their own terms, and that reflects the specificity and complexity of the final stage of life. This absence of the coherent conception of old persons in society is often concealed or disguised in modern cultures by treating old age as a social problem that should be conceded and avoided (Davies 2020; Gilleard and Higgs 2020). While the question of whether the ageing population presents a threat to modern society will be discussed in Chapter 3, here we will continue our exploration of the complexity of the process of ageing and search for the factors that shape the experience of old age and dying.

First, to fully explain the diversity and complexity of experiences at the end of life, there is a need to overcome the shortcomings of many cultural narratives of the old age by taking into consideration the role of subjective characteristics in shaping the expectations and quality of the end of life. The incorporation of subjective meanings given to later life and death can provide a platform for seeing both the potentials and the ordeals of old age and approaching death. The inclusion of individuals' subjective experiences, seen as linked to cultural and structural limitations, brings to our attention the importance of values, dispositions and attitudes in shaping the features of the last stage of life (Ray Karpen 2017). People's subjective experiences of being old differ, and these differences are subsequently reflected in people's diverse attitudes to mortality. For some, old age 'isn't a battle, it is a massacre', as a central protagonist in Phillip Roth's (2007: 156) novel, *Everyman*, observes; others, because of their different values and character traits, manage to inhabit the last stage of life without such desperation. Yet our perceptions of age are not only to a degree subjective and to a degree culturally conditioned, but it is also to a degree age-dependent. When the time comes for 'all the theatrical props of old: the pills and sticks, the shrieking hearing-aids and dental weaponry, the tricks for countering the loss of names and threads and glasses for circumventing insomnia' (Miller 2010: 5), we cannot continue to overlook the consequences of our chronological age.

In other words, the subjective characteristics and the chronological age are both essential factors in any conceptualization of ageing as a complex and multi-factorial process leading to death. The impossibility of total detachment from the chronological age and the role of subjective characteristics have been confirmed by the findings of several empirical studies. These investigations demonstrate that the subjective experience of ageing is indeed a multidimensional and multidirectional phenomenon – but only until a certain stage of ageing (Keller et al. 1989; Stevernik et al. 2001). These studies found the coexistence of both negative and positive experiences of ageing, from the acceptance of ageing as a new stage in life, with new freedoms, interests and feelings, through the toleration of ageing as a natural and gradual process without remarkable features, to experiencing ageing as a period of loss and decline (Stevernik et al. 2001). Thus, with advancing age, the ageing experience is increasingly framed in terms of physical vulnerabilities and social loss (Stevernik et al. 2001). In other words, the multidirectionality of ageing is not sustained with increased age, as the experience of ageing becomes less positive and less related to life-satisfaction as people get older.

The importance of chronological age, which reveals people's degrees of physical and mental frailty, cannot be overlooked. This still holds today, despite the fact that older people's experience of transitions across time has become more fluid and boundaries between the life-stages are now more blurred than they were in the past (Grenier 2015). Even though the significance of our chronological age in our lives now seems to be diminished, as many current processes of cultural, social and medical change led to greater flexibility in the relationship between chronometric time and ageing (Baars 2015), the ticking of time cannot be ignored for too long. Although transitions between life stages are now less clear, nonetheless the chronological age always 'marks a time when our body's changes are more prominent than before, no matter how healthy we are and when our perspective on time alters' (Holstein 2015: 14). Moreover, people generally seem to recognize the realities of their ageing bodies. The unlikelihood of escape from chronological age and from its impact on our body is well illustrated by Miller's (2003) observation that inhabitants of old age are, collectively, easily recognized as

> deaf, blind, severely breathless and arthritic. There have been broken hips and arms and pelvises, mismanaged cataract operations, glaucoma and recurring leg ulcers. There have been multiple bypasses and the insertion of stents. And, of course, cancer of several kinds and a stroke or two. (Miller 2003: 3)

Thus, there is a need to recognize that ageing is both a social and biological construct. To capture contemporary accounts and meanings of old age as lived in time, there is also a need to acknowledge the impact of chronological age on people's experience of later life. Old age, no matter when we draw its beginning, always unequivocally, inevitably and irreversibly leads to deterioration in the organism and subsequently to 'terminal decline' (Small 2007: 21). When older people cross a boundary into the last stage of life, the beginning of which can be defined by their chronological age combined with a deterioration in their functional health, there is no escape from the inevitable ingredient of the human condition: mortality.

Recently, apart from a greater flexibility in the relationship between chronometric time and ageing the picture of the period between active living and biological death has also been complicated by changes in the dying trajectory of the aged and the increasing length of the end of life. These developments have exposed an ambiguity where ageing ends and disease begins, and the role of each in human decline and mortality (see Part III for more details). The growing profile of this protracted period in life has brought to public attention a need a for a clearer focus and understanding of the period between the onset of major illness in old age and death, a period that can last for months or even years. This is the stage that Carr and Luth (2019) label 'the end of life'. The emergence of this distinctively contemporary life-course stage is a result of two centuries of changes in when, where and from what cause people die. For example, medical advances have contributed to death occurring later and later in life, while the medicalization of death means that dying after a long life tends to take place in institutions, and comes in a variety of ways. While more on changes to the nature of death, places of dying and the various trajectories of death in old age will be discussed in Chapter 8, here it is worth pointing out that the end-of-life experiences are shaped by socioeconomic structures and interpersonal relationships. Because of the high costs of increased longevity and the medicalization of later life and death, as well as the problematic nature of many new choices of medical procedures and technologies to prolong life, end-of-life experiences are affected by socioeconomic factors, gender and educational, economic and ethnic characteristics, and they reflect older people's physical and mental conditions.

Yet there is considerable imprecision in defining the relationship between being old and the end of life; given that not everybody lives to this age, death is not always connected with old age. Hence, we can view old age

> as a contingency, though of a rather impure sort. It is not just a matter of circumstances coming to the agent from outside him or herself; nor is it just a matter of subjectivity, psychology and feelings. It involves both, but is, strictly, neither. (Small 2007: 4)

Even though the end of life is distinct from being old (at once inevitable yet not at all inevitable), there is a large overlap between later life and the end of life since most people now experience the end of life during old age. Potential tensions caused by the imprecision and elusiveness of defining the relationship between old age and the end of life may lead many to ask, 'How old is old?' This question places the complexity of the notion that 'old' becomes fully visible in a broader historical and cultural context.

One consequence of the limited life expectancy experienced by most people in the past, when – as discussed in the previous chapter – far fewer people reached older age, was that the qualifying age for the inclusion to the category of 'the old' was set rather low. For example, when the first old age pension was introduced in the United Kingdom in 1908, life expectancy at birth was 40 years for men and 43 for women, and only 24% of people reached state pension age (which was 70); the pension was only claimed for an average of nine years (Osborne 2020). Since 2020, the qualifying age for state pensions has climbed to 66 and by 2017, 85 percent of people were reaching the state pension age and were living for another 24 years after claiming their state pension (Osborne 2020). The lifting of the qualifying age for the status of 'old' can also be illustrated by the fact that being a centenarian is no longer so unique, although it is still sufficiently exceptional to be recognized by a card from the monarch. In the United Kingdom in 1914, the probability that someone born that year would live to 100 years of age was just 1%, and one person was enough to take responsibility for the monarch's cards; however, by 2016, the number of centenarians had increased by 70%, and it required seven people to send the Queen's cards that year (Grant and Scott 2016).

The above examples illustrate not only that increased in longevity has been changing our perception of what it means to be old, but that the chronological age is useful for policy and statistical purposes as well as for the country's acknowledgement of its elderly people. The usefulness of chronological age, however, can sometimes be questioned; this is because the public judgement about 'how old is old' can reflect ageist attitudes or can result in avoidance of the elderly so as not to be reminded about death. For example, Doris Lessing (1984: 72), in her novel *The Diary of a Good Neighbour* (written under the pseudonym Jane Somers), shows how Janna, 'a woman of fifty who is physically not near death', realizes that for her old people did not exist on the streets because she was 'so afraid of old age, of death'. Janna's new awareness of her avoidance of older people resulted from her accidental friendship with 'a woman of over ninety who is near death', which led her to question the distancing mechanisms used by society to 'get the old out of the way, out of sight' (Lessing 1984: 74, 21). Lessing's (1984: 32) portrait of average people wondering why the old people did not die out and asking the elderly, 'What is the point of their being alive still?' illustrates how the ordinary adults protect themselves from facing death by marginalizing older individuals and by refusing to recognize the realities of ageing bodies.

To sum up, in response to the changes in contemporary societies' demographic structures, the earlier chronological distinctions, which associated old age with being between 60 and 74 years old, and later with being over 75 years, have been replaced by a new category that recognizes 'the oldest old, typically after the age of 80' (Carr and Luth 2019: 515). While remembering that old age is more than a stage defined in chronological terms, here we view ageing as multifaceted and integrated within the life-course process, with its own ups and downs and with its own interactions between the body, self and society. Such a conceptualization of old age as a cultural category configured by societal values and orientations, as well as age-related deterioration, brings to our attention the fact that ageing is a complex process whereby continuity and change take place in the context of knowledge of finality and increasing bodily vulnerability. It means that we look at the old age as the later years of a long life, when 'an inevitable and irreversible deterioration in the organism as a consequence of its age' brings us closer to the end of life (Small 2007: 3). While not forgetting the consequences of older age's alterations to body and mind, in what follows we focus our attention on how people's awareness of death changes with ageing.

Age and the awareness of mortality

As Freud argued, we cannot imagine our own death and even 'in our relation to death we fantasize about survival' (Hägglund 2012: 114). The majority of not very old people tend to go through most of their lives believing that death is something that happens to other people. However, people's awareness of mortality may differ in dramatic times, such as pandemics, and their approach to death can also be altered by such factors as religion, cultural contexts and our subjective characteristics. Among the personalized features that play an essential role in altering people's perceptions of their mortality is the person's age. The sense of time in old age is different than it is in youth, hence facing a diminishing future is one source of the older person's distinct awareness of mortality. While the extension of life due to advances in medicine and public health makes death appear somewhat less proximate and central to our daily concerns, still there is a moment when, for the aged person, death becomes 'no longer a general, abstract fate' (de Beauvoir 1972: 440) and when they become aware of this personal event that is close at hand. Yet confronting mortality does not translate into one specific and stable attitude towards death (Adams 2020; Ardelt 2013; Clarke et al. 2012; Zimmermann 2012). While recognizing the inconclusiveness of the relationships between older people's sense of mortality and their attitudes to death (discussed in Chapter 7), here we focus on the relationship between chronological age and awareness of mortality – and facing the latter 'paradoxically implies being alive, questioning how to live, raising moral issues' (Brombert 2013: 165).

While proposing the inclusion of human temporality to help understand our approach to death, we acknowledge that the chronological age is not the only factor that needs to be taken into account when explaining how awareness of finitude impacts people. First, ageing is distinct from death – even though old age does come at the end of life, and even though in old age death is not an unexpected event, the risk of death is not limited just to this category of age. Moreover, age is not the only factor that needs to be considered when explaining the role of the awareness of finitude because this awareness is situational (for example, associated with people's experiences of illness and death), and this is only partially determined by age. Yet, even though preoccupation with death is not necessarily connected with chronological age (for instance, young persons' self-perceived health or the death of friends can lead to thoughts about death), there is a certain age-related focus on death (Marshall 1980). Not only is death at a young age seen to be tragic in itself, while at the other end of life it tends to be perceived as 'natural', but the manner of an older person's death matters less than that of a younger person, which is generally deemed premature and heartbreaking. Various empirical studies support the notion that age-related conditions and circumstances – for instance, illness or the death of a spouse – 'lead to cognitive work to make sense of the newly relevant fact of mortality' (Marshall 1980: 103). Moreover, as the total number of days spent in hospital increases with age and as people who die aged 75 years or older often spend several days in hospital in the last year of their life (Dalrymple et al. 2020), the elderly are under the pressure of illness and deterioration, and therefore have a clearer awareness of and feelings about the impending death. In general, it can expected that people's awareness of death increases with age as they become more conscious that their allotted time is running out.

In other words, the issue of mortality takes on greater urgency as we get older, with the weariness of one's body and the pervasiveness of death in one's social circles, and with more and more ageing friends and acquaintances dying. Although there is no common timeframe to which we can all relate, there is no escape from our embodied existence or the directionality of life, which means human 'existence means existing in time' (de Beauvoir 1972: 361). Moreover, we 'do not simply persist in time: we age, and our perception of being-towards-death is situated and quantified and scrutinized as well as psychologized in the language of ageing' (Small 2007: 6). With our growing understanding of the irreversibility of time, we seem to be colluding in our own demise as we know that 'each moment leads to another moment, this one to another and so on; that each moment destroys itself and that it's no use trying to hold back' (Sartre 1965: 85). The realization that the passing of time suppresses every moment, and as the moment ceases to be, the experience of loss is revealed, which brings us closer to death (Hägglund 2019). Hence, as we move through our lives, our need to make a sense of death and our understanding of mortality are both changing. In other words, as time does not remain identical throughout the life-course, anxiety about death occurs differently throughout the life-cycle and older adults can be expected to have different relationships with time and mortality than younger people do.

Looking at a lifelong journey from childhood to old age, results of empirical studies show that today's children, despite the variety of individual circumstances, are faced with two common factors shaping their relationship with death. First, children's awareness of mortality is now influenced by an overwhelming parental refusal to discuss the possibility of death with children. Second, young people's understanding of death comes from history lessons about fallen heroes who sacrificed their lives for the nation (Mahon 2011). While in the past most children learnt about death by witnessing death of their siblings or parents, during the contemporary childhood, as recent studies show, the idea of death seems to be presented as an issue for the distant future. Apart from glorified dead war heroes or other dead celebrities, it is seen as better kept suppressed or hidden (Walter 2017). Hence, on one hand, children's anxiety about death is smooth and calm down by telling them that death is not yet their problem for a long time to come, while on the other hand, by being taught about the worthiness of the death on the battlefield and how proud they should be of dead people's achievements, children are educated to be respectful when confronted with death: 'In short, we learn at a very early stage to be hypocritical about her ridiculing her with one turn of the face and then becoming deeply reverential with another' (Black 2018:4). Generally, for the majority of contemporary young people, the question of mortality remains fairly opaque (Bauman 2006).

As the journey of life continues, the transition to the teenage years brings 'an appreciation of the biological reality of death and their culturally transmitted understanding of an afterlife' (Adams 2020: 185). Adolescence, which is full of tensions, ambiguities and interest in risk-taking, is characterized by range of attitudes towards death, from strong death anxiety to total indifference. However, as the life-cycle perspective asserts, teenagers can become preoccupied with death and can experience death anxiety (Walter 2017). A fear of one's own non-being can be particularly marked in adolescence, and although today's teenagers have access to various professional resources to help them with death anxiety, there is a high rate of suicide in this age cohort (Walter 2017). Yet, as the years go by, adolescent death concerns are pushed aside by the two major life tasks of young adulthood – pursuing a career and beginning a family – and in the early adult years the issue of mortality is often deflected into the distant future.

While the majority of mature adults remain indifferent to death, some because of their work and others because of their life circumstances cannot avoid the issue. First, many middle-aged people encounter death daily in their professional roles; these people include doctors, nurses, undertakers, paramedics, policemen and firemen, all of whom witness death frequently – some on a daily basis. Their stories illustrate how, through their professional working lives, they come close to death and how much they have learned by dealing with situations that most of us spend our lives avoiding (Clarke 2020; Terkel 2003; Ware 2012). Second, in middle age, people are often faced with the death of their elderly parents or relatives, and even friends, and such new situations challenge them in terms of how to think about the death and how to talk about someone who is no longer there. Lydia Davis (2007), in a short story that describes how she faced the death of her father through using a linguistic consideration, illustrates how we hesitate over the words we use when talking about death as we try to avoid facing the truth of the situation. The narrator of the story, feeling confused by the gap between the truth of her father's death and the words she speaks, tries to remember that to know him is a present-tense enterprise but still wonders how to deal with someone who was so present and now is not. The surprise that comes with the realization that death changes the tense – once he has died, we now longer 'know' him but 'knew' him – illustrates how even not-so-young people are unprepared to face death. Moreover, middle age does not just expose people to the ambiguousness of language about death and dying, but also to steady changes in their own body, appearance and emerging signs of ageing – all signals of approaching a new stage in life.

Arriving at the end of a lifelong journey does not necessarily mean people in this phase of life are automatically concerned with mortality. Even if it is true that, as we are grow older, we spend more and more time thinking about what it implies to be mortal, it is also true that at the same time we 'spend a great deal of time trying, more or less strenuously, *not* to think about that fact and what it implies' (Small 2007: 21). Since it would be destructive to live with the continual awareness of our own mortality, we go to extraordinary lengths to repress our awareness of death, and this repression is a protective mechanism that often works right until the end of life. While in her late seventies, Jane Miller (2010: 1) opened her book about old age by saying 'I am old and feel and look old', but immediately stressed that people like her, although knowing that 'they likely to be dead within the next several years ... give little sense of being haunted by death or dreading it' (Miller 2010: 3). Moreover, it 'is difficult for people of advanced years to start remembering they must die' (Spark 1961: 39) and this is not only because of their death denial or their lack of meditation on mortality, but also because of declining mental capabilities that are often connected with dementia and other illnesses. With the passing of time, and with fewer people experiencing older age with chronic illnesses, and still enjoying very good physical and mental health, at some point for everyone, 'the positivity of the news about human ageing beings to crumble' and it can mean that sometimes the end of life is accompanied by a loss of agency (Baltes and Smith 2003: 128).

All the advances in medical technology and more flexible relationships between biological time and calendar time (as discussed in the previous chapter) have increased the variability of being old and the capacities to control and anticipate mortality. However, despite these new opportunities to confront ageing and death, older people's time horizon, in contrast to young people's firm focus on the future, is limited. For this reason, older people often experience a sense of having run out of time (May 2018). Older people know that as time accelerates, the exit is coming closer – or 'Unresting death, a whole day nearer now' (Larkin 1977, in his poem 'Aubade'). The acceleration of time in later life results in feeling that 'as the years go by our future shortens, while our past grows heavier' (de Beauvoir 1972: 361). Life speeds up as you get older, to use the title of Draaisma's (2004) book, because physiological clocks happen to run more slowly in an old body than they do in a young one, so as we grow older objective slowing down creates subjective speeding up (Draaisma 2004: 224). The acceleration of time further increases the ambivalent relationship with time in older age as the past 'seems subjectively to have become nearer instead' while the future wanes (Draaisma 2004: 224).

The topic of older people's awareness of mortality is therefore rather complex and difficult to address, even as death sooner or later becomes inescapable, although it cannot be foreseen as occurring on a definite date. Unsurprisingly, the issue of death seems to attract total silence in dominant cultural narratives and self-help books on ageing, which operate on the assumption that the last phase of life itself prepares the elderly for the acceptance of death. Although this notion of acceptance is never elaborated and explained, it seems to be rooted in the long-established idea that older people are more tolerant of death, a view supported by at least two philosophical traditions. The first perspective asserts that older persons understand that from the moment of birth, 'nature has condemned us to death' (Socrates, quoted in Choron 1963: 65), so they learn to accept that death is not a matter of choice. This binary perspective views life and death as inextricably connected parts of the same continuum and also asserts that such an understanding comes naturally with the passage of time, as we grow older. The narrative of a trajectory from birth to death assumes the 'unity of a life', while at the same time treating the last phase of life 'as of minor importance' (Small 2007: 2). By being concerned not with the essence of being but with the transitory and perishable essence of huma conditions, this approach 'focuses on passing', and argues that we 'are in death while you are in life' (Montaigne 1987: 103–5). Living with this sense of transition, in contrast to our frequent assumption that the best remedy against the fear of death is to pretend that death does not exist, suggests that the best protection against death anxiety is in fact awareness that our time here will not last forever.

Equally important for the acceptance of mortality in old age is the argument developed by the Stoics, ancient philosophers who appreciated the role of the elderly in helping us to reconcile ourselves with mortality. This long philosophical tradition asserts that older people embrace their finitude without fear, as in old age death is more desired than later life, as death enables older people to avoid the disabilities and miseries of old age. Moreover, the Stoics argued that old age gives courage in the face of death, so fear of death is unfounded (Choron 1963: 45). For example, an ageing Cicero observed that, 'When a man has reached my age, he ought not to be repining at the approach of death' (quoted in Choron 1963: 65). In other words, both approaches – the binary perspective that views death and birth being a part of the cosmic order of things and the Stoic position that asserts death is not a threat for older people – assume that old age helps elderly people to view their mortality without fear.

Although many people would like to believe that death in old age can easily be tolerated and accepted, the existing empirical studies construct a more complicated picture. They show that older people's relationships with mortality are flexible and open to deliberation and change (Adams 2020; Ardelt 2013). While some studies indicate that older people – especially those with multiple morbidities and numerous encounters with the deaths of others – may be more accepting of death (Lloyd 2000; Siddell 1993), other empirical investigations suggest that for many older people, death is not a matter of indifference (Fortnert and Neimeyer 1999; Hockey 1990; Howarth 1998; Marshall 1975, 1980; Neimeyer and van Brunt 1995). Nonetheless, it is the conceptualization of older people's awareness of mortality as increasingly insistent yet flexible that is revealed in recent studies. Such a perspective is behind the need to negotiate feelings about 'the end of times' that are increasingly prominent in modern Western societies. While continuing to fear death, and despite strong in individual differences, 'older people are still able to move forward into manageable relationship with their mortality' (Adams 2020: 198). Longitudinal studies that have explored perceptions of nearness to death in people older than 70 years show that these individuals have an accurate idea of how close they are to death (Kotter-Gruhn et al. 2010). However, older people's awareness of the nearness of their death does not necessarily result in a single, stable attitude towards death (Clarke et al. 2012). Ardelt's (2013: 151) observation that older people have more exposure to the death of other age cohorts comes with the discovery that being afraid of death does not appear to be related to accepting death, and that neither wisdom nor a sense of purpose in life appears to be required for accepting death. Additionally, Terkel's (2003: 39, 206, 339) in-depth conversations with older people offer considerable evidence that older people's relationship with death is consciously negotiated, often changing and ranging from 'being afraid of death' through 'I have absolutely no fear of death' to 'I think about death all the time. Then I pretend I am not thinking about it and I pretend it does not exist.' This ethnographic work also discloses that although the majority of older people do not want to discuss mortality, 'as is something that we can't possibly understand', others want to be prepared for death, as

> anybody who says they are not afraid of death is kidding themselves, I do not know whether we fear death itself, I do not know, either we have any understanding about the death itself that is what we fear about it. (Terkel 2003: 63)

A general conclusion from this new investigation that demonstrates the inconclusiveness of the relationships between older people's sense of mortality and their orientations towards death is that a variety of death attitudes exist (Adams 2020; Ardelt 2013; Clarke et al. 2012; Zimmermann 2012). In short, the realization of one's mortality does not necessarily translate into one specific and immutable way of coping with the proximity of death.

Moreover, most studies also seem to suggest that all varieties of awareness of finitude – from being unreconciled to mortality, through seeing it as natural and not dwelling on it, to waiting for it, are contingent on a person's religion, social values, contacts, cultural context and resources. For a very long time, religion has been one of the most important factors determining one's awareness of mortality. With the idea of our finitude playing a central role in many religious scriptures, religious beliefs in an afterlife often help people to face death. In the past, religion provided a framework for beliefs and ritual actions that gave meaning to death and taught us that people should not fear death. Traditionally, people's search for ways of responding to consciousness of mortality led to religion, seen as a way to mediate suffering and redemption from the awareness of finality. For example, Christianity, which bestows scared meaning upon suffering and offers hope of an after-life, equips people with 'the cultural resources to live through and beyond this experience' (Wilkinson 2005: 33). In contemporary Western societies, with the decline of the role of religion in mediating experiences of mortality, people have explored various ways to deal with the issue of death without the past religious support to negate our nothingness. In today's increasing secularized societies, 'where most of us believe that death ends everything' (Small 2007: 136), the end of life is often characterized by an individual struggle to make sense of things. However, as the study of the elderly in the world's most secular society – Denmark – shows, the absence of the support of religion does not necessary mean that people cannot confront mortality with remarkable calm and acceptance (Zuckerman 2008).

Another important resources in helping older people to negotiate their finitude is connection with family and friends. These relationships are a source of help, comfort and reconciliation with the anticipated death. Literary diaries and novels show how feeling of despair evoked by the approaching death can be alleviated by close bonds with others. For example, both Heilbrun (1997) in *The Last Gift of Time: Life Beyond Sixty* and Diski (2016) in her book *In Gratitude*, while illustrating the subjective feeling of regret connected with one's mortality, demonstrate that characteristics of such emotion involve not only regrets about 'their disappearance from these stage', but also sadness that the people close to them who would be left with the loss and a need to deal with her absence. They also are grateful to others for their love and want to protect them from suffering and grief. Hence, it is possible that our wish to spare our loved ones the anguish of mourning 'can help us to accept our future death as a loss with which we strive to reconcile ourselves in advance' (Ricoeur 2004: 359).

Since 'there is remedy for everything except death' (Cervantes, quoted in Bauman 2011: 388), the acceptance of death 'remains a task we must all engage in, and one that we face up to more or less successfully' (Ricoeur

2004: 358). To engage in this task means bridging a gap between wanting to live and having to die through the acceptance of death, and in doing this we rely on various supportive resources, including religion, family and social networks. Under normal circumstances, and in more certain times, older adults have a choice of various ways to negotiate and work on the acceptance of death. However, the COVID-19 pandemic has introduced new risks and created deep uncertainty about the care and conditions of the end of life. Hence, the final part of this chapter will consider the impact of the pandemic on the emotional mood, narratives and reality of dying during COVID-19.

COVID-19 and ageist prejudices

The COVID-19 crisis has exposed and activated ageist prejudices that are deeply embedded in British society. There are many consequences of the ageism of the COVID-19 policies, with the two most tragic outcomes of these policies being connected with the UK Government's decision to discharge older patients from hospitals into care homes without being tested, which contributed to the high level of mortality among care home residents, and with the abuse of 'do not resuscitate' orders, applied to care home residents without regard for their wishes or welfare (Calvert and Arbuthnott 2021; Horton 2020).While these two examples of COVID-19 ageism will be discussed in Chapter 9, here we focus on the UK Government's initial consideration of allowing the majority of the population to become infected with coronavirus to build 'herd immunity' and its later decision to label all those over 70 as 'vulnerable' and to ask them to self-isolate. Both policies – the considered strategy of a herd immunity, which viewed older people as 'expendable' members of the herd (Clarke 2021) and the policy of 'the chronological quarantine' (Fletcher 2020) – can be seen as cases of age discrimination. They could have, or indeed have, led to the worsening of the aged people's physical and mental health. Moreover, as the COVID-19 pandemic policy supplemented existing discrimination against older people with the narratives of herd immunity and lockdown, it put older people at risk of internalizing the idea that being older means being vulnerable, as well as being a burden on the rest of society.

Although there is still little research into the pandemic's impact on ageism and the mental health of older individuals, there are some discussions about the worldwide emergence of ageism in the context of the COVID-19 pandemic (Ayalon et al. 2020) and there are the previous studies of the impact of stereotyping on older people's wellbeing (Levy et al. 2009), as well as some investigations of the pandemic's impact on older people's physical and mental health (Age UK 2021; Corcoran and Wood 2021). Even though we are interested mainly in the UK case, it is worth mentioning, as Ayalon et al. (2020) illustrate, that during the pandemic, ageist prejudices spread throughout the world via social media, traditional media and public announcements. By scrutinizing articles from many countries about the responses to COVID-19, Ayalon et al. (2020) demonstrate that 'in public discourse is an increasing portrayal of those over the age of 70 as being all alike with regard to being helpless, frail, and unable to contribute to society'. One of the most revealing illustrations of how older adults' are portrayed as helpless, frail and unable to contribute to society in any important way is provided by the words of a German professor in law science who said:

> Every life has equal value, but that civil society should invest the same energy … to provide additional months or years to a 95-year old … is much of an imposition for common sense. (quoted in Ayalon et al. 2020)

The impact of ageism on older people's physical and mental health in the United Kingdom during the COVID-19 pandemic began from the outset of the pandemic and was connected with the herd immunity strategy, which was considered by the government despite its questionable ethical dimensions. This strategy, though officially denied, was at the centre of the controversy over how we could best protect the vulnerable in the first stage of the pandemic. The main assumption of the idea of a herd immunity – that is, the idea that the population as a whole could block transmission, even if some individuals were still susceptible – can be questioned on various grounds, from scientific to ethical to practical ones (Kucharski 2020). The strategy of herd immunity would have been particularly disturbing for older people, not only because they could have seen it as an extremely unhelpful tool for disease control, but also because they would have been afraid that the herd immunity policy could have entailed the sacrifice of the old, or those deemed less worthy of saving.

In the first three months of the pandemic – that is, until the delayed lockdown (23 March 2020), the UK Government, which at that time still enjoyed a high level of social trust, briefly contemplated herd immunity as a preferable way of handling to the COVID-19 emergency. This first initial response to COVID-19 seems to have due to governmental planning being for an influenza pandemic; hence it was guided by the argument that, as with flu, 'the herd immunity is the right response of you haven't got a vaccine' (Calvert and Arbuthnott 2021: 106). The strategy of herd immunity was also central to the government's plans in late February and early March 2020 because it was argued that this would protect the economy and preserve jobs as the younger generations could continue to work in a normal way. Moreover, by postponing a general lockdown while allowing the young and fit to acquire immunity, herd immunity could delay the peak of the pandemic until summer (Calvert and Arbuthnot 2021).

Nevertheless, herd immunity was 'a big gamble', given that there was no clear evidence at the time that those people who contracted the virus actually retrained any lasting antibodies (Calvert and Arbuthnott 2021: 176). The supporters of the policy of herd immunity were not concerned with this strategy's ethical dimensions or the fact that this policy could have increased risks faced by the old, and that many of the aged could needlessly die. Yet such disregard of ethical standards could have practical consequences that were clearly pointed out by Chris Whitty, the United Kingdom's chief medical officer, who said, 'If I as an individual increase my risk, I increase the risk to everyone around me ... sooner or later the chain will meet people who are vulnerable or elderly' (quoted in Burch 2020: 22). Hence, Age UK called on the government to 'resist the ageist siren calls to shut older people away' in order 'let the virus rip' (Age UK 2022). This urgent plea was supported by many other voices, with more than 200 British scientists and academics signing a letter condemning the considered policy (Calvert and Arbuthnott 2021: 194) and with many doctors and the WHO pointing to the value of getting test-and-trace working properly (Clarke 2021; Francis 2021). The increasing criticism of the considered strategy pointed that the concept of herd immunity effectively meant that 'the weakest in society – the ill and the elderly – are left to perish' (Calvert and Arbuthnott 2021: 106). Although some advocates of the herd immunity policy asserted that it did not imply older people were dispensable, they still argued that if people did not want to shield, 'this should be their choice' and viewed old age as 'the rational time to take up a dangerous sport' (Burch 2020: 22). Despite of the growing disapproval and denunciation of the herd immunity as being 'toxic politically' (Calvert and Arbuthnott 2021:106), the government, with the support of proponents of protecting the economy, remained intent on pursuing the herd immunity policy.

At least to some degree, this government willingness to continue with such a dangerous experiment was made possible because the statistical data could assist the argument that the high death rates from COVID-19 were not a social problem. With the great majority of deaths from COVID-19 occurring in the elderly – which is true of 'virtually all other causes of death too' – it has been 'easier to lose sight' of the issue of death of the aged (Chrisakis 2020: 302–3). COVID-19's pattern of mortality allowed us to ignore the issue of the risk of COVID-19 to the elderly and to disregard the fact a herd immunity policy could have left them feeling that they were expendable. The problem of risk faced by the elderly from coronavirus was not too hard to discount because, for example, the data that the median age of coronavirus victims (83) actually exceeded UK life expectancy at birth (81) could be presented out of context to argue that the high mortality rate from COVID was not a social issue as it was only the elderly who were dying with the disease, and they were 'people who would have died anyway within a short time' (Spiegelhalter and Masters 2021: 103).

When the strategy of herd immunity was made public, it became obvious that British society did not support the government's project. The public's rejection of the idea, together with the increased criticism of herd immunity within the scientific community, the medical world and the charity sector, made it clear that the government had to give up on its policy of herd immunity (Calvert and Arbuthnott 2021). Despite the government's denial that it had considered adopting policies of 'prioritising the young over the old', public attention was drawn to the ethical dimensions of a herd immunity strategy (Reisz 2020: 3). Newspapers and social media accused the government of thinking about adopting this policy to 'let old people die' in order to 'protect the economy, and if that means some pensioners die, "too bad", the criticism which was the quickly rejected by government as being 'highly defamatory fabrication' (Walker 2020). Although, from the outset of the epidemic, Downing Street was officially denying media claims that the prime minister's aide said 'let old people die', newspapers reporting on the government's policy of 'sacrificing' the elderly and rationing health resources in a way that would negatively affect the elderly were alarming (Butler 2020: 33). Articles about the elderly being abandoned to the worst the virus could do, about 'callous betrayal of our most vulnerable' and asking the disturbing question of whether 70-year-olds had as much right to live as 20-year-olds (Ellen 2020: 27) revealed the price the elderly were expected to pay for the normal functioning of the economy. Of course, not all media were critical of the herd immunity policy: some social platforms proposed tackling the pandemic by 'letting old people die' (Walker 2020), while others cultivated ageism by suggesting that 'people in their late 70s weren't worth the economic cost it would require to save them' (Hattenstone 2020). This grim rhetoric about older people was possible mainly on social platforms that functioned without traditional editorial gatekeepers, able to monitor the content or impose self-discipline policies.

With the main media exposure of the herd immunity potential impact of the elderly and with the rest of Europe starting to go into lockdown, the UK government was forced to abandonment the policy of the herd immunity. While describing the herd immunity 'as a scientific concept, not a goal or strategy', the government introduced the first lockdown at the end of March 2020 (Calvert and Arbuthnott 2021:106). The lockdown, which is our second example of the impact of ageism on older people's physical and mental health in the UK during the COVID pandemic, started with older people being collectively written off as a homogenous group that is at risk as it was announced that over-70 were to self-isolate to protect them from the virus, while whole society was asked to protected these 'more mature citizens' (BBC News).

More specifically, the British government's guidance on social distancing for the first lockdown stated: 'We are advising those who are at increased risk of severe illness from coronavirus (COVID-19) to be particularly stringent in following social distancing measures. This group includes those who are aged 70 or older (regardless of medical conditions)'. There are several problems with the whole group of the population, those over 70, being treated as a homogeneous group, and being 'defined to be at risk, and labelled as vulnerable' (Evans 2020). Firstly, the older cohort is a very heterogenous group, as we will show in more detail in a next chapter. Secondly, many older people have been deeply upset and distressed about that label as it associates old age with vulnerability and as such is prejudicial. The referral to the chronological age has left many older people upset and angry. Thirdly, older people had a miserable time in lockdown, when shielding in their homes or secluded in care homes, they were full of fears, confusions and worries. All of which together have impacted on their mental and physical well-being.

Moreover, during the first lockdown, while telling the over-seventies to stay at home, the government did not come with any offer of protection to those who were most vulnerable. Labelling the elderly as vulnerable was not accompanied by any acknowledgement of the physical and mental limitations of ageing and any recognition that these conditions become more threatening when the elderly lack resources and social support. In other words, during the health crisis, while being informed about the risk of death from the coronavirus, older people, were not cautioned about the risks of isolation, loneliness or COVID-induced fears of a loss of social connectedness and risk of death, and were not made aware of frailty as the classification method that was helping to work out which patients should be denied acute care. Rather, the fact that the assessment of frailty could be used to define their suitability for medical assistance was hidden from them (see Chapter 3). During the first lockdown, older people, who were classified solely on the basis of their chronological age to determine risk, were asked to live in social isolation and were left alone with their fears. This policy showed 'that the old, and particularly the materially and physically vulnerable old, have been regarded, with their carers, as little other than an inconvenient cost' (Evans 2020).

Finally, the reliance on chronological age as sole criterion for defining risk has been questioned not only in terms of its discriminatory value but also because it is an arbitrary and imprecise, rather than scientifically sound, criterion. The introduction of the rule of self-isolation based on the criterion of chronological was not accompanied by any explanation for why and on what kind of medical and legal basis such 'age-based apartheid' was proposed (Fletcher 2020). Hence, it resulted in the articulation of different positions. For example, the British Society of Gerontology (BSG) described the government response as ageist, while the former president of the British Geriatrics Society (BGS) rejected accusations of ageism and instead depicted the policy as an instance of evidence-based pragmatic discrimination (Fletcher 2020). Similar objections were raised in other countries, which voiced the argument that using chronological age as the sole criterion for determining risk was behind 'the current pandemic of ageism' (Ayalon et al. 2020). For example, a critical debate about ageism animated by COVID-19 took place in Poland, where the government legislation, which made it mandatory for all those 70 years of age and above – that is, for four million people, or more than 10% of the whole population – to stay indoors from 24 October 2020; it was evaluated to be unconstitutional and to violate the human rights of old people (Kaczorowska 2020). Moreover, the Italian Society of Anaesthesia, Analgesia and Intensive Care's announcement early in the crisis, suggesting that intensive care treatment might be restricted by age to maximize the life-saving effectiveness of limited resources was criticized as ageist, while the Canadian Association on Gerontology was negatively judged for using arbitrary age cut-offs, thus reinforcing negative age stereotypes and prejudices (Fletcher 2020).

In the United Kingdom, the arbitrariness of chronological age as a criterion for self-isolation has been exposed further with the fluctuation of the age marker during the following waves of the pandemic and with the lack of clear definition of who is 'old', and how old is 'old'. The instability of the age category and the confusion over the definition of 'old' can best be illustrated by a quick look at the language of official health announcements during the pandemic. From the beginning of the COVID-19 crisis, the governmental strategies of coping with the coronavirus relied on a set of confusing definitions of 'old'. For example, while the first lockdown asked all people over 70 to shield, in the second wave of the pandemic it was proposed that people over 60 should 'be especially careful and minimize their social contacts, but there will be no return of a formal request to shield themselves' (HM Government 2020). In further discussions of the second lockdown, the term 'clinically extremely vulnerable' was used interchangeable with the notion of 'elderly', or those over 70 years of age, in a very confusing way. Moreover, when the 2020–21 winter was approaching, the NHS informed the public that it had 'the flu vaccine in stock for patients over 65', while the first announcement of the UK Vaccine Task Force, in December 2020, promised that a COVID-19 vaccine would be available for the 'old' – that is, people aged over 50. Yet in early December 2021, it was announced that all people over 40 years of age were eligible for their booster jabs, or their third vaccinations. The coronavirus has highlighted some flaws, inconsistencies and prejudicial confusions in our understanding of how old is 'old', who is 'old' and how they are at risk.

By associating old age with vulnerability, the pandemic has not provided the general public with vivid images of the elderly, but rather confirmed the message given by a road sign encouraging drivers to look out for elderly pedestrians, which features two bent figures with sticks. The COVID-19 pandemic, during which the British media were full of narratives and images of elderly residents of care homes, presented us mainly with pictures of just one, very distinctive stage in the ageing process: the fourth age, which is viewed as some kind of 'an imaginary black hole' filled up with illness, immobility and sufferings (Higgs and Gilleard 2015: 17). The fourth age – in contrast to the third age, which is characterized by fitness, activity and productive lifestyle – is represented by ill-health, incapacity and dependence on others (Laslett 1989). By associating older people solely with the decay and dependency, such images acted to reinforce comments on some social platforms about older people being a burden to society and suggestions about how older adults could be 'managed' (Ellen 2020). With the coronavirus generating high levels of uncertainty, and with daily reports of deaths in care homes, as well as with media information that older people 'were withering away', certain sections of social media – and the presence of social media is what made this epidemic different from its predecessors – were 'all busy stockpiling either ageist prejudices or paranoiac visions about the young wishing the old dead' (Ellen 2020: 27). Such statements, prejudicial stereotypes and images of old people, which were allowed to resurface on social media during the pandemic, revealed the existence of ageism, with its assumptions that the death of old people did not represent a great loss to society.

Our discussion of the United Kingdom's initial responses to the coronavirus has shed light on the underlying ageism of COVID-19 policies, which could be seen as a manifestation, or even an exacerbation, of the country's long-existing institutional ageism. The pandemic has exposed the pandemic policies' lack of an ethical sensibility in relation to old age and the absence of any considerations of the likely adverse effects of COVID-19 strategies on older people's wellbeing. Following the research that found self-perceptions of stigmatized groups can negatively influence their longevity (Levy at al. 2009), it is clear that the COVID-19 policies not only had negative effects on older people's mental and bodily conditions but that these responses to the threat of coronavirus could also have adversely affected older individuals' self-perceptions, in turn impacting their longevity. This argument is in line with the results of extensive, longitudinal and cross-cultural research that suggests internalized stereotypes of the old can influence older people's beliefs about their own ageing, and that such stereotypes could detrimentally impact older people's health (Levy et al. 2009). Those who internalized less positive self-perceptions of ageing as a result of stereotypes and stigmatization of the old can expect more health problems and shorter lives than those who did not internalize negative age attitudes. Moreover, this disadvantage caused by negative age beliefs and their harmful effects on older people's health remained after age, gender, socioeconomic status, loneliness and health were controlled (Levy et al. 2009).

Remembering the effects of ageist stereotypes on longevity, it can be argued that in order to tackle the COVID-19 ageism, we need to uncover the stereotypes of old aged that underlined the state's responses to the pandemic and recognize them as presenting threats to older people's wellbeing. The depth and breadth of stereotypes of ageing transmitted to older individuals by the COVID-19 policies have impacted the wellbeing of those older people studied. For example, older people polled in the 'Lived Experience, Voices of Older People on the COVID-19 Pandemic' study reported high levels of anger, frustration and distress about the assumptions made about them during the pandemic. While knowing that, for them, the risks of catching COVID-19 were higher, these older individuals were also aware of the policy's underling suggestions that they had outlived their usefulness (Corcoran and Wood 2021).

The Age UK research on how the COVID-19 pandemic has impacted older people's physical and mental health also shows that older people were worried about the practical, physical and emotional effects of the pandemic. In particular, those who had long-term health conditions reported that the pandemic was an extremely challenging time for them. The study found that because of the pandemic's required isolation, many older people were enduring increased levels of anxiety, and experienced physical and cognitive decline. Summarizing the results of the study, Caroline Abrahams, Age UK's charity director, said that 'this pandemic has hit the fast forward button on ageing for millions of older people' (Age UK 2020). Research carried out by the Mental Health Foundation and Independent Age showed that the coronavirus pandemic had damaged the mental and physical health of many people over the age of 65, with a large proportion of the United Kingdom's 12.5 million older people suffering as a result of their loneliness, worsening mobility and grief (Corcoran and Wood 2021).

On the basis of these studies, it can be argued that the COVID-19 pandemic has not only increased the visibility of death in old age, but has also exposed stereotypes, prejudice and discrimination against older adults that are deeply embedded in UK society. The COVID-19 crisis and the policies adopted to handle it have impacted elderly people's wellbeing, their levels of anxiety connected with defying the image of being vulnerable and frail, and the quality and conditions of end-of-life care.

CHAPTER 3

The ageing population as a threat to society

When the aged are seen as a problem

The chapter explores the argument that the ageing of modern society presents developed nations with a threat to their productivity and wealth, and creates a generational divide. Recently, as a result of the demographic shift that has occurred, many contemporary societies have seen the re-emergence of the use of divisive intergenerational rhetoric. Yet the history of relationships between generations shows that there is nothing new about conflicts between older and younger generations. By rejecting chronological age as the sole explanatory factor behind people's interest, and by showing the diversity and divisions that exist among the aged population, this chapter questions the assumption that increased longevity necessarily creates conflicts over intergenerational inequality. The following section, by including the role of the body as a marker of division and difference, illustrates that age-related frailty and dependence are sources of fear and burden. Finally, the chapter analyses how the COVID-19 pandemic has made elderly people increasingly vulnerable and exposed them to negative experiences, ranging from loneliness to death. It also shows how the pandemic has constructed the bases for both generational divisions and the opening up of new intergenerational exchanges that could reposition care of the old as an opportunity rather than solely an obligation. The chapter concludes by arguing that in order to learn a lesson from the recent health emergency and to realize the importance of social solidarity in managing the processes of ageing and dying, we need to understand how to eliminate the fears faced by the elderly.

Before we discuss how and why the aged are now constructed as a social problem, and before we explore how the recent demographic shift has contributed to the perception of the old as a burden to modern society, we need to recognize that ageism has always existed in many countries, not just in the West, and that tensions between the generations have a long history (Calasanti 2020). Throughout history, there have been various ways of confronting the elderly and their imminent death, ranging from older people's recognition of the need to accept their fate, through senicide – that is, the extreme institution that existed in many cultures in the past – to the separation of the elderly from society in residential facilities, which is a modern phenomenon. The first type of approach can be founded in the premise from antiquity that human worth is aligned to productivity. The idea that the old should not reject the opportunity of ending their lives when they are no longer useful for society was expressed by Socrates, when he argued – as reported by Plato – that old people who are not productive citizens ought not to fear of death but accept their fate as their responsibility to the state. Socrates, who showed an enormous courage in accepting his sentence to die at the age seventy two, knew that 'when a man has reached [his] age ... the fragilities of old age will be realized'. He believed that since the man's greatness consists in accepting his human conditions with responsibility, when he cannot be a productive citizen, he should acknowledge it and accede to his death (Socrates, quoted in Choron 1963: 43–6).

Senicide, or geronticide – that is, killing or abandonment of the elderly to the point of death – was one way to solve the problem of who should live and who should die. It was a practice of killing the elderly who were already at an age of perceived uselessness, and was usually performed by members of their tribe or family (Holland-Batt 2020). Such practices illustrate the potential for violence in any society as soon as 'any category of humans is placed outside the pale of those whose life has value, nothing more natural than to kill them' Simone Weil (quoted in Rose 2022: 60). Geronticide was done in various ways: in many societies in the past, old persons were simply neglected or abandoned so that they would die without becoming a burden on their families. For example, in the period from 400 to 800 CE, a Germanic tribe known as the Heruli killed the sick and elderly (Pyali

2017). The killing of the old was also practised in Sardinia, where women known as *accabadoras* (terminators) would bludgeon or suffocate the elderly until they died. In Japan, the apocryphal practice of *ubasute* involved abandoning elderly relatives on a mountaintop to die of exposure (Holland-Batt 2020: 20). Likewise, in the Arctic regions of Greenland, Canada and Alaska, the Inuit used to practise senicide by leaving their elderly on the ice to die. Senicide among the Inuit people was, however, rare except during famines; the last known case of an Inuit senicide occurred in 1939 (Pyali 2017). The only place where some cases of senicide are claimed to still occur today is the southern district of the state of Tamil Nadu in India. Although *thalaikoothal*, a practice whereby the elderly are given cold oil baths to reduce the body temperature, then fed coconut water and milk to prompt renal failure, is unconstitutional in India, apparently it can still be found in some places. Soumya's report from 2016 notes that the only difference between a few recently observed cases of *thalaikoothal* and past practices was that 'earlier the family conducted it as a ritual, now it is more of a silent affair' (quoted in Pyali 2017).

Senicidal thinking, expressions and symbols can also provide a conceptual framework for an extreme form of ageism. For many centuries, such a perspective has been present in various cultural expressions, extending from folk legends through novels and dystopian literature to folk horror films. For example, the fictional tradition of *ättestupa*, which according to Nordic legends and sagas refers to sites where ritual suicides of elderly people took place during prehistoric times, came into use in the 2019 movie *Midsommar*. Likewise, a popular Japanese folk tale refers to a fictional ritual of *obausteyama*, in which old women are abandoned on the tops of mountains by their sons (Danely 2015). Fictional visions of senicide can be found in dystopian novels, where the ruling generation typically justifies overt violence towards the aged through the lens of economic rationalism; the elderly are viewed as 'burdensome "parasites" who are expensive to maintain' (Cruikshank 2003: 23). For instance, in Trollope's science fiction novel, *The Fixed Period* (1882), which is set on the island of Britannula off the coast of New Zealand, in the then-distant year of 1980, the elderly are separated for retirement at age 65 then, so they do not have to endure the indignities, weakness and selfish misery of extreme old age, they are euthanized at the age of 67 years and six months. This radical solution of executing all older citizens is proposed by the enlightened rulers of Britannula who, when faced with the problem posed by medical progress – that is, a growing ageing population – chose to prioritize the quality over the quantity of life. In Huxley's *Brave New World* (1932), the elderly are killed at the age of 60 then cremated and recycled into fertilizer. The subject of the cost of longevity is also explored in Lionel Shriver's recent novel, *Should We Stay or Should We Go* (2021), which asks how long we want to live and how we wish to die. The novel argues that for anybody 'to survive in a state of advanced decay is unnatural', laments that the ageing population is a 'burden on younger taxpayers' and makes the aged 'feel literally guilty for living and also dying for too long' (Shriver 2021: 48). By raising the issue of potential conflicts of interest between older and younger generations, this work of fiction has exposed the growing cost of the expanded lifespan in terms of societal ageism.

In many Western countries, the prediction of the approaching 'demographic agequake' has added to the intergenerational tensions, which began in at least the 1990s and were later enhanced by the financial crisis of 2008. With the 'silver tsunami' causing concern to politicians, the ageing population has been defined as the greatest threat to today's society. Viewing the aged as a social problem, as several studies show, has been on policy agendas or parties' manifestos in the United Kingdom, United States and Australia (Bristow 2019; Calasanti 2020; Walker 2018). In other words, scapegoating of the older generation, justified by the demographic change, has been used by policy-makers as a way to cut back on welfare entitlements. As the rhetoric around the old has changed, 'old people have moved from being seen as deserving and entitled to being viewed as undeserving dependants, especially those who are the most economically vulnerable' (Calasanti 2020). However, this recent ageism, which has been brought to the surface by fears and threats signalled by the metaphor of the 'silver tsunami', would have not been possible without the presence of long-established stereotypes, prejudices and negative attitudes towards the aged in modern society.

The demographic shift has forced Western societies to realize that over the next several decades, they will be facing many new ordeals. These forthcoming challenges are seen as a result of the expected very unbalanced age structure, with huge numbers of elderly people – especially those over age 85 – and small increases in the population aged below 64 years. It is projected that in the United Kingdom by 2066, there will be a further 8.6 million residents aged 65 years and over, taking the total number in this group to 20.4 million and making up 26% of the total population, while in the United States the number of people aged over 85 is expected to nearly quadruple over the next four decades (Colby and Orman 2015). Moreover, it is estimated that in the United Kingdom in thirty years' time, around 20% of people aged over 80 will have some form of dementia (Lloyd 2000), which means that many people dying in old age will spent several years in poor health and will require extensive care. For many Western countries, the challenge of an increasingly larger share of retired people who are not contributing to the labour market and whose demands for medical and social care will continue to increase poses an urgent financial problem. As we all live longer, the question arises of whether we can afford pensions that need to last more than twice as long as when they were first introduced at the beginning of the twentieth century. Thus, the quality of provision to older citizens and their post-retirement welfare are rapidly becoming a real social problem for all nations in contemporary times (Grant and Scott 2016).

However, the answers proposed by the political elites to solve this very real problem facing developed countries have, as many policy scholars suggest, been neither adequate nor correct (Bristow 2019; Calasanti 2020; Walker 2018). While concerned about the expected arrival of this 'demographic time bomb' and fearful of its consequences (increased health costs, social care costs and pension costs), governments have constructed a narrative of generational inequality in which the aged are defined as a social problem or a burden on the public purse (Bristow 2019). While claiming that this expanded longevity has brought new costs and problems for the state, political and cultural elites of many developed countries have employed the generational war rhetoric of 'baby boomers' versus 'millennials' to justify welfare cuts (Bristow 2019; Filipovic 2020; Gibney 2017). From the first decades of the twenty-first century, with the post-war baby boomers (the generation born between 1946 and 1956) coming of age and with the 'golden cohort' (the generation born between 1925 and 1934) slowly leaving or being hidden away in care homes, it has been the generation of baby boomers that has come to be seen as an unwanted burden for millennials (the generation born between 1981 and 1994 – or, in some classifications, as late as 2000).

By constructing divisive intergenerational rhetoric and using it to call for welfare reforms, policy-makers and campaigners for intergenerational equality have attacked older adults as 'the entitled generation' that damages the economy, undermines the standard of living and makes societies dysfunctional (Gullette 2015: 25). In media, the baby boomers have often been represented as greedy, self-indulgent individuals with gilded pensions and overpriced houses (Bristow 2019). In several books, it has been claimed that, by meeting all their own housing, healthcare and financial needs at the expense of their children, the baby boomers have forced the next generation to take a back seat (Willetts 2011). The baby boomers have been labelled a 'generation of sociopaths' who have 'mortgaged the future' and 'betrayed America' (Gibney 2017: 12). Some writers, while pitting the young against older people and painting a picture of the baby boomers as a selfish generation responsible for many contemporary problems, from climate change to depriving younger generations of many benefits, 'exacerbate generational warfare, arguing that older people in need of life-saving measures should be permitted to die in favour of younger people' (Holland-Batt 2020: 22). With the duty-to-die campaign's argument that the older people should 'go cheaply' by refusing medical treatment gaining notoriety and moving out of the field of bioethics, the generational gap between millennials and the baby boomers has been expanded even further (Gullette 2015: 25).

As these representations illustrate, by making the baby boomers guilty of 'stealing' the future from younger generation, policy-makers and campaigners for intergenerational equality have constructed a narrative of an intergenerational divide that suits their political agenda. Political elites, together with champions of intergenerational equality, have blamed baby boomers for failing to protect the interests of future generations and demanded that 'politics must act to address that' (Willetts 2011: 34). By declaring that younger people's economic problems, unsatisfying jobs and inability to afford houses can be solved just by 'mugging grandmas' who do not deserve what they have, they have inflated intergenerational conflicts over resources without offering any real solutions to these societal problems

(Bristow 2019): 'Policies couched in the language of "intergenerational equity" do not seek to redistribute resources from old to young; rather, they aim to curtail the entitlements of older people in order to cut public spending overall' (Bristow 2019: 214). In other words, intergenerational equality calls for fair treatment of young people should be viewed with suspicion, as in reality these demands for improvement of intergenerational equality are simply arguments designed to reduce spending on pensions and healthcare for elderly people (Bristow 2019; Calasanti 2020; Walker 2018). This divisive rhetoric of intergenerational divide wants us to believe that there is conflict between old and young; thus, in order to activate and stir generational frictions, it accords the lower value or status to older people. This rhetoric of a generational 'war' has made ageism into a newly acceptable prejudice (Bristow 2019) and consequently the scapegoating of the aged has become very harmful experience for the elderly. With 'boomer' becoming a term of abuse and with the setting of young people against the older generation, many baby boomers sense that 'everybody hated old people; it was acceptable, encouraged even because of your paid-off mortgage and your free education and your ruination of the planet' (Wood 2020: 34). They feel that, by being blamed for forgetting about the younger generations and forgetting to 'act their age', they are scapegoated and forced to accept their declining status and social invisibility (Miller 2016: 18). While this type of narrative is unacceptable when used with regard to other groups in society, it is apparently still acceptable to discriminate against baby boomers.

Nonetheless, even if the stigmatization of the baby boomer generation – which is no coincidence, but rather constructed for political purposes – is socially acceptable, it still means the intergenerational conflict is really felt by the two generations concerned. Researchers have documented that although young do not see anything positive in being 'old', they 'hold very different, even positive views of elder family members' (Calasanti 2020). Of course, younger people do not have much knowledge about ageing, but they do not necessarily accord the lower value to older people (Chung and Park 2019). Empirical studies also show that there are vital bonds across generations, that young people do not see their grandparents as responsible for their economic fate and that young adults do not accept discrimination against older people as a remedy for their difficulties (Bristow 2019).

Furthermore, the interests of old and young are not necessary entirely opposed – for example, in the United States, 13% of grandparents provide care on a regular basis to grandchildren, while 62% help children and grandchildren financially (Calasanti 2020). Moreover, the interests of old and young are not necessarily in conflict, not only because older generations often provide essential support and help to their children and grandchildren, but also because all groups can suffer equally from politicians' use of the intergenerational argument to justify austerity politics and welfare state reform. As the propagated divisive rhetoric does not explain social issues in terms of structural and other divisions, such racism, gender and ethnicity, it leaves many real problems unaddressed.

In conclusion, the existence of conflicts between generations can be questioned because of the imprecision and misuse of the concept of generation itself, which makes it rather problematic to identify generational interests. The notion of a generation is 'a muddled concept', rarely defined beyond chronological age and often used interchangeably with age (Bristow 2019: 65). However, despite the confusing status of this notion – mainly because of the symbolism attached to generations – it can be used to sell specific political programmes by blaming a selected age cohort for problems that might more realistically be handled by addressing class or other divisions. Yet the notion of generation, understood as something more than merely collections of a people of the same chronological age, can be of the significance. This importance of the concept of generation is connected with the uniqueness of each generation in terms of its historical and cultural context of experiences that occur during its members' formative adult years. In other words, generations only make sense 'when we try to define them, not by the dates in which they happen to be born, but by the social events that characterized the time at which they came of age' (Bristow 2019: 74).

Such a conceptualization of generations explains the specificity of each generation in terms of their respective social, economic and cultural circumstances. Without denying that there are many differences in each demographic cohort in terms of its social composition, aspirations, expectations and experiences, the uniqueness of generational experience can contribute to some common shared features of members of a given generation. Unique generational participation in the same historical and social circumstances can endow 'the individuals sharing in them with the common mentality and sensitivity' (Mannheim 1973: 291). The distinctiveness of generational context translates itself into a set of embodied practices and tastes, attitudes, preferences and dispositions, which are sustained by collective memories and enforced by control, through rituals of exclusion, over access to collective resources (Misztal 2003). The uniqueness of generational experience is reflected in generational differences, ranging from differences in health and life expectancy to variances in attitudes. For example, those in the 'golden cohort', in contrast to the previous generations, were exposed to rationing in their adolescent and early adult years (between 1940 and 1954) and had specific health, eating and smoking habits (Murphy 2009). In comparison to the 'golden cohort', the baby boomers have lived in more stable and affluent societies with a culture defined by the proliferation of television. By the virtue of their sheer demographic power, they have impacted their respective countries' economic and cultural life more than the previous generation. At the same time, when an older generation comes to be identified with nothing more than chronologic age, ageism easily surfaces on the basis of a distorted notion of generation. By ignoring differences of class, gender, ethnicity and race, this can facilitate the rhetoric of generational conflict.

This brings us to the final argument behind our questioning of seeing the aged as a social problem. More specifically, the rhetoric of intergenerational divide is flawed because demographic characteristics or chronological age cannot be seen as the sole explanatory factors behind people's interest. In other words, this rhetoric is based on an incorrect assumption of the uniformity within age groups, as if the differences between generations were greater than those within them. Especially critical for us here is the misleading assumption of the homogeneity of the old cohort as a group: the elderly. Today's increasing heterogeneity of a growing group of older adults includes structural inequalities and subjective differences. In modern societies, later life becomes a site of growing diversity that is constituted by 'both division and difference where discourses and practices oriented toward choice of autonomy, self-realization and pleasure are becoming as prevalent as those oriented toward decline, hardship and inequality' (Gilleard and Higgs 2020: 5). To fully grasp the heterogeneity of the aged, we need to recognize subjective differentials, and social divisions such as gender, class, ethnicity and race, as well as diversities that are structured by social relations of after working life, type of household and the fluctuations of the economies of contemporary developed societies (Gilleard and Higgs 2020). Given the ways advantages and disadvantages add up over the life-course, 'it comes as no surprise that we observe the greatest disparities in old age' (Calasanti 2020). For instance, in the United States the greatest income inequalities exist among the older population (Calasanti 2020). Although now, in contrast to the past, the living standards of pensioners and those of the general population in the majority of modern nations are similar (Gilleard and Higgs 2020), differences of wealth remain within the aged cohort. Moreover, although some older people are quite wealthy, a large proportion of elderly people are financially insecure. In the United Kingdom, for example, the proportion of elderly people living in severe poverty is five times what it was in 1986, and this rise, from 0.9% of the elderly population in severe poverty to around 5%, is the largest increase among Western European countries (Ravallion 2015), while in the United States a 62% of beneficiaries rely on social security for 50% of their incomes (Calasanti 2020). Apart from differences in financial wealth, education, occupation, gender, ethnicity and race, identity and subjectivity also play a critical role in sourcing social difference. While social divisions imply an externally ordered hierarchy of resources, power and status, subjective factors can shape life styles, cultural interests and the level of engagement in paid and in unpaid work – for example, one-third (36.5%) of older citizens in the United States spend between 100 and 499 hours each year volunteering (Calasanti 2020).

However, the heterogeneity of the aged goes beyond these factors, as the body creates new differences in health and frailty in later life (Gilleard and Higgs 2020). With ageing, the body acquires much greater importance as both site and source of social divisions. Thus, in addition to the structural accounts of social, the body should be included in our consideration of the heterogeneity of the aged cohort. Given the role of the body, with its health and frailness, as a marker of division and difference, in what follows we will explore the corporeal signs of frailty and infirmity in old age.

When the body's failure is a source of division

In this section, by including the body as a marker of division and by acknowledging that the cost of an ageing population also needs to be understood in terms of age-related health inequalities, we explore how older people's health predicaments – particularly frailty and social death – become forms of exclusion. With advanced age, when the body ceases to be a shelter and instead becomes a threat, with the risk of frailty and irremediable illnesses, the 'fourth' age arrives, encapsulating the 'bleaker aspects of old age' (Gilleard and Higgs 2015: 268). The features of the 'fourth' age as a period where 'human agency is no longer visible' (Gilleard and Higgs 2015: 268) will be explored further in the final chapter of this book. Here, we focus only on the single aspect of the 'fourth' age: the frailty of people who are in this 'horrific, disgusting and tainted by mortality stage' (Gilleard and Higgs 2015: 137). The assessment of frailty, which divides 'too old' (the 'fourth' age) from those who are merely 'older' (still in an earlier period of ageing – the 'third' age), is used as a tool for rationing care in in later life (Gilleard and Higgs 2017, 2022). After discussing frailty as a source of distinction and exclusion in later life, the chapter explores the fears that are often connected with frailty, particularly a fear of social death. Even though frailty and social death can overlap, social death – because it marks the end of independent and socially rewarding life –should be discussed by itself as the extreme case of a further separation of those who are very old from those facing the proximity of death.

When I started writing this part of Chapter 3, the world's oldest person celebrated her 119th birthday in a Japanese nursing home. On 3 January 2022, Kane Tanaka became the oldest of a large and growing group of centenarians in Japan, one of the fastest ageing societies on Earth, where life expectancy has reached 87.74 for women and 81.64 for men. It is also a nation that annually celebrates Respect for the Aged Day (McCurry 2022). Mrs Tanaka, like the majority of centenarians, experiences the weaknesses of her body – for example, she 'reportedly uses gestures to communicate with nursing home staff', on whom she totally depends for care (McCurry 2022). Her case illustrates not only the increased longevity that is occurring, and that women make up the vast majority of centenarians, but also that this expanded longevity comes with the limitations of the body and the loss of autonomy. In other words, despite the medical advances and despite generally better health conditions and an expanded lifespan, in later life older people face many challenges, ranging from an increased risk of frailty through the deteriorations of cognitive and physical powers to social death.

At present, frailty – which accumulates with age – starts later and proceeds at a slower rate than in the past, thanks to medical advances. Consequently, only around 10% of people aged over 65 and between 25 and 50% of those aged over 85 live with frailty (Age UK 2022). The baby boomers, who in 1965 were singing 'I hope I die before I get old' (Wolpert 2011: 222) and approved of Dylan Thomas's advice that 'Old age should burn and rave at close of day', are not a topic of this section because on they have not generally reached the 'fourth' age (Wolpert 2011: 222). The majority are still in the 'third' age, which embraces a narrative of 'good' or 'successful' ageing, and offers the possibility of a rewarding social life and inclusion. Here we are interested in those who are already in the 'fourth' age – that is, in people who have failed to 'age well', or have aged beyond that point, and who now suffer from chronic and degenerative diseases of ageing and experience a fear a loss of social agency and exclusion. Typically, these people are aged over 85 and, although even this group's health and frailness vary, they mostly experience the body's incapacities to some degree, creating new health difficulties and inequalities.

While the baby boomers are seen to be a social problem, those older and frail people tend to be perceived as a burden, or as bed-blockers whose claims on life-extending health and social care from public resources are questioned. With the growing applications of the term 'frailty' as a major source of 'social division, separating those who are merely older from those who are too old' (Gilleard and Higgs 2017: 1681), there is increasing evidence that very old people are often seen as the subjects to the age-related rationing in healthcare (Lloyd 2000). Such a rationing of healthcare is presented as 'fair' approach on the basis that rationing should favour the young 'because the old will already have experienced enough good health in order to each old(er) age' (New and Mays, quoted in Lloyd 2000: 174). However, it is difficult for the public to accept that not everybody who needs care gets it, especially when is clear that old people are blocking beds in hospitals in the United Kingdom mainly because Britain's social care is in crisis and the health system is overwhelmed (Lanchester 2021). For the last twenty years, despite seventeen white papers, green papers and reviews of funding concerning social care (Clarke 2021), the systematic crisis of the health and care system has caused daily problems and the reality of rationing health services is becoming increasingly acute. It is only very recently that efforts and calls to address the issues in the health and care system have been recognized (see Chapter 9 for further discussions of the governmental proposal to tackle the health and care crisis). As the age-related body's frailness and incapacities divide those who are fit and 'ageing successfully' from those who are already frail and not 'ageing successfully', the United Kingdom's poorly functioning health and social care system means health inequalities becoming more noticeable (Gilleard and Higgs 2017).

The potential for divisions and inequalities in treatment is constructed with a help of the application of the category or notion of 'frail' and development tools for its assessment. As an increased reliance on frailty poses challenges to today's older people and the health and care system, it is important to examine the potential impacts on health policies as well as on shaping older people's status and self-perception. The notion of frailty has been the focus of various theoreticians and practitioners concerned with services for older people for a couple of decades now. For researchers in age studies, the term 'frailty' exists alongside 'successful ageing' as one of 'the leading paradigms of our time' (Grenier 2020: 2338). In such debates, frailty, as the symbolic marker between activity and decline, refers to functional decline and general weakening, risk of falling and diminishing capabilities. The simplest illustration of the body's deterioration due to aged-related physical impairment is the case of older persons' vulnerability to falling, which is a 'powerful metaphor of decline' (Kingston, in Katz 2015: 168).

As subsequent injuries from falling can result in death, and as the fall rate and cases of death by injury increase with age, it is not surprising that dying from injuries connected with falling among people aged over 75 is one of the most common causes of death in the United Kingdom (Katz 2015: 166).

Yet, despite the growing interest in the application of this term in many settings – including clinical ones – the notion frailty is still a problematic concept as there is an absence of a universally agreed definition of frailty and as the term originated from 'lay' or everyday language. Moreover, the concept of frailty has a long history in 'lay' language, which goes back to 'Middle English when frailty was used to refer to weak morals' (Gilleard and Higgs 2022: 207). Today, according to many dictionaries, frailty in everyday language stands for infirmity, being weak, delicate, failing, feeble, debilitated, incapacitated, crippled and wasted, while Wikipedia defines it as a state that 'embodies an elevated risk of catastrophic declines in health and function among older adults'. All non-clinical or 'lay' definitions, like clinical ones, stress that frailty is a condition associated with ageing; however, they also tend to add that frailty is 'something to be feared'(Grenier 2020: 2345). Unsurprisingly, older people do not identify themselves with the word 'frail' or with the phrase 'living with frailty', even though living with frailty does not necessarily mean one is incapable of living an independent and socially rewarding life. Elderly people reject these expressions because such phrases resonate with their deep fear of losing independence, dignity and control over their lives – in short, with a fear of social death (Britain Thinks 2015).

This lack of relevance of the notion of frailty for older adults themselves was observed in *Frailty Language and Perceptions*, a report by Britain Thinks for Age UK and the British Geriatrics Society. The report discovered that older people themselves do not use the word 'frail' or the phrase 'living with frailty'. The term 'frailty' is not part of older people's vocabulary, as they worry about the negative connotations of this notion. They resist the stigma and stereotypes of older age and therefore express a rather strong aversion to the term 'frail'. Moreover, clinical attempts to assess frailty do not resonate with older people (Britain Thinks 2015). Subsequently, older people's unwillingness to accept the label 'frail' was addressed in the International Association of Gerontology and Geriatrics' (IAGG) Global

Aging Research Network (GARN 2016) report *White Book on Frailty*, which was accompanied by a promotional video, *Beware of Frailty*, designed for public and educational awareness (http://frailty.net/frailtynews/internationalinitiatives/beware-of-frailty). While presenting professionally identified risks of frailty and identifying older people's resistance to so-called 'frailty services', the video warns older people about frailty and tells them that 'solutions are available, so do talk to your doctor'. *Beware of Frailty* cautions older people about the risks and perils of frailty (i.e. weakness, weight loss, slow walking speed, fatigue), and asks the elderly to seek medical help when required (Grenier 2020: 2345).

In contrast to older people's resistance to the term 'frailty', the Britain Thinks (2015) report notes that the notion of frailty is accepted and increasingly used by professionals and specialists in health and social care to describe a physiological state resulting from a combination of age-related comorbidities. Despite the recent reliance of the notion of frailty in geriatrics and other clinical disciplines to address medical issues and the production of frailty assessment tools, the concept of frailty is not always precisely defined. Yet, despite a multiplicity of meanings, most clinicians agree that frailty comprises three fundamental elements: 'that it is a condition or syndrome rather than a disease'; that it 'results from a multi-system reduction in reserve capacity'; and that 'this failure results in the decline of physiological systems' (Gilleard and Higgs 2022: 205). For example, in geriatric medicine, frailty is defined as a 'common clinical syndrome in older adults that carries an increased risk of poor health outcomes including falls, incident disability, hospitalization and mortality' (FrailtyPrevention 2022). Professionals and specialists use the term 'frailty' in clinical settings to describe a 'spectrum of physical and mental health states and to assess risk or to put together a care plan for elderly persons' (Britain Thinks 2015). For geriatricians and care professionals, frailty describes those people who are approaching the end of their lives, malnourished and highly dependent on care. In contrast to' lay' older people, they also have knowledge of the Comprehensive Geriatric Assessment (CGA) or the Clinical Frailty Scale (CFS) – that is, the tools used to identify frailty in older patients to provide an acute frailty service that will ensure appropriate care for frail older people.

The increasing prevalence of the usage of the term and employment of the frailty assessment methods in general practice in England's NHS raises questions about the unintended consequences of the appropriation of a lay term, with its potential to facilitate stereotyping of older age for the way patients are viewed. As there are now many written instructions to support the care of frail older people in an NHS setting, some specifying that people aged 65 and over should routinely be screened for frailty, it is essential to know how healthcare professionals use and make sense of the term 'frail'. Gilleard and Higgs' (2022) qualitative study, which explored how health professionals perceive frailty, discovered that they s negotiate an 'ideological dilemma' – a tension between contradictory sets of meanings and consequences for action – based on their 'lay' and clinical experience of the term 'frailty'. Their investigation shows that the appropriation of a 'lay' term into clinical practice with a specific clinical meaning and viewing 'an entire person through a lens of frailty' resulted in the creation of an ideological dilemma that 'could have a negative impact on the assessment of frailty depending on the system of assessment used' (Gilleard and Higgs 2022: 204). Hence, Gilleard and Higgs (2022: 220) 'recommend that frailty at the very least be used with a critical appreciation pertaining to its lay connotations and its impact as a negative label'. While the participants in this study found the term 'frailty' useful to communicate quickly with professional colleagues, their shared knowledge of its stigmatizing connotations rendered it a term they were uncomfortable using with patients themselves, for fear of causing offence or making a patient feel 'bad about themselves'.

In other words, since the labelling of the patient as frail can profoundly challenge someone's sense of self, perhaps there is little justification for the assessment of the elderly in this way for their eligibility for care, especially as the assessment tools for frailty are not perfect and can be used without any consultation with elderly patients or their knowledge. Such labelling can also be potentially damaging in terms of health outcomes and can negatively impact how older people are perceived by others. Even though they often lack any knowledge of the classification practices connected with in the clinical use of the term 'frailty', older people are nonetheless afraid of the stigma associated with the term. Moreover, in the context of today's extended longevity, ageing raises the risk of developing not only frailty but also deterioration of cognitive capabilities and dementia; thus the fear of a potential loss of autonomy, independence and dignity is more strongly felt. Although living with frailty does not necessary mean being incapable of living an independent life, nonetheless as frailty and social death can come simultaneously, their potential overlap increases older people's deep fear of being powerless and without social agency. Such a fear of loss of social agency can be seen as one of the factors behind the widespread fear of social death that is often associated with dementia in later life.

The notion of social death describes older people's fear of being denied the benefits of living in society and of being treated 'as if they were already dead' (Glaser and Strauss 1965). The term 'social death', which since the 1960s has been used to describe the opposite of wellbeing (Kralova and Walter 2016), refers to a situation in which the person is treated as if they were already biologically dead (Sudnow 1967). Social death implies a distinction between physical and social death; it is not the same as physical death, as it does not always occur at the same time. The notion of social death is sometimes understood as reflecting the dehumanizing consequences of dying in modern hospitals (Sudnow 1967), and is mainly defined more broadly as the social practice of treating the elderly as a being socially dead (Glaser and Strauss 1965). However, in both conceptualizations of this notion, the term 'social death' preserves its relevance for detection of any inequality or denial human rights. When the individual is biologically alive, but when others – by implying that the older person has no choice or does not fit into the social context in an acceptable way – confer upon them the status of social death, such a change in social relations can be detrimental to the wellbeing of the elderly. In other words, people who are judged and treated by others as close to physical death can become aware of dying; together with their subsequent withdrawal and rejection of social interaction, when interpreted again by others as indicating social death, this can move them even closer towards biological death (Caswell and O'Connor 2015).

The term 'social death', in all its meanings, is about the marginalization of old and very frail people at the end of life. By capturing older people's social exclusion and changes in the nature of their social relations and their disempowering experiences at the end of life, the notion of social death allows us to grasp the level of discrimination and unfairness that exists in the treatment of elderly. The status of social death is imposed by others and comes with painful consequences, as it increases the awareness and fear of a dying person of becoming irrevocably lost to themself as an active agent, which determines the nature of social interaction (Glaser and Strauss 1965). Much the fear of social death 'settles on the loss of agency that is associated with frailty, particularly mental frailty and the perceived abjection of an undignified journey towards non-existence' (Gilleard and Higgs 2015: 267). The increasing fear of loss of social agency in later life, and thus a fear of undergoing a premature social death, is especially linked to a fear of dementia. Today in the United Kingdom, over 907,000 people live with dementia and the number of dementia cases is projected to increase by 75%, to almost 1.6 million by 2050 (Gregory 2022a). As 'all people with dementia, or all those who appear to be frail and elderly, are also socially dead' (Caswell and O'Connor 2015: 250), the significance of social death among older mentally frail people cannot be overlooked in any attempt to challenge unfair and unequal treatment of the elderly. As age is the biggest risk factor for dementia, and as older and frail people with dementia are often seen as being 'as good as dead' (Caswell and O'Connor 2015), the fear of social death is a feeling that grips many in later life. Several studies have identified the elderly as a group that is particularly prone to undergoing this kind of social death, especially in the context of care and residential homes (Gilleard and Higgs 2015).

Social death is a form of exclusion, exemplified by the symbolic role of the nursing home. In the United Kingdom, only around one-third of people with dementia live in residential care settings, while the majority lives in their own homes and are often cared by members of their families. However, when the condition progresses and full-time care is required, many people with dementia are moved into care and nursing homes, with the average prevalence of people living with dementia in care homes being 63% of men and 71% of women (Alzheimer's Society 2022). Moreover, in both cases – living with dementia at home or in residential care – inequalities and precarity in the care process affect all because of a lack of sufficient support for family caregivers and because systems of care are often fragmented. For example, in the Unites States, national level policies and programmes that support family caregivers are limited, while in the United Kingdom, policies are also often inadequate (Mong 2020).

Social death is about attitudes of families, friends and medical professionals towards people judged to be at the end of life. As people living with dementia are progressing through stages of a terminal illness, their isolation and separation from loved ones have an irreversible impact on their condition, especially as some of them are not continuously in periods of social death. Moreover, the fate of people with dementia in residential homes across the United Kingdom was disproportionately disrupted by the COVID-19 pandemic (see Chapter 9). However, while old people with dementia fared worst of all during the coronavirus crisis, the wellbeing of other groups was also impacted.

The pandemic and generational divide

In the United Kingdom, the COVID pandemic did not just negatively impact the health and mental condition of the older population; it also disrupted the daily lives, routines and opportunities to develop and participate in education, work and social life of younger generations (Lee 2020). During the COVID pandemic – as all crises – the concept of who 'shall be saved and who shall die is settled by institutions' (Douglas 1986: 56); hence, the psychological and socioeconomic scars inflicted by COVID-19 policies on both old and young reflect the state's decisions about who should suffer and who should be spared in this recent health crisis. In the United Kingdom, the government's handling of the pandemic has contributed to intergenerational tensions as both groups – old and young – believed that their own generation was abandoned to its fate in order for another generation's problems to be dealt with. In what follows, we explore what psychological and socioeconomic legacies COVID-19 policies may have left on younger and older generation, and whether COVID-19 has worsened the relationship between the generations. After illustrating the expansion of the intergenerational divide in the context of the coronavirus epidemics, it will be argued that the

COVID-19 pandemic has also provided new opportunities for debate about how to overcome intergenerational divisions and improve the relationship between old and young.

At the beginning of the COVID-19 pandemic in the United Kingdom, we were warned that the virus did not discriminate and that 'everyone is at risk'. The underlying narrative about threats posed by the coronavirus was that 'we are all in it together', or 'we are on the same boat' (Cooper and Szreter 2021: 7–13). Yet it was quickly discovered that the risk of dying from COVID-19 doubles with every six years of age, which means that people over 75 years are 10,000 times more at risk than those who aged under 15 (Spiegelhalter and Masters 2021; Woolhouse 2022). Subsequently, the aged were marked as vulnerable and frail by two decisions: one introducing frailty tests and another regarding lockdown. Even days before the first lockdown, without any wider consultation, the Clinical Frailty Scale (CFS) was adapted by the National Institute for Health and Care Excellence (NICE) to help decide whether patients should be offered or denied acute care during the COVID-19 crisis. The NHS staff in England were asked to follow the NICE guideline saying that on admission to hospital, all adults should be assessed for frailty, and that other comorbidities and underlying health conditions should also be taken into account (Owen 2020). As the COVID-19 pandemic has sharpened and made it more difficult to negotiate the 'ideological dilemma' involved in the clinical use of the term 'frailty', the use of the Clinical Frailty Scale (CFS) to assess which patients should be denied acute care and the emergence of illegal 'do not resuscitate' notices in care homes and hospitals has been criticized by many bodies, including the healthcare regulator, the Care Quality Commission and various charities. Subsequently, the UK healthcare regulator branded such a procedure and related actions unacceptable. However, even though in 2020 the National Institute for Health and Care Excellence (NICE) issued a new guidance in which it advised NHS trusts to 'sensitively discuss' with old and frail people the possibility of their acceptance of 'do not attempt cardiopulmonary resuscitation', it did not assure many old and frail people that they, like people under the age of 75, would not be denied lifesaving COVID-19 care, such as ICU care (Owen 2020; see also Chapter 8).

While the introduction of the frailty scoring system could have made elderly people feel as if they were being labelled and assessed in terms of their eligibility for care, the announcement of the first lockdown (23 March 2020) added to their psychological suffering and discomfort. Although the policy of self-isolation of older people was presented as being grounded in the available scientific evidence, and therefore could not be seen as being discriminatory, many elderly people felt lonely and abandoned. The UK government, aiming to construct and preserve a spirit of intergenerational solidarity and in order for its health policies not to be seen as contributing to intergenerational tensions, undertook attempts to enhance a cooperative mood with a help of a new catchphrase, 'Don't Kill Granny with the Virus'. From the end of August 2020, this slogan called on younger groups to take into consideration that the elderly were more susceptible to the COVID-19 risk, and therefore older people needed to be protected. The 'Don't Kill Granny' campaign, by asking younger adults to keep their distance, wear masks and not to take the virus back home to vulnerable relatives, appeared to lower of the level of risks and threats confronted by older people. By telling younger people to 'protect their grannies', this message expected them not to think about old people as expendable and emphasized the value of solidarity between the generations.

Nonetheless, many young people who thought COVID-19 would not affect them, and who hoped for a return of 'normality', were angry about a forceful front-page message warning them not to 'infect their grandparents'. Other millennials rejected the governmental instruction as incorrectly assuming that they might 'want the elderly to sicken and die' (Ellen 2020) and as propagating the idea that younger generations acted irresponsibly. Feeling that they had 'more than shouldered the burden of this pandemic', young adults refused to accept the official narrative that they not 'done their bit' (Chetwynd-Cloison 2020). With the growing fatigue and negative consequences of the lockdown, a social mood in England was slowly becoming more complex. One the one hand, there was societal recognition of the 'golden cohort' generation, members of which are always admired for their war and life efforts, as illustrated by the public admiration and knighthood bestowed on Captain Tom Moore, the British World War II veteran who raised more than £33 million for the NHS by walking daily in his garden in 2020. On the other hand, the main rhetoric of solidarity underwent substantial erosion until it was ultimately replaced by narratives of ageism.

In contrast to the admiration for Captain Tom Moore in the official media, social platforms, such as the hashtag *#boomerremover*, undermined generational solidarity. While the facts remined the same (i.e. COVID-19 is a far greater threat to the elderly, frail and infirm than to the young and healthy), certain sections of social media were 'all busy stockpiling either ageist prejudices or paranoiac visions about the young wishing the old dead' (Ellen 2020: 27). Analyses of Twitter data posted through four months of 2020, and related to older adults, showed that ageist content was prevalent on Twitter in the context of the pandemic (Xiang et al. 2020). While the daily average of ageist content was less than 20%, almost three-quarters of jokes were aimed at older adults – half of which were 'death jokes' (Xiang et al 2020). Jokes targeting older people were also circulated on other platforms – for example, in the context of the coronavirus pandemic there was a widely shared a photo of a bus full of older women and men with the text, 'To save the economy, the government will announce next month that the Immigration Department will start deporting seniors (instead of illegals)'. By presenting older adults as nothing more as than 'a living symbol of time running out' (Martens et al 2004: 1534) and as susceptible to the negative effects of COVID-19, such jokes, cartoons and messages on Twitter and other social platforms justified pushing older people aside as not a particularly important problem. Moreover, by misreporting risks and acceptable ways of controlling the pandemic, these messages indicated that the older generation puts unreasonable pressure on an already stressed healthcare system. At the same time, by portraying younger persons as immune to the virus, and hence as not representing any cost to society, social media could negatively impact the solidarity between generations.

However, it was not just public discourses on social media platforms that contributed to the expansion of the generational divide. With growing warnings about the grave economic fallout from the pandemic, official narratives that accelerated the intergenerational tensions in the United States ranged from the Lieutenant Governor of Texas's assertion that 'it would be better that older people die in the pandemic if that would protect the economy for younger people', through phrases such as 'saving old lives just to ruin young ones', to frequent complaints about the pandemic policy doing 'the harm to our children' (Calasanti 2021). In the United Kingdom, a Conservative MP suggested that, in order to save the future of younger generations, we should rank life according to who was most 'deserving'. After accusing the government's lockdown programme of aiming to 'abolish death', he said, 'We should accept that death happens, that old [people] died; at some stage we need to accept that people of 80 or 70 died' (Charles Walker, Conservative MP, on *BBC Newsnight*, 12 October 2020). In this spirit, a group of Conservative Party members of the House of Lords voiced their rejection of the lockdown restrictions as imposing totally unnecessary limitations on individual freedoms and claimed that, 'Anyone who wishes to resume normal life, and take the risk of catching the virus, should be free to do so' (Ridley 2020).

The COVID-19 crisis did not just deepen already existing intergenerational tensions and insert new stereotypes, prejudice and discrimination against older adults; it also added to social inequalities, disparities between regions and ethnic groups, poverty levels among children and pensioners, and an increase in domestic violence, as well as much longer hospital waiting lists (Inman, 2021). However, the public attention was not so much directed to the pandemic trapping more people in a situation of poverty and making their already difficult economic and health conditions much tougher. What worried the public was COVID-19's threat to drive a 'war of the generations' in the post-pandemic decade. This new risk of intergenerational tensions was exposed by the younger generation's criticism of long lockdowns across Western Europe for imposing misery on them (Butler and Bannock 2021). In this process of questioning the consequences of lockdowns, young adults were joined by experts in public health.

For example, claiming that the British long lockdown did more harm than good, Woolhouse (2022: 8) points out that, as a result of that policy, 'children and young adults ... were robbed of their education, jobs, and normal existence, as well as suffering damage to their prospects, while they left to inherit a record-breaking mountain of public debt'. Following this type of argument, the public was informed that:

> COVID has involved an upturning of the contract between the generations: children have been conscripted to protect adults, and have paid the price. To protect people from a disease whose median victim was 83 years old, children missed 18 months of interacting with one another, at the stage of life when they need it most. (Lanchester 2021: 13)

With the growing realization and evidence of difficulties, suffering and misery indirectly caused to younger people, the issue of the increase in intergenerational unfairness has been brought to the attention of the public. Because of potential psychological scars of COVID-19 on teenagers, and because of worries that the pandemic may have had a lasting impact on young people's mental health, they are often now seen as 'a sacrificed generation' (Butler and Bannock 2021).

Much evidence and studies from many countries illustrate that, despite the fact that they are the least likely group to become ill from COVID-19, teenagers and younger people suffered disproportionately during the pandemic. They experienced the biggest educational disruption in modern history, a surge in unemployment and the psychological effects of lockdown isolation. All recent studies from developed countries show that many months of lockdowns destabilized their mental wellbeing, education and job prospects. For example, an investigation by Alayon et al. (2020) suggests that younger adults were at greater risk of psychological distress and loneliness during COVID-19 lockdowns than older adults. A study by the European Union documents that 64% of young Europeans are at risk of depression, up from 15% before the pandemic (quoted in Butler and Bannock 2021). The British studies also documented that during the pandemic, young people's mental health deteriorated, and the impact of loneliness, academic stress and chronic insecurity meant many teenagers and young adults felt ' burnout' and experienced very high levels of anxiety connected with worries about their future (Butler and Bannock 2021). While accusing the UK Government of failing them, some young adults said that their 'whole generation has just been pushed aside as a problem to deal with later'. Young people from other European countries also expressed their misery and disappointment due to not receiving financial support for lost jobs and feeling like 'the lowest priority' or simply that they had been abandoned by their governments (Butler and Bannock 2021).

At the end of the pandemic's second year when, even though vaccines worked, restrictions were still in place, many people experienced a growing 'Corona fatigue'. In November 2021, when tougher restrictions were introduced due to the threat of new variants, thousands of people – especially non-believers in the vaccination programme – took to the streets in several European cities. For example, Brussels, Copenhagen and Rotterdam saw demonstrations and protests against new constraints and rules, such as COVID passes and mandatory vaccination. Although among protesters there were also young people who felt disadvantaged, depressed and convinced that their interests and needs did not count, the major factor motivating demonstrators was not the intergenerational conflict or ageism, but rather their anti-vaccination stand or frustration with the restrictions. The majority of younger people not only accepted the importance of following COVID-19 measures and regulations as they recognized that vaccines alone would not stop COVID, but they also slowly came to realize that in many respects the pandemic had presented both them and older generations with the same difficult challenges.

The growing recognition by younger adults that they share with older people the feeling of being left alone to deal with negative experiences of loneliness and mental vulnerability has offered a chance of new understanding and a link between the two generation. Despite the pandemic imposing separation between the older and younger generations, 'the two groups at either end of the age spectrum could be bonding because both feel disfranchised by the government's response to COVID' (Hill 2021). Older people were not cautioned about the risk of isolation and were not told to be beware of frailty as the classification method helping authorities to work out which patients should be denied acute care; rather, they were asked to shield themselves while the threat of various COVID-19 related disruptions to young people's lives and subsequently to their mental conditions was not properly assessed. In short, for both generations the deepest cost of the pandemic came in the area of mental health. And because of this shared experience, the pandemic, despite COVID-19 presenting a higher risk to the elderly than to the young, and despite the crisis having exposed intergenerational tensions, bases for mutual understanding have also been established.

Post-lockdown, with the threat of COVID-19 still present, the generations found they were mixing more than in in normal times as in this transitional period old and young often worked together, especially in the UK voluntary sector (Hill 2021). In the second part of 2021, both groups were often actively engaged in charity projects designed to overcome various problems that emerged during the pandemic. This working together has helped to mediate negative stereotypes and led to new bonds between the generations. Such an 'unusual bonding between those in their 60s and older, and those in their early 20s and younger, has been partly galvanized by the enforced separation of the generations during lockdown, leading the age groups to value each other in a way they had not previously' (Hill 2021). It can be said the pandemic has enhanced opportunities for the generations to get to know each other, and thus facilitated alliances and links between them. Hence, perhaps the COVID-19 pandemic, by both potentially exposing many intergenerational tensions and showing the importance of fostering intergenerational allegiance, could help us to rethink obligations toward the old and enhance a search for the quality care of the elderly from a moral perspective. To seize this opportunity and prevent the risk of returning to the same crisis situation, various questions have been proposed for further examination by the proposed public inquiry into the government's handling of the pandemic. While some call for 'national discussion about how the old are going to make it up to the young' (Lanchester 2021:13), others, including the independent Joseph Rowntree Foundation, request public inquiry into the pandemic's impact on levels of poverty and ethnic inequalities in the United Kingdom, while the Bereaved Families for Justice group demands justice for elderly victims of the COVID-19 policies. It seems that unless we also openly discuss the issue of generational obligations and relationships, claims of COVID-19 having an unequal generational impact will continue to undermine a mood of social cooperation and solidarity.

To conclude, the COVID-19 pandemic has not only shed light on the consequences of the generational divide; by burning down old stereotypes and signalling a need for the elimination of fears faced by both the young and the elderly, it has also demonstrated that an opportunity exists for the construction of new intergenerational bonds. In order to learn a lesson from the recent health emergency and to realize the importance of social solidarity in managing the processes of ageing and dying, there is a need for further discussions of intergenerational obligations and responsibilities.

PART II

Encounters with death

CHAPTER 4

Meeting death – places and occasions

Living in the world of obituaries and funerals

The second part of this book seeks further explanations of the specific relationship the elderly have with mortality. There is nothing like increasing age to make someone aware of their own mortality, but there are also some indirect consequences of ageing that advance older people's awareness of death's inevitability. Older adults are conscious that the 'calendar is just about up' (Clarke et al. 2012), not only because of their age and their falling bodies affected by multiple chronic conditions, but also because of their numerous indirect encounters with death. They visit death's own territory, such as cemeteries, attend the rites of passage, such as funerals, and deal with variety of techniques of memory-preserving, such as obituaries. Apart from indirect meetings with death in the private sphere, older persons are also frequently confronted with 'the problem of death' in public discussions and media representations. Hence the elderly live increasingly in the shadow of death, and consequently learn to handle grief and bereavement. Moreover, during the pandemic, when the risk and visibility of death increased dramatically, older adults – with worries about their loss of control over the end of life and anxiety about a lack of contacts with loved ones in the final moments – were challenged to reflect on death and dying due to new fears about their own vulnerability.

While recognizing that obtrusive encounters with mortality at the old age are often a result of the declining body, Chapter 4 focuses mainly on older people's frequent but indirect meetings with death in the course of their private lives. First, looking at how older adults are immersed in the world of funerals and obituaries, it reveals how death intrudes on the elderly's everyday experiences and practices. Second, it explores older people's everyday life in the shadow of death, which is illustrated by experiences of people living in residential facilities. Finally, the chapter demonstrates how older people's experiences of the vulnerability and risk they faced during the COVID-19 crisis have affected their relationship with and ownership of death. It shows how pandemic, with its new risks and new rules, presented the elderly with a magnified burden and made their encounters with death more unsettling.

'People's anticipatory images of death are shaped by peculiarities of societies at a particular stage of development and so with a particular structure' (Elias 1985: 84). However, although people's experiences of death often depend on culture, 'death is not only culturally produced, it is never simply reducible to some particularly culturally determined meaning' (Holmberg et al. 2019: 6). Furthermore, even though adults' knowledge about death often does not come through concrete, direct and personal experience, for the elderly death is not completely beyond the realm of life. Thus, while recognizing the role of cultural schemas, religion and traditions in the process of constructing meaning, it can be argued that the older people's awareness that they have been overtaken by time also plays an essential role in shaping images of death. Here we are especially interested in how, when we are getting older, our more frequent indirect encounters with places, occasions and situations connected with death, gradually narrow our options by providing a reminder that time 'is gnawing at us', creating an awareness of mortality and giving a new meaning to death (Coetzee 2005: 11).

Of course, people of all ages confront death indirectly all the time – through objects that once belonged to dead relatives, through news, media and various artforms, from literature to film. However, while knowledge of and relationship with mortality are shaped by indirect encounters with death in all stages of life, the presence of death in older people's everyday experiences and practices is of a different significance than it is in the lives of younger generations. Getting older, which comes with increasingly exposure to things that represent death, places connected with death and the deaths of other people, leads people to reflect and act on their feelings about mortality. Older people's indirect confrontations with death are not only a general reminder of the inevitability of death; such encounters at later stage of life can also give life a special value and focus by instigating a more direct question regarding for whom the bell will toll next (to paraphrase John Donne's famous poem 'For Whom the Bell Tolls').

While grief and mourning after the death of loved ones will be discussed in the next chapter, here we look at how living in the world of funerals and obituaries can influence older adults' thinking about their diminishing future. Since older people's attendance at funerals and their readership of obituaries of their peers are among the most important indirect encounters with death at that stage, it can be argued that the older person's awareness of their own impending death is influenced, although not necessarily in the same way, by these two indirect encounters with death. The significance of funerals in old age is different from that in other stages if life because being older means that people around you – people who lived with you through the main part of your life – are gone. Although the death of others is a reminder of human mortality for people of all ages, for older adults the death of their peers presents a special emotional and spiritual challenge. When people get older and when the number of people dying around them increases, they don't just start reading newspapers from the obituaries pages, as the main characters in Muriel Spark's novel *Memento Mori* do, and become acquainted with funeral rituals; they also realize that one day they 'will be the star of that show' (McGinnis, quoted in Kemp 2019: 7) and that they could expect much more from life: 'nothing will be given to [them] again expect [their] funeral' (Blythe 2000: 254). Most importantly, by helping older people to accept that death is something that inevitably happens – something to be expected – funerals can prepare them for their own death or even normalize death.

The rich literature about funerals, from historical to anthropological, illustrates that funerals have always played an important role in society and asserts that religion and the socioeconomic status of the dead have shaped funerals throughout human history (Arnold 2008; Frisby 2019; Walter 2017). All researchers agree that funerals have been a public spectacle for centuries and that funeral customs and traditions have been among the most extensive, elaborate and obligatory of all human ceremonies. The function of this rite of passage has always been the promotion and maintenance of 'the emotional well-being of the individual as well as the social cohesion and structural integration of the group' (Fulton 1995: 195). While different cultures and religions view the relationship between the living and the dead differently, they all recognize the significance of funerals in helping people to manage dead bodies and grief (Irish et al. 1993). Moreover, they also recognize the social importance of burials, as it is hoped that by prompting mourners to think about their own mortality, funerals can make them more responsive to bonds with others. Funerals have also been known for reinforcing social divisions and schisms as the role of participants in a funeral reflects their position in society and reaffirms their status (Fulton 1995; Simmel [1910] 2007).

Across the centuries, funeral ceremonies have shaped our links with the deceased as 'there has always been the powerful underlying need for connections with the dead' (Frisby 2019: 3). In the past, religious faith offered the answer to the questions of how best to memorialize the dead, how to make sense of their death and how to come to terms with the loss (Aries 1981). Since the nineteenth century, funerals and grieving rituals have begun to change, although customs continued to help the bereaved to come to terms with their loss (Howarth 2007). Over the last several decades, funeral rituals have undergone a major transformation as older customary forms have replaced rituals and practices for disposing of the dead as well as for coping with death (Parsons 2018; Walter 2017). Yet, despite these changes, the burial practices and ceremonies are still important in contemporary Western societies (Laqueur 2015). Although today there are not many funeral processions moving through towns and mourning dress codes are not often observed, nonetheless the importance of funeral rites continues to be appreciated and recognized by people (Peterson and Jacobsen 2019).

The growing diversity in the ways in which funerals, cremations and memorial services take place, and where this occurs, have been followed by changes to ways of coping with grief, with the recent development in mourning practices being a response to advances in digital technology. The significance of today's changed funeral practices and mourning rituals reflects contemporary people's search for a more personalized, environmentally responsible and ethical expression of grief. The importance attached to funeral ritual sometimes expresses itself in pursuit of the replacement of traditional rituals, leading to their integration into new ways of closure (Walter 2017). While in the past the funeral was a part of a long process of events, including final vigils, wakes and visits to the family after the funeral, now it is often a singular personalized ceremony (Toolis 2017; Walter 2017). Moreover, while in the past funerals looked forward, 'helping the deceased's souls on its way', today in Western societies, funerals increasingly 'look backwards, celebrating the life that was lived on earth' (Walter 2017: 59).

Although contemporary funerals are not the same as they were in the past, 'when the village funeral [was] a great coming-out occasion for old' (Blythe 2000: 253), nonetheless they are still important celebrations of the relationship between the living and the dead. Since the 1990s, people's choices regarding how funerals, cremations and memorial services take place have been expanded beyond the traditional churchyard burial. Among members of the baby boomers generation, there is a strong a trend towards cremation. This group is also not satisfied with the impoverished practices of the past, especially those exposed in Jessica Mitford's (1963) book *The American Way of Death*, which criticized the language of professionalism employed by funeral directors and raised questions about profiting from the death of others. Mitford's study not only made it to the top of the *New York Times* best-seller list; it also shaped the terms of public debate over the funerals in the United States. The book represented a turning point in American attitudes toward the funeral industry and to its commercialization and exploitation. The subsequent investigations of funeral industry and further negative evaluations of death care industry and funeral rules have contributed to increased diversity and changes in the way people personalize their mourning and commemoration (Landrman 2003).

In the contemporary United Kingdom, people look for more personalized funeral or memorial services to commemorate the lives of their loved ones (Parsons 2018; Walter 2017). More people are choosing cremation, after which they can opt to scatter remains out at sea, in the backyard or in a number of other places. They can select humanist funerals or more environmentally responsible and ethical means of grief, such as the natural funeral – also known as woodland, green or ecological burial (Clayden et al. 2015; Davies and Rumble 2012). They can decide to have funeral services in person or via the internet. Yet the choice is costly: in the United States, the cost of a funeral is around US$7,000, while in the United people are expected to pay £3,700 for a funeral (Landrman 2003: 23; Walter 2017: 63). In England, funerals are commonly held in a church, crematorium or cemetery chapel, while the memorial service typically takes place at a funeral home after cremation. In the United States, unlike the United Kingdom, there is a visitation ceremony before the cremation or burial at the funeral home, where people can view the body in an open casket. Everywhere, though, the best funeral is one that is 'full of stories' (Miller 2016: 223). Now, with the internet offering new ways for a person's story to be told, both funeral homes and individuals have taken to sharing memories and life stories online. The same trend towards digitalization has been responsible for the emergence of online obituaries, or death announcements accompanied by brief biographies, which alongside the traditional newspaper obituary, death notice and local radio announcement, are prominent sources of information about recent deaths and funerals.

With their growing attendance at funerals, an older person often becomes 'a connoisseur of funerals and memorial services' (Miller 2016: 223). Empirical studies that confirm old people tend to attend funerals also suggest that the deaths of their relatives and friends frequently prompt the aged to dwell on their own mortality. For instance, Clarke et al. (2012) conducted in-depth interviews with men and women aged 73 to 91 years with multiple chronic conditions; his results illustrate that the older adults not only have more exposures to death, but also reflect more on death and dying, discuss the prevalence of death in their lives more frequently and express their anxieties about their impending death more often. Clarke et al. (2011) discovered that many of the elderly interviewees could provide the exact number of the funerals they had attended. They recorded that a 75-year-old man said:

> Last summer I went to nine funerals. This year I've been to three funerals. And it does affect you – profoundly ... Like I've gone to so many funerals over the last three years ... And you look around – we're all going there. I mean that's the ultimate destination, I guess. And you look around and say, 'Well, the next one could be yourself.' (Clarke et al 2011)

While this man confessed that attending funerals helped him to accept death as a necessary and natural event, other interviewees observed that attendance at funerals assisted them in adopting a more pragmatic attitude to death. In particular, they pointed out that the enriched knowledge of sermons, orations, eulogies, music and flowers may prompt them to think about how to organize their own funeral (Clarke et al. 2011).

Attending funerals does not just help elderly people to assess what works and does not work at burials, however; it can also give rise to feelings of total terror and paralyzing thoughts that 'it cannot be me yet'. For example, another elderly person interviewed by Clarke et al. (2011) said she stopped going to funerals because funerals were bringing 'the thought of death to her mind' and although she knew that 'the older you get, the nearer to the front of the church you get', she preferred to suppress such paralyzing thoughts (Clarke et al. 2011). Apart from the denial and insistence that 'it cannot be me yet', another feeling that often accompanies attendance at a funeral, where normally conversations about conditions of the death take place, is a fear of losing control over one's body and especially about the means of dying. Consequently, in order to avoid the fate of their diseased friends, some people may try to organize how and when they die and are buried. One such attempt is portrayed in Ian McEwan's (1998) novel *Amsterdam,* where a suicide pact between two friends is presented as their way to secure some control over the end of their lives. The anxieties and fears of death of Clive and Vernon, the novel's main characters, are brought up to the surface at their mutual friend's funeral, where they learn about the terrible suffering she faced at the end of her life and her undignified death. After attending her funeral, the two men decide they are prepared to do anything to avoid a loss of control at the end of their own lives, which could rob them of their autonomy in death. For both Clive and Vernon, it is very important to preserve dignity until the end, so in order to control the unpredictability of life, they make a suicide pact. Yet their unconventional personal euthanasia pact results in tragic and unpredicted consequences as they have not foreseen that, even when accepted, death remains frightening.

Attendance at funerals is directly associated with the readership of obituaries. Like funerals, obituaries serve to bind people together as they are composed to celebrate or reaffirm community values (Norman 2019). They, like funerals, also serve to sustain social divisions by reaffirming public recognition on the selected 'notable dead' (Bonsu 2007). Moreover, like funeral rituals, obituaries have evolved over the course of the last century. In the golden era of obituary writing, before the spread of social media and newspapers' downsizing, the obituary typically only offered an account of the lives of the rich, male and famous. While the first modern obituaries in newspapers appeared in 1731 in the London-based *The Gentleman's Magazine*, since the 1970s the nature of obituaries has changed significantly (Fowler 2007). The revolution in obituaries has democratized who is mourned and how, and although still some lives are more greatly and extensively mourned than others, there is now less gender and class bias and a more informal and direct style of presentation. Thus, by the 1980s obituaries had become more diversified, had been opened up to women, ethnic and other minority groups, and were written in a less formal and celebratory style (Fowler 2007; Phillips 2007). Since then, in Britain and many other Western nations, newspaper obituaries of ordinary people as well as celebrities have attracted a significant and growing readership. Also popular are the paid obituary notices that have come to be considered to be a family's and community's final tribute to an individual on their death (Norman 2019). Moreover, it is today commonly 'accepted that the emphasis on obituary composition should be on capturing life rather than death' (Starck 2007: 373). Now, with increasing access to and a growing role of social media, families often post online obituaries and digital memorials, while funeral homes' websites report on the recently departed. Unlike printed versions, online obituaries and information about funerals can be shared everywhere instantly.

Since the ageing baby boomers generation is relatively digitally literate, the popularity of obituaries and information about funerals has been increasing their attendance at the funerals of their peers (Davies and Rumble 2012). Initially, the attendance of one's peers at a funeral announced online could feel a bit like a class reunion. However, with more funerals on the horizon, the realization slowly dawns that there are fewer people to talk to and that one's own demise looms (Miller 2016). The issue of mortality takes on urgency as older adults, by reading obituaries and attending funerals of their friends and acquaintances, become aware of how the age gap between them and the diseased keeps narrowing. As the narrator in Erica Jong's novel *Fear of Dying* (2015: 10), a retired actor, witnesses her friends' and colleagues' deaths, she becomes painfully aware that:

> As you get older, the losses around you are staggering. The people in the obits come closer and closer to your own age. Older friends and relatives die, leaving you stunned … it gets harder and harder to deny your own death.

Reading obituaries and attending the funerals of one's peers may prompt older people to reflect on their own mortality. However, while presenting older persons with the magnified burden of sadness and frightening distress, these indirect encounters with death do not necessarily uniformly shape their thinking about their diminishing future. Older people's reflections on their relationship with mortality can be also influenced or shaken by some events and experiences in everyday life.

Everyday experiences in the shadow of death

Getting older does not just decrease the probability of living in the world of funerals and obituaries; it also multiplies the number of encounters with things and places that represent death in everyday life. With time passing, when it is impossible to avoid the failings of one's body and when faced with a growing number of indirect encounters with death, the issue of mortality intrudes into older adults' thoughts and daily lives, and becomes an essential part of their attempts to make a sense of life and death (Clarke et al. 2012). In turn, older people's awareness of the shortening of time influences many of their practical decisions and shapes their everyday lives. For example, older adults' understanding that many 'things' will outlast them (as illustrated by elderly people's typical sayings when buying things – 'this sofa will see me out') and their practice of 'decluttering' suggest that 'the end of any life amounts more or less to a tidying up; you no longer feel the urge to throw yourself into a new project, you are content just to dispatch day-to-day matters' (Houellebecq 2006: 329).

Among events and experiences in older people's everyday lives, which can be of significance in the process of negotiation of their relationships with death, are indirect encounters with death when they are patients in hospitals in the proximity of dying people, when they are carers for their dying partners or relatives and when they are residents in care homes for elderly people. While it is important to recognize the diversity within the older population in terms of health conditions, and to acknowledge that getting older does not inevitably mean greater demands on hospitals beds or on places in residential facilities, we need to realize that in general the total number of days spent in hospital increases with age and that – as all studies document – multimorbidity ('the presence of two or more long-term conditions, which are those that cannot currently be cured but can be managed through medications, lifestyle or other treatments') increases with age (NICE 2016).

In the case of those aged 75 years and over, the prevalence of chronic and long-term conditions increases the number of people admitted to hospital as well as the number of those living with complex health and care needs and in significant need of care and support. Because of the NHS hospitals' very high bed occupancy rates, open bays and limited single rooms, a significant number of older people who are hospitalized are often surrounded by others who are dying and experiencing age-related problems (Oliver 2018). In England in 2017, there were 16.6 million hospital admissions for people of any age; among them, 3.5 million (22.2%) were aged 75 years and older, despite this age group only representing 8.2% of the population. Older people who are admitted to hospital tend to develop mobility issues, dependence, disability, dementia, delirium, incontinence and sensory impairment; they also tend to stay longer in hospital than those in younger age groups (Oliver 2018). With around two-thirds of NHS hospital bed days taken up by people aged over 65, and a quarter of bed days taken up by people aged over 80, older patients – even when they are not in specialist geriatric units – 'may be near others who are close to death or who show confusion and behavioural symptoms, which can be disruptive or upsetting, though in no way the patients' fault' (Oliver 2018). Moreover, there were a total of 0.8 million admissions to hospital for people aged 75 years and older in the last year of life. These admissions accounted for 23.7% of all admissions for people aged 75 years and older, and only 5% of all admissions of people of any age (Gov UK 2020). As a substantial proportion of people aged 75 years and older are hospitalized in the last year of their life, and as many of them tend to die in hospital, older adults cannot not avoid indirect encounters with death when in hospital, and they learn that whatever the original affliction may have been, 'in the end, the dying come to resemble each other far more closely than those who, with similar diagnosis, continue to live' (Clarke 2020: 194).

A totally different source of familiarity with death is associated with performing caring duties for a partner or relative at the end of life. With the growing longevity in our society, the number of older people unable to perform routine, everyday self-care tasks, including walking, feeding, toileting and bathing, was 1.7 million in 2075; it is expected to increase by 69%, to 3 million, by 2040 (Wittenberg et al. 2018). Subsequently, with the growing number of older people living at home who are in need of healthcare and rely on it for their partners or other relatives, many older people are themselves carers: 12% of those aged 65–74 years, 9% of those aged 75–84 years and 8% of those aged 85 years and over provide care to others. Women are more likely to provide informal care and support than men up to and including the 75–84 years age group, while for the 85 and over age group, this is reversed (Age UK 2020; King's Fund 2018). While caring for elderly members of their family until the end, older adults become very acquainted with the biological processes of deterioration and dying. Being older persons themselves, and caring for dying elders, they cope with the daily demands of the chronically sick person in their care. Older carers, who are concerned primarily with helping their dying loved ones, try to observe the arrival of death without anguish, even though they dread what they know is looming for themselves. By weakening any refusal to acknowledge our finitude and by prompting people's individual thinking and their own ways of confronting mortality, such experiences can have an enormous impact on older people's experience of death (Dessaix 2020; Higgs and Gilleard 2015).

Totally different indirect encounters with death take place in aged care residential facilities. Before we discuss this further, it needs to be stressed again that today's prolonged longevity does not necessary mean living in care homes, as older people now increasingly live independently longer – on average into their mid-eighties in the United Kingdom – and older American adults, for example, spend as much as 80% of their time at home (Ray Karpen 2019: 4). Yet in the United Kingdom, the number of people aged 85 years and over with low 'dependency' (less than daily care) is projected to increase by 148%, while the number with high 'dependency' (twenty-four hour a day care) will increase by 92% (Kingston et al. 2018). In the United Kingdom in 2021, 548,000 older people received long-term care and there were also 231,000 episodes of short-term care. After moving into a care home in the United Kingdom, half of all people die in a year and three-quarters die in three years. In England, where an estimated half a million physically disabled elderly were living in care homes, more than half (56%) of newly admitted people to a nursing home could be expected to die within twelve months (Pocock et al. 2021: 1638). Since, according to the Alzheimer's Society, around 70% of people living in a residential or nursing home have some form of dementia, and it is one of the main causes of their death, we explore this issue in Chapter 9, which looks at death and dying in care homes. Here we illustrate everyday encounters with death in care homes, the ways in which residents of care homes cope with the presence of death and its impact on their everyday experiences and practices.

The decision to enter into residential care is the turning point in many elderly lives. This 'big move', to use the title of Waytt-Brown's (2019) book, normally takes place because of the frailty of the elderly person and the multiple chronic conditions they are experiencing. It is one of the most determinant moments for negotiation of death, as care homes or residential homes are seen as places of exit from life. There are numerous studies and reports about the functioning of such institutions, yet given that an exploration of ongoing everyday life in care home requires attending to people's individual perceptions of and feelings about them, we are here interested in the subjective experience of everyday life in care homes and its contribution to residents' interpretation of their situation. Such subjective experience, defined as people's individual ways of making sense of and interpreting their social world, is constituted by the tensions between expectations and opportunities; it is also marked by contradictions between the perceived 'banality, triviality [and] repetitiveness' of everyday experiences and the realization that, in another sense, 'nothing could be more profound' (Lefebvre quoted in Ferguson 2009: 39). As death is part of ongoing everyday life in care homes, subjective experience of everyday life in such facilities shapes attitudes to and apprehensions of death and dying, which are an essential part of the sense-making practices. To understand older people's everyday experience of living in the shadow of death, we will look at the diaries of two residents in such facilities and at one reflective work from an older writer based on his visits to a nursing home. Rather than seeing only the limitations of nursing or care homes, these three writers, whose works will be discussed below, describe their subjective experiences of encounter with residential facilities. Their observations deepen, enliven and enrich our understanding of ageing and dying.

One such personal story that expands our comprehension of the impact of exposure to death on the elderly is Anne Waytt-Brown's tale (2019) *The Big Move: Life Between the Turning Points*. Waytt-Brown, a well-known humanist gerontologist, moved to a continuing care retirement community in Baltimore in the United States because of her husband's heath needs when she was only 71 years old and still a healthy person. Her account is very interesting because it combines both her 'inside', or subjective, experience of the place with her professional, or 'outsider', knowledge. When they moved into the retirement community, she discovered that 'being a humanistically inclined gerontologist did not help [her] initially negative feelings about [their] new dwelling' (Waytt-Brown 2019: 16). As she struggled to adjust to life as a resident, she was helped neither by remembering that 'the rest of the world tends to dismiss those of us who no longer live in ordinary housing' nor by the fact that the average age of residents was 85 and not many of them were in good shape physically (Waytt-Brown 2019: 21, 15). Only when she realized that if one reaches out to others, it takes less time to feel at home, Waytt-Brown gradually began to find ways of getting to know other residents and coming closer to understating their attitudes towards death.

The residential facility, which consisted of three different levels of care, was a continuing-care community, thus 'residents may stay here, regardless of worsening health, until they die' (Waytt-Brown 2019: 12). Living there meant continuously facing many things that reminded her and other residents 'how tentative our plan – and our lives – really are' (Waytt-Brown 2019: 17). However, despite the fact that 'painful signs of the future, consisting of disabilities, decline, and death' could be seen everywhere, many residents did not want to talk about death, while staff tried to 'postpone death as long as possible' (Waytt-Brown 2019: 22). Observing the residents of the community, Waytt-Brown (2019: 19–24) realized that people came to the place with all their strengths and weaknesses, and that some had learned to adjust while others felt overwhelmed, unable to accept their own frailty and scared of what the future might hold for them. People who made their final years frightening and burdensome were unable to face death and the fear of being forced to confront images of their demise, but at the same time they felt they had lost control of their own lives. Those residents who engaged in conversations with others about death and were consciously and deliberately reckoning with life and death tended to experience a better end-of-life quality. Waytt-Brown (2019: 23, 24) did not know how long she and her husband could live independently and what problems might in time upset her equilibrium; however, she knew she had friends there with similar experiences who could support her. By being able to talk to them, by sharing her fears about the nature of changes and discussing death, she found the strength to for care for others and to help them at the end of their lives as well as to reflect on her own life and its purpose, and to engage in a further search of its meaning.

Also a diarist, Hendrick Groen (a pseudonym – the real name of the author is Peter de Smet) was initially overwhelmed by moving into a community of mostly disabled, chronically ill and very old people. In his fictional work, *The Secret Diary of Hendrick Groen, 83 1/4 years Old*, Hendrick Groen illustrates many negative consequences of this turning point in his life but he also presents old age as not only full of death, but also full of life. Suddenly confronted by the end of independent living, Hendrick struggles to accept his status as a resident of a care home and wonders how to live with an awareness that there is 'nothing that will stop decline' and that 'genuine improvement is not on the cards, ever' (Groen 2017: 8). He realizes that the care home, connected to a nursing unit for seriously impaired geriatric patients. is 'a constantly revolving door of the living and the dead' and that there is only one exit from this institution (Groen 2017: 85). Hendrick works out that in the care home there are around 50 deaths a year: 'If you grow to a very old age in here and remain on your feet, you may have to attend as many as 500 burials or cremations in the last 10 years of your life. A lovely prospect' (Groen 2017: 85).

However, despite knowing that the care home is where he 'will remain until your final departure for the churchyard or crematorium', and despite his dislike of its residents' habit of 'sitting in their little rooms and waiting for death', he is still determined not to allow death to deter him – 'at least not other people's death' (Groen 2017: 81, 221, 267). Although Hendrick acknowledges that the time is running out and that 'the real problem is insoluble', he still does not give up on his trust in the future and is confident that there is still something meaningful to look forward to (Groen 2017: 74). Confronted often enough with death and decay, he realizes the value of friendship and starts searching for contacts with others. Despite his contempt for the majority of care home residents, Hendrick soon learns that even in the care home, the loss of professional standing, occupational status and family roles can be managed by the construction of many substitutions in the form of new passions, habits and interests. Therefore, by getting to know, meeting and relating to other residents of the care home, he tries to help them to overcome the discontinuity associated with the loss of their previous identities and reconstruct their image of the future. However, even when the residents in the care home are eager to engage in new projects, to form new interests and cultivate new friendships, they are – as Hendrick soon realizes – always presented with difficulties that limit their forward-looking plans, contacts and ventures. This is because death is always on the horizon; thus, even as he and his new friends drink to 'friendship, until death do us part', they are aware that death is not 'an abstract concept for any of [them]' (Groen 2017: 371).

Hence, while being thankful for every day, Hendrick knows that he always needs to be prepare for things getting worse. In this spirit, he helps his friend Grietje, diagnosed with the beginning of Alzheimer's disease, to cope at least with the first stage of the sickness. By developing a well-researched programme of routines, Hendrick makes her feel as if she has some control over her fate. Although the whole process of discussing, planning, preparation, training and structuring routines does not prevent the illness from developing and 'Grietje is slowly and almost imperceptibly going downhill', at least for some time Grietje, despite becoming 'muddled about time and place', getting confused about many things and losing memory, was still able to 'laugh about it herself, though not very heartily' and to say, 'Every fine day is one more day' (Groen 2017: 253, 367). Hendrick also shares the experience of death with his dear friend Eefje, for whom there is no hope of a long survival. Hendrick and Eefje decide to confront together what will happen to her in six months to a year. As Eefje 'seems to be sinking slowly to death, Hendrick helps her achieve "a peaceful death"' (Groen 2017: 345). He sits next to her, reads to her and sometimes caresses 'her old cheeks' (Groen 2017: 358). When 'Eefje is slowly, gently, slipping into death', Hendrick stops reading to her but still visits and holds her hand (Groen 2017: 366, 358). Through these meetings with death, Hendrick realizes that he wants to control and own his death; he is more afraid of losing physical independence and becoming increasingly dependent on others than he is of death, which he wishes not to prolong, as he does not want to 'end up as a sputtering toddler in a nappy' (Groen 2017: 74).

Living in care homes can make older people 'feel more aged, more useless and more depressed' (Higgs and Gilleard 2015: 112) as they experience a loss of autonomy, preferred spaces and lifestyles. For many, it involves a reckoning with mortality as they feel they have become superfluous, redundant and needless and realize that there is only one type of exit from care homes. Even visiting these places – especially for an older person – can have an impact on people's way of thinking and experience of death. For example, visits to a nursing home induced Australian writer Robert Dessaix, himself nearly 80, to realize how much he desired to control or possess his own death, the awareness of which he has always seen as giving a special value and meaning to life. Expressing his feelings from indirect encounters with death in his book *The Time of Our Lives: Growing Older Well*, Robert Dessaix (2020) wonders what is left of the inner life when one approaches death. Even though he knew a lot about the ageing process and was aware of the difficulty and ambiguity of older people's everyday life, Dessaix was not prepared for the sight of older people in a nursing home. He was shaken by 'decrepitude and dementia everywhere he looked'. Although he knew not to expect the high quality of everydayness, the 'sounds of madness rustle and reverberate up and down the corridors, the smells of sickness hang in the air. Even the sane seem slightly gaga, the healthy hunched and tilted. It shakes me every time I see it' (Dessaix 2020: 67). While observing that in nursing homes death tends to arrive slowly, from a multiplicity of ailments rather than a single and specific disease, he reflects on the contradictions and complexities of old age and dying. The realization that although we know about death all our lives, 'when you come face-to-face with it, it shocks you, it claws at your heart' provokes Dessaix to ask many questions about how to live amidst such endless suffering and how to find a pathway through it (Dessaix 2020: 74). The visit to and experience of the nursing home led him to recognize that everybody needs to individually navigate the final stage by, on the one hand, trying to preserve 'a sturdy mental core' to the end and, on the other, by accepting the reality of the falling body and the inevitable end (Dessaix 2020: 69). For Dessaix, who fears cognitive impairment, nothing could be more essential at the end of life than the preservation of an awareness of an approaching death.

All indirect encounters with death, from attending funerals or reading obituaries of one's peers to living in nursing homes, lead people to experience an emotion of sadness that is very difficult to overcome. Sadness is the existential despair that is linked to the ontological condition of being aware of the end (Ricoeur 2004). It is the emotion connected with the growing consciousness of mortality, the experienced of loss and 'the work of mourning' (Ricoeur 2004: 496). Sadness is inherent to the last stage in life, when people understand that they are at the end and that death is imminent, and when they know that their choices are limited and their opportunities are restricted. The feeling of sadness can ease our fear of mortality as its full force may help us to reconcile ourselves to the fact that everything human must die (Ricoeur 2004). Since it is 'so sad that one must leave all this, that one must prepare to go', sadness of older age, although being a more general and more passive emotion than grief, is an integral part of the work of mourning (Ricoeur 2004: 504). As the work of mourning 'definitively separates the past from the present and makes way for the future', sadness may lead older people to accept that no one is immune to death (Ricoeur 2004: 499).

It is worth noticing that sadness is an emotion experienced from within, connected with the awareness of mortality – and one that is difficult to avoid and evade. Such an emphasis on the subjective aspect of sadness implies that it is a rather solitary and private feeling; however, as the coronavirus pandemic illustrates, this private emotional state can be influenced by external factors. In what follows we look how the recent health crisis, by making the lives of older people more lonely and risky, as well as by increasing their indirect encounters with death, impacted their feelings.

COVID-19 and new risk situations

There are many illustrations of how our awareness of death can be influenced by some external factors and situations framing our indirect encounters with death. For the most of today's older adults, one of the most significant factors that has furthered their indirect contact with death and hence has impacted their thinking about death, is the recent pandemic. For example, during COVID-19, the simplification of funeral rites and the reduced nature of mourning services, such as the limitations on the number of people permitted at crematoria and cemeteries, presented older people with the magnified burden of sadness and frightening distress (Sherwood and Pidd 2020). As the new reality of funerals during the COVID-19 lockdowns affected members of families of diseased persons in particular, we will discuss it in a next chapter, which deals with mourners and grief, and the impacts and consequences of direct encounters with death. In what follows, we examine how the pandemic, by multiplying external indirect encounters with death, has made the life of older people riskier and has left them feeling more vulnerable.

It is often observed that the recent pandemic is a part of a long human history of living with risk and that every generation has its own epidemic. Thus, it can be argued that for today's older generation, the recent pandemic was especially a step 'into the unknown' and into a risky situation (Bresalier 2020: 11). The pandemic, the most traumatic exposure to the risk for older people in contemporary Western nations, has presented the elderly with a new visibility of death in the public arena, particularly with the deaths of their peers, and has left many older people to deal with the loss of their loved ones. The COVID-19 crisis unleashed anguish and anxiety among many older people and it taught many to take the risk seriously.

In modern societies, the idea of risk is attributed with more significance than ever before, as risk is now seen as the common denominator of our times. Although our history is full of extreme risk situations, such as plagues or wars and natural hazards, which all caused collective and individual traumas and a sense of loss, it is claimed that in late modernity risk has become 'something of an omnipresent issue, casting its specter over a wide range of practices and experiences' (Mythen 2004: 1). According to this perspective, as developed and popularized by Beck, we now live in a risk society – that is, in a society where political conflicts and divisions are no longer defined by a logic of the distribution of goods but 'are becoming defined by the distribution of "risks"' (Beck 1992: 7).The idea of a risk society maintains that the process of the intrusion of humans into nature has resulted in humanly produced risks, and that the consequences of these 'manufactured risks' give rise to radical changes in social structure, politics and culture (Beck 1992: 9). Human-made disasters, such as Chernobyl, and the growing destructive power of natural hazards, such as Hurricane Katrina or the 2004 Boxing Day tsunami, are seen as evidence that contemporary societies cannot cope effectively with the risk produced by modern development, and cannot deal with climate change and resolve the complexities and contingencies of environmental challenges.

We live in an increasingly complex global society, in which risks will continue and in which 'there are no bystanders anymore' (Beck 1996: 32). In the risk society, everyone is vulnerable and everyone depends on specialized scientific knowledge to define risks and ways of dealing with them (Beck 1996). Since we are not competent to evaluate scientific opinions on risk prevention, we cannot protect ourselves against the danger without accepting the scientific view in advance of encountering the risk situation. Viewing the COVID-19 pandemic in the context of the risk society allows us to say that insuring against the coronavirus without the help of science has been impossible just as insuring against exposure to environmental risks without relying on science is impossible.

Throughout the pandemic and in its aftermath, despite vaccination, the risk of COVID-19 remained high for thousands of older people, especially those deemed clinically extremely vulnerable to COVID-19, for whom 'living with COVID-19 seems to include accepting a very high death rate' (Clinically Vulnerable Families UK spokesperson, quoted in Thomas 2022). Although the risk faced by elderly people during the COVID-19 pandemic was lower than it may have been for clinically vulnerable people, all older people – even those without underlying health problems – were asked to shield at the onset of the health crisis. The impact of these many days of isolation on their mental health cannot be overlooked, as many of them felt vulnerable, lonely and unsafe. The pandemic was difficult for many older people because of the risk of the virus, but also because the COVID-19 crisis brought them into direct encounters with death, as some of them lost their partners, relatives or friends. Yet even indirect encounters with the COVID-19 crisis, such as reading and watching records of death, numbers of infections, statistics of admission to hospital and figures for vaccination, may have unleashed feelings of anxiety and anguish. For example, many older people were worried by headlines about high rates of cases and deaths among elderly people, especially in care homes. However, for the majority of older people it was living in isolation and feeling very vulnerable and lonely that were the most painful experiences connected with the pandemic. Moreover, for many older people the end of lockdown restrictions did not make much difference, as many older people have never really emerged from twenty-two months of lockdown. This means the feelings of isolation and loneliness still mark their lives.

Even though, in the context of COVID-19 epidemic, older people were cautioned about the risks of contact with others, at the same time they were not warned about the potential negative impact of isolation and loneliness on their physical and mental health. Isolation and loneliness are both risk factors, as studies carried out by charities such as the Mental Health Foundation and Independent Age have demonstrated. This research, while arguing that the coronavirus pandemic has already damaged the health of people over the age of 65, discovered the additional impact of coronavirus on the older people's mental and physical health (Corcoran and Wood 2021). The studies concluded that the coronavirus pandemic may have resulted in further deterioration to the heath of many of the 12.5 million older people in the United Kingdom because of its effects on their mental wellbeing. For the research, the charities interviewed a number of older people who lived totally on their own for almost two years and often did not talk to anyone for days. One man in his seventies said that 'the worst thing has been the loneliness', while a woman in her late eighties observed, 'To be in this flat entirely on your own – I mean, I don't know what I'd do without my little iPad' (Corcoran and Wood 2021).

Although Omicron has led to significantly lower numbers of deaths than previous COVID-19 waves, the removal of COVID-19 restrictions in England from 27 January 2022 (for example, making masks no longer mandatory) was criticized by several charities, such as the Alzheimer's Society and the MS Society. They all said it was too early to drop basic measures which helped to protect vulnerable members of society without any assessment of the risks to those who were most vulnerable to the effects of COVID-19. The charities also warned that clinically vulnerable people 'have just become collateral damage in political considerations' (Charlotte August, CEO of National Voices, quoted in Thomas 2022). Even though the UK cases of COVID-19 infection and death were falling and there were high immunity levels, around five million people still had not been vaccinated by January 2022, so without some infection control measures, such wearing masks on public transport, older people faced too much risk to be able to really get on with their lives. As the pandemic lowered older people's capacity to carry out normal lives, there was no 'return to normal' for many older people. Their physical and mental health was affected by the pandemic and they faced the risk of the virus, in addition to loneliness and isolation. In short, the pandemic left many older people feeling vulnerable, which can induce feelings of powerlessness and lower resilience.

Feeling vulnerable is connected with the experience of fear, uncertainty, anguish and a lack of safety and control. Such a combination of feelings can reduce people's capacity to protect themselves against danger and is typically caused by exposure to risk situations (Erickson 2006; Perrow

2006). For example, studies show that while people normally tend to treat the world around them as 'safe', those who have experienced some risky situation in the past, such as a natural disaster or health crisis, tend to feel vulnerable because they have lost 'an illusion that they are safe', which is one of 'the bargains men make with one another in order to maintain their sanity' (Erickson 1994: 234). Hence, by highlighting the older people's vulnerability, the COVID-19 crisis – like other catastrophic situations – may have lowered their capacity for resilience. Lessons from other major calamities suggests that 'instead of focusing only on preventing disasters and coping with the aftermath – which we must continue to do – we should reduce the size of vulnerable targets' (Perrow 2007: 1). Thus, in the case of another health threat in the future, our task should be to reduce older people's vulnerabilities and make sure that older people are not left feeling fearful, full of anxiety and without any of control over their fate.

When feeling vulnerable and hopeless about the future, people tend to seek safety and security. During the pandemic, while trying to gain some control over their health and survival, many people looked for information about the COVID-19 threats and vulnerability to the risk of infection and illness from the virus. Studies show that during the pandemic, instead of trusting the official data, increasing numbers of people searched the internet for information about the virus and for advice on how to protect vulnerable groups (Freeman et al. 2020; Geddes 2020; Henley and McIntyre 2020). The peak of informational demand was in March 2020, at the beginning of the first lockdown, when people searched online for the coronavirus update five to six times a day on average, while in April 2020 'UK coronavirus deaths' were people's top concern (Geddes 2020). This reliance on new media for information about the coronavirus can be seen as an expression of a distrust of the scientific and governmental consensus on the pandemic, a distrust that was widespread in many countries. For example, 38% of Americans, 36% of Hungarians, 30% of Italians and 28% of Germans believed that the death rate of the virus had been 'deliberately and greatly exaggerated' and did not trust scientific advice for the value of crucial health practices (Henley and McIntyre 2020),while in the United Kingdom, 60% of adults believed that the government and scientists were misleading the public about the cause of the virus to some extent (Freeman et al. 2020).

Because of the capacity of digital platforms to spread ideas and information efficiently and easily, the coronavirus epidemic created 'a perfect storm for conspiracy theorists'(Uscinski and Enders 2020). As one of the main problems during the pandemic was the large amount of contradictory and unstable information circulating, it was very difficult to dispel the rumors that COVID-19 was a hoax and to silence the voices supporting the anti-vaccination movement (Galchen 2022). In other words, today's main problem is not information deficit but rather the content of messages that aim to cause 'feelings of extreme anxiety, powerlessness, and stress, which in turn encourage conspiracy beliefs' (Uscinski and Enders 2020). Moreover, as more recent studies – particularly of Twitter – have shown, scare stories spread further and faster than reliable data (Galchen 2022). Another research study based on a representative sample of 2,501 adults found that in the United Kingdom, conspiracy beliefs were not confined to the fringes and such ideas were associated with less compliance with government guidelines and greater unwillingness to undertake future tests and treatments (Freeman et al 2020).

In the United Kingdom, despite being exposed to confusing information, older people – as their very high level of vaccination indicates – have not refused COVID-19 vaccines. Nonetheless, the exposure to incoherent messages may have undermined their feelings of safety and security. Moreover, as older people can be a relatively easy target for misinformation, their reliance on mass media to inform themselves about new risks could have been counter-productive – that is, it may not always have led to lowering the level of risk (Berman 2020). For example, there is evidence that older people in the United States were particularly impacted by the dissemination of misinformation and fake news, which exploited their anxieties and vulnerabilities (Uscinski and Enders 2020). Many elderly people, especially those experiencing cognitive decline or those who were digitally illiterate, were easy targets for the spread of fake news, such as questioning the severity of the virus and doubting the safety and usefulness of the vaccine, and misinformation such as that the virus was manufactured on purpose and that it might be a bioweapon. As higher levels of coronavirus conspiracy thinking 'were associated with less adherence to all government guidelines and less willingness to take diagnostic or antibody tests or to be vaccinated' (Freeman et al. 2020), the virus could have been transmitted faster and further. All these coronavirus conspiracy theories further undermined people's trust in the authority of science and government. In other words, by choosing to forgo crucial health practices, such as social distancing, frequent hand-washing and wearing a mask, people believing in coronavirus conspiracy theories put not only themselves but also others at risk.

The essential role of new digital media during the COVID-19 pandemic is just one of the features that distinguish this health crisis from previous epidemics. The coronavirus crisis, in contrast to the HIV/AIDS epidemic, which created a new stigma of a dangerous dead body (Troyer 2020), has unleased older people's fear of a virus over which there is no control and exposed their anxiety about how they could have died – in hospital, without their family, attended in their final minutes only by medical staff. Admissions to care and nursing homes remain below pre-pandemic levels as some older people have deferred their entrance into care facilities. For example, in the United Kingdom in April and May 2020, fewer people were placed into homes by their families, which meant occupancy of care homes fell from 88% to 79%, while weekly admissions fell from twenty-two per 1,000 residents on 29 March 2020 to eight per 1,000 by 31 May 2020 (Duncan and Booth 2020). Moreover, many older adults who felt vulnerable and tried to avoid hospitals, seen as overburdened with the COVID-19 emergencies and with delays to scheduled procedures, stayed at home or with relatives, and these actions could have led to a higher number of deaths. Because a substantial number of people who would normally have been in hospitals stayed at home instead, between March and October 2020 in Britain there were 61,000 excess deaths above the five-year average, with 30,000 the total number of excess deaths happening in people's homes across the country (Duncan and Booth 2020).

There is yet another significant difference between the COVID-19 pandemic and other risk situations. While other crises, from Hurricane Katrina to the 2004 Asian tsunami, compelled people to work together to provide support and aid to one another, the COVID-19 epidemic required us to take on the individual responsibility of protecting ourselves by remembering to wear masks, and by social distancing and self-isolation. However, this personal responsibility has also been an expression of collective responsibility because, by protecting ourselves, we have also been protecting others. Thus, it can be argued that the recent pandemic has reinforced the message from other risk situations: that there is a need for social solidarity to fight the invisible threat.

CHAPTER 5

Facing the death of loved ones

The experience of loss in later life

This chapter examines various forms of coping with irretrievable loss and provides insight into the various ways in which bereaved older people experience grief in normal times and how they faced it in the period when, due to the COVID-19 pandemic, mourning and funerary rites were disrupted, often leaving the dying and the bereaved to suffer alone. Following the discussion of indirect encounters with death in Chapter 4, here we explore how personal losses force older people to confront the irreversibility of the flow of time and mortality. The chapter argues that people's direct encounters with death, when they experience the loss of loved ones, can result in questions about the existence and the imminence of death. Although, through their long lives, older people could have experienced the deaths of many of their close friends and members of their family, regardless of their past encounters with the deaths of others, 'they all need to prepare for their own death' and grief due to the loss of someone they loved can lead them in this preparation (Stillion 1995: 319). The final part of the chapter shows that grief following death from COVID-19, which was unexpected, untimely and lonely, has been fundamentally different from mourning and grieving under normal circumstances.

Grief is an integral part of human experience that, while being a very private emotion, is also socially shaped; hence 'grief is deeply interwoven in historically changing socio-cultural contexts rules and norms' (Peterson and Jacobsen 2019: 195). The nature of grief and Western practices around mourning have been changing for millennia (Aries 1981; Howarth 2007).

For centuries, the religious promise of salvation and redemption offered people a hope that they would see their loved ones again in the afterlife: 'The religious traditions of consolation were able to situate individual suffering within wider frame and to offer a grieving person an account of where an individual life fit into a divine or cosmic plan' (Ignatieff 2022: 12). While in the past grief was primarily the domain of pastoral and communal care, with the coming of the twentieth century, with its secularization and celebration of science, death became privatized and invisible and was seen as a taboo. Subsequently, grief became less subject to social norms than in the previous centuries (Aries 1981). In Britain and the United States in the1960s, the space where death could exist was reduced and grief was hidden, partly as a result of the increasing pressure of a new 'ethical duty to enjoy oneself' and new imperative to 'do nothing which might diminish the enjoyment of others' (Gorer 1965: 45). In the first two decades of the twenty-first century, after losing its traditional institutional settings, such as churches, synagogues and mosques, grief has become an even more problematic, difficult and intensely private experience, often treated as an illness from which we need to recover.

In contemporary Western societies, with their detachment from tradition, place and kin, and where religion does not provide a powerful script for mourning and source of solace for the living as it did in the past, mourners are at liberty to decide how they want to grieve. Under such conditions, grief can be very personal experience of loss; however, that freedom can be confusing, and grief can become problematic (Peterson and Jacobsen 2019). Additionally, because today's norms about how to respond to bereavement are often contested, grief is often invisible, taking place behind closed doors (Walter 2017: 84–85). Furthermore, because modern society celebrates success and does not value failure or loss, and finds it difficult to face death and deal with grief, today grief is a 'difficult emotion' (Ignatieff 2022; Peterson and Jacobsen 2019). Moreover, grief becomes a more complex phenomenon also because, as a result of the evolution of scientific approaches, it is seen as an illness that requires diagnosis and treatments. Now, as the world has lost meanings that once were rooted in religious traditions, if we want help in times of grief we seek it from therapeutic professionals. Finally, by increasing the complexity, difficulties and anguish of grief, the coronavirus pandemic further problematized the nature of grief and changed the context of bereavement.

While recognizing that grief needs to be understood in the context of cultural scripts, social norms and personal styles (Kellehear 2002; Murry et al. 2015), this chapter searches for aspects of grief common to older people who outlive their loved ones. It asserts that although each person's grief is different, there are still some similarities in the ways in which older people live through and express their grief. Generally, elderly people have coped with many death and losses across their many years of life, but it is the loss of a spouse that is the major source of sorrow of most older adults (Howarth 2007). By bringing the realization that their own death is becoming ever more imminent and inescapable, this grief also forces them to face their own mortality. Hence, exploring what is specific to older people's experience of loss is an important step in developing of our understanding how universal truth about how mortality becomes very personal.

Before we start searching for specific aspects of grief common to older people, there is a need for a quick clarification of the meanings of three words that describe responses to loss: grief, mourning and bereavement. While all three terms refer to the pain and suffering that occurs after experiences of loss, and while these notions are often used interchangeably, their connotations and significance differ. Furthermore, it is not easy to clarify their distinctive meanings as they are defined in a variety of ways; moreover, some definitions are confusing, with grief seen by some as a source of creativity and strength, and by others as a pathological problem that can be 'solved' or as mental illness to be privatized, specialized and treated by professionals and councilors (Granek 2010). Nonetheless, there seems to be a consensus that grief is an all-encompassing concept, as it is almost a universal condition of human life, which crosses all historical periods and cultures. Although expressed differently by people from different societies, religions or cultures, grief as 'synonymous with inner turmoil' is 'the most overarching' human response to loss (McManus 2013: 125). In short, it is an internal process of giving meaning to the experience of loss (Clarke 2020; Samuel 2017; Wolfelt 2011). Grief as the emotion or activity of grieving is very lonely, non-negotiable and without previous experience (Clarke 2020; Hockey et al. 2007; Katz 2001; Woleft 2018).With the emergence of scientific interest in the notion of grief, the religion-based understanding of grief and the conceptualization of grief as an emotional human impulse have been supplemented by the idea of grief as a transitional state of repairing the emotional, psychological and social bonds shattered by death (McManus 2013: 130).

Although our understanding of grief has been changing, as the shift from the religious discourse for making sense of loss to the scientized approach to grief illustrates, grief always tends to refer to what is felt after a loss. Subsequently, such a definition of grief always reinforces the same distinction between grief and mourning, where grief is seen as the emotional reaction to a loss, while mourning refers to what is done (Lofland 1985; Walter 2017: 84). The other important difference between grief and mourning is that grief happens and can be more or less passive experience of loss, while mourning is the act of dealing with grief, and required attention to the socially prescribed practices that are activated by bereavement (McManus 2013: 125). Hence grief is a part of mourning, but mourning is not necessary a part of grief (Howarth 2007: 195).

In short, grief is an internal feeling of the pain of loss, while mourning is culturally prescribed behaviour appropriate to those who have been bereaved, which aims to take the individual beyond the passive reactions of grief. In the past, mourning was 'a vehicle for social communication through the cultural and/or public display of grief through behaviours' (Howarth 2007: 219). This traditional function of mourning was supported by such rituals as dressing in black garments, covering all mirrors in the house or visiting the grave. Yet today we do not only prefer the bereaved to not show their grief and to 'move on' quickly or achieve 'closure'; we are also not well equipped to communicate grief, navigate it and support the bereaved in such a way as to allow them to function effectively (Berns 2011; Samuel 2017). With the emptiness of places such as churches, where once people comforted each other in collective rituals of grief and mourning, now people seek professional help (Ignatieff 2022). Mourning has 'to a large degree been removed from public space, the days of the funeral procession moving at a leisurely pace were now over, mourning clothing went out of fashion and comprehensive mourning rituals were gradually replaced by science and denial' (Peterson and Jacobsen 2019: 198). Like mourning, bereavement is the cultural referent for grief, as both bereavement and mourning are 'the means through which the objective event (death) is socially noted and a acknowledged' (McManus 2013: 125).While the purpose of active processes of mourning is to enable the living to overcome the passivity of reactions of grief, bereavement refers to the time period immediately after the loss, or to the state of having lost something (Walter 2017: 84) or the situation of a person who has recently experienced the death of a loved one (Katz 2001: 3).

The grief theory, which emerged as a topic of scientific study within psychology in the early twentieth century, has kept developing in step with changes within the discipline of psychology (Granek 2010).The psychological perspective, which dominated studies of grief until the 1990s, was originally conceived by Sigmund Freud (1953) in his work 'Mourning and Melancholia'. Within Freud's psychoanalytic and non-pathological framework, mourning is seen as a serious departure from 'the normal attitude to life' initiated by the need to detach from the lost object. It comes to a decisive end after a certain period of time when the subject severs its emotional attachment to the lost one and reinvests the feelings in a new object (Freud 1953: 245–56). In his conceptualization of grief, Freud does not see a need to refer grieving persons for medical treatment; rather, he proposes grief work as something that would free the ego from attachment to the deceased and, in so doing, would allow new attachments to be formed.

From Freud, through Eric Lindemann (1944), who focused on 'grief work' and described sensations of somatic distress occurring in waves and analysed pathological or distorted grief, to Bowley (1969, 1981), who promoted attachment theory, all theorists of grief saw the detachment from emotional pain caused by the loss of loved ones as the main aim of mourning (Rando 1995). The scientific theories of grief, including theories of attachment and loss, stage theories and meaning-making theories, objectified grief in the language of psychology. All these classical psychological approaches assumed that the task of grief is the reassimilation of the individual into life by leaving the deceased behind and forming new attachments. In the earlier conceptualizations of grief within a biomedical model, grief was framed as an illness from which one can recover quickly by detaching oneself from the deceased through the working through of feelings (Bowlby

1969, 1981; Parkes 1972; Raphael 1984). In later clinical approaches, grief work was seen as also encompassing the overcoming grief's symptoms, including 'such diverse physical and mental feelings and activities as; sleeplessness, restlessness, loss of appetite, frustration, hallucinations, "irrational" behaviour, shortness of breath, heaviness, in the chest, nausea, headaches, uncontrolled weeping, sadness, despair, hopelessness, apathy an irritability' (Lofland 1985: 172).

Among clinical theories of loss, which focus on the stages of accommodation grief demands from the bereaved person, the most influential has been Kübler-Ross's (2011) stage theory of grief. In *On Grief and Grieving*, Kübler-Ross defines the five stages of grief – denial, anger, bargaining, depression and acceptance – through which people are supposed to progress and emerge out of their grief with a feeling of having left the deceased behind. Kübler-Ross's model has been the predominant way for counsellors and professionals to approach grief for many decades. However Kübler-Ross's conceptualization of psychological of pathways through grief has been criticized for being too prescriptive, linear, rigid and individualistic in its assumptions (Howarth 2007). Since grief is a very personal emotion, which can come in various forms, from 'large griefs' to 'little griefs', and in different guises, ranging from prolonged – even incurable – grief to repressed grief, searching for these many faces of grief cannot be restricted the viewing grief as a diagnostic category (Peterson and Jacobsen 2019: 195). However, as a psycho-social transition where people are passing through stages of grief (from four to twelve stages of grief, depending on the writer), grieving still continues to be seen as relevant by many psychological theorists of grief. Some, dubious about the limited view of the ending in the model of transition through grief, propose viewing grief as a condition that may deepen our understanding of the meaning of life – for example, in his book *Finding Meaning: The Sixth Stage of Grief*, David Kessler (2019) adds one more stage to the process of grieving: meaning.

No person's grief occurs in a social vacuum, so new theories have attempted to enrich psychodynamic theories of attachment, which generated stage and phase theories, by incorporating the acknowledgement of the role of social factors. Parkes' (1972) observation that mourners' adjustment to their new status – for example, the status of a widow – prompts them to change their social expectations was followed by Stroebe and Schut's (1999) assertion that grief is not a linear process but rather an ongoing fluctuation between the pain of loss, and the cost and tensions involved in the construction of a new life. Their dual process model of grief also emphasizes the importance of social context in which people move back and forth between the emotional pain of loss and efforts to reconstitute their social life. Moreover, traditional models of grief have also been challenged by Klass et al. (1996), who have argued that people do not necessary relinquish their attachments to the deceased in order to attach to others. This new approach to grief and its model of 'a continuing bond', while arguing that mourners can retain ties with the dead, has undermined several assumptions of classical theories of grief, such as their claims about linear and individualistic features of grief.

By bringing into focus the importance of social context and human interdependence, the new theories encourage the development of a more sociological approach, which rejects the universalism of grief expression, recognizes cultural diversity of grief and stresses that grieving tends to take place in the presence of significant others and that it is most often shared with others who also mourn the loss (Howarth 207; McManus 2013; Peterson and Jacobsen 2019; Walter 2017). By taking into account historical changes in the social context of grief, bringing together psychological and social aspects of grief and focusing on the social construction of loss and its cultural diversity, such a sociological perspective is more inclusive and interpretative, and allows us to grasp the complexity and contradictions of people's experiences and relations. For example, Walter (1996, 1999, 2017), who examines bereavement as an ongoing process of negotiation and meaning-making, shows how changes in societal culture and social norms impact the grieving process, seen as aiming to construct a story that places the dead within their lives. The construction of such a story, capable of enduring through time, or a durable biography, 'enables the living to integrate the memory of the dead into their ongoing lives; the process by which this is achieved is principally conversation with others who knew the deceased' (Walter 1996: 7). Walter's definition of grief – as the articulation of personal biographical narratives that include the deceased – also emphasizes the ongoing relationship between the living and the dead. According to Walter, this type of grief process is particularly necessary today as our attitude to grief has changed because of alterations in our social, family and emotional lives. Since today's context is more culturally diverse and offers more freedom of choice about how to mourn, and because the baby boomers are more affluent, individualistic, emotionally expressive generation than their predecessors, we can expect more personal, spiritual, humanistic ways of addressing loss (Walter 2017: 84–86). This shift towards interpretative, subjectively oriented accounts of loss and grief that encompass both letting go and keeping hold of the dead has been also endorsed by other theorists of grief (Hallam and Hockey 2011;Valentine 2008). The new model of grief offers a more flexible understanding of the experience of loss as 'exercises in interpersonal meaning-making through the construction of narratives' (McManus 2013: 133).

Studying grief, which is an intensely personal as well as 'a social affair', is a very difficult task as it requires a multidisciplinary approach and relies on the diversity of research methods (McManus 2013: 135).We will start here with sociological studies of older people's grieving process, which take account of today's cultural and social contexts, and recognize that grief is age and gender specific. Surprisingly, despite the fact that spousal bereavement in later life is a common event, there are not many empirical studies looking at personal grief in older age and relatively few sociological studies of widowhood in old age. All investigations of how bereaved older persons respond to grief and the ways in which their social roles affect the loss experience share several discoveries about the nature of grief in old age.

First, sociological investigations of bereaved older people bring to our attention the significance of the cultural scripts by which people grieve, the social support mechanisms available to widowed people and changes in their social relationships and social status (Bennett 1997; Bennett and Bennett 2000; Bennett, Smith and Hughes 2005). Second, the studies of personal grief in older age show that the loss of a spouse is of major importance in the lives of elderly people (Bennett 1997; Bennett, Smith and Hughes 2005; Littlewood 2001). Furthermore, research looking at older bereaved people makes us aware that while the experience of loss is as important to older people as to people widowed at a younger age, later life bereavement differs in terms of adaption patterns, coping mechanisms and resilience (Parkes 2010). The studies also point out that older people's grief may differ according to gender and social expectations. The studies of the nature of grief in old age show that learning about how grief should be displayed and handled, how social ties and location change and what they are entitled to can be different for a wife when she becomes a widow than for a husband when he becomes a widower (Bennett 1997; Stroebe and Stroebe 1991).

Turning our attention to more detailed discoveries of empirical investigations on widowhood, we can observe that several studies of how widows and widowers respond to grief recount that widowers report depressive feelings significantly more often than widows (Bennett, Smith and Hughes 2005). The investigation of bereavement in males found that the loss of a spouse was 'the most stressful life event' (Howarth 2007: 196) and that widowers are more likely than widows to die of a 'broken heart' during the first year of bereavement (Parkes 2010: 9). On the other hand, because of their assumed lack of practical domestic experience, widowers received more support than widows (Bennett 2009). Nonetheless, the effects of bereavement on older women are also very profound. The significance of bereavement in older widows' life is due to women tending to live longer than men; thus, with approximately 51% of woman over 65 (compared with 14% of men of the same age) widowed at least once, the death of male partner in later life among women is a high-probability life event (Stillion 1995: 316). Interestingly – probably because of women's longevity – there are more studies of how widows handle loss than investigations of how widowers cope with loss.

The exploration of the experience of widowhood from the perspective of older women, based on interviews with widows, indicates that the average widow takes many years after her spouse's death to regain her former level of life satisfaction (Bennett and Bennett 1999; Bennett and Vidal-Hall 2000; Biswas-Diener et al. 2004). The study of older widows indicates that their partner's death has long-lasting effects on both their mental health and their morale (Bennett 1997). Another investigation explains that the strength and longevity of the impact of the loss of a husband for older women results from the fact that the identity and feeling of security of elderly widows are bound up with their wedded status, thus they do not seek to 'move on' or detach themselves from their deceased husbands (Littlewood 2001). In addition, the impact of bereavement on females is reinforced by the fact that becoming a widow often follows overseeing the care and death of their partner. While facing many challenges regarding domestic duties and sustaining their independence, the widows often elaborate narratives of the events that led up to their husband's death and the death itself. Preserving the memory of these events, which had an emotional impact upon them, is important for the widows as a means of coping and surviving, and as a means of demonstrating respect for their husband (Bennett and Vidal-Hall 2000). There are also some indications that, in addition to the effects of loss, that the older widows are also impacted by living alone, the process of ageing, and lower social status and lack of support, while the widowers received more formal support than the widows (Bennett 2009).

More generally, studies of widowhood seem to suggest that no one who outlives a spouse is spared the anguish of grief. The depressive feelings associated with non-coping in older widowed people are connected not only with gender, but also with socioeconomic status, social networks and health. As the elderly 'do not have the luxury of time between losses or unlimited time to set new directions for their lives' (Stillion1995:316), being widowed in old age comes with higher levels of depression; hence, emotional and practical support at the time of a spouse's death is important for helping older bereaved people to come to terms with their loss.

While enriching our understanding of grief as the experience of reckoning with the shift in personal relationships and social status after the death of loved ones, sociological studies so far do not tell us much about frequent, although not so often discussed, responses to death of loved ones, such as intensive pain and suffering, delayed sorrow, suppressed grief, fear, numbness or a sense of disbelief. From this type of research, we learn about older bereaved people's cultural and social contexts and their experience of reckoning with the shift in personal relationships and social status after the death of loved ones, but we do not learn much about the complex nature and reality of grief. To fully grasp this complexity of grief, we need to turn to diaries and memoirs of bereavement that describe the feared loss and mourning. In the next part of the chapter, we will give voice to the depth of grief as expressed in literary works that portrait the workings of bereavement and grief.

Stories of grief

There are many confessional memoirs of grieving with titles such as *Shattered: Surviving the Loss of a Child* (Roe, 2017), *Surviving the Loss of a Loved One: Living Through Grief* (Brown, 1999), *Surviving Death: How to Overcome the Loss of a Loved One* (Mulpagano 2017) and *Must You Go? My Life with Harold Pinter* (Fraser 2011). There are even more self-help books offering advice to their readers on how to come to terms with grief and bereavement, such as *Grief Day by Day: Simple Practices and Daily Guidance for Living with Loss* (Warner 2018) or Gary Roe's series of six books on how to understand one's grief after losing one's parents, partner, child or friend – for example, *Comfort for the Grieving Spouse's Heart: Hope and Healing After Losing Your Partner* (Roe 2019). Here, though, we are not interested in self-help manuals or confessional memoirs because to learn more about grief as an intimate, unpredictable deeply personal emotion, it is essential to explore the content of literary bereavement memoirs and diaries of grief. In other words, we will focus only on notable books by older writers who are reflecting on the death of their beloved spouses and who, with enormous imagination, accuracy and skills, disclose their experience of bereavement.

A few literary works about grief experienced by older widows or widowers that can help us grasp some universal aspects of grief are C.S. Lewis's (2020) *A Grief Observed*, Joyce Carol Oates' (2011) *A Widow's Story*, Joan Didion's (2012) bestselling *The Year of Magical Thinking and* Julian Barnes' (2013) *Levels of Life*. Even a quick comparison of Lewis, Barnes, Oates and Didion's memoirs after the deaths of their spouses reveals that there are many common topics that run through the diaries of grief experienced first-hand after the loss of a beloved spouse. These overlaps in the books' portrayals of grief, such as the confrontation between the image of grief, or 'mad midnight moments' of contemplating grief (Lewis 1961: 55) and its reality as a prolonged process of sorrow (Barnes 2014), illustrate that to grasp and express the core, deep, common features of grief is a very difficult process that requires honesty and precision. All these diaries of grief, in very carefully chosen words, explore the tensions underlying the experience of grief and the issues of time and meaning in context of the experience of loss.

The authors of these memoirs, while trying to express extreme emotions, confess to their lack of preparedness for the trauma of the loss and admit to their initial misunderstanding of the nature of grief. Lewis (1961: 5) opens his diary, which he kept after his wife's death, with a sentence: 'No one ever told me that grief felt so like fear.' While revealing the depth of his love for his late wife, he admits feeling lost for words when trying to express his sorrow: 'I thought I could describe a *state;* make a map of sorrow. Sorrow, however, turns out to be not a state but a process. It needs not a map but a history' (Lewis 1961: 55, italics in original). Barnes (2014), when his wife of thirty years died, felt as if nothing had prepared him for it. Eight years after his spouse's death, although still unwilling to recover from his grief and still not wanting to accept any consolation, Barnes describes and enacts his wife's absence and tries to articulate his continuing anguish. Like all the grieving people who 'rarely know what they need or want, only what they don't, offence-giving and offence-taking are common', Barnes (2011: 134) is rather irritated with his friends 'for their inability to say or do the right things' and for their attempts to heal his grief. As he knows his grief cannot be shared, Barnes is instead interested in being comforting to others or in doing 'grief work'.

Unlike Barnes, Joan Didion (2012), completed a book about the death of her husband of forty years within twelve months of his death. She also acknowledges that the reality of grief was unknown to her. She admits that it was only after her loss that she realized people were unable to understand grief until they had lost what they valued, and she cannot comprehend her own previous optimism: 'Grief turns out to be a place none of us know until we reach it' (Didion 2012: 188). In the version of grief we imagine, we are expected to heal by giving up our loved one because they are dead (Didion 2012: 188). However, this 'healing' model of grief does not prepare us for the shock of grief to be so 'obliterative, dislocating to both body and mind' (Didion 2012: 188). We do not expect to 'be literally crazy, cool customers who believe that their husband is about to return and need his shoes' (Didion 2012: 188). Yet the reality of grief is not a movement forward; rather, 'the burning raft' is a more accurate representation of the place to which grief takes the bereaved (Didion 2012: 75). When a friend asked her about her feelings, Didion (2012: 171) answered, 'I just can't see the upside in this.' By this she did not simply mean, as was suggested to her, that she 'couldn't see the light at the end of the tunnel'. It was much more: Didion did not have any *hope* for the light at the end of the process of grieving. She wanted to walk through the storm of grief, even if it took her down. Didion (2012: 198) expressed her awareness of our mortality without any anger by saying:

> We are imperfect mortal beings, aware of that mortality even as we push it away, failed by our complication, so wired that when we mourn our losses we also mourn, for better or for worse, ourselves. As we were. As we are no longer. As we will one day not be at all. (Didion 2012: 198)

The model of grief as 'pure, solemn and elevated' feelings that ensure personal growth is also questioned by Oates (2011: 111). After the death of her husband of 47 years, she feels 'very mute', believing that at the centre of grief 'there are no words', that grief is silence and emptiness (Oates 2012: 153). Like Lewis, Barnes and Didion, she realizes that she knew nothing about the ongoing pain of having loved entirely and lost entirely, and that she was not told that grief is 'not Mozart's Requiem Mass', but rather feels like 'crude gravel that hurts to walk [on]' (Oates 2012: 153). Moreover, Oates (2012: 300) questions why everybody says grief can be healed and 'wants to imagine the widow strong – stronger than she is, or can hope to be' (Oates 2012: 300). Generally, she seems to be more and more 'convinced that there is any inherent value in grief; or if there is, if wisdom springs from the experience of loss, it's a wisdom one might do without' (Oates 2012: 407).

Oates (2012: 300) believes that older widows cannot solve their grief because when we are 'a certain age and alone', there is not likely to be 'any improvement in our situation'. Being aware that her capacity 'for suffering edges towards self-annihilation' and with suicides thoughts trapped in her head, Oates (2011: 275, 299) realizes that she is 'danger of [her] life'. Full of fears that she would be unable to bear being 'an unloved woman no longer young', she thinks about ways to end her life; 'There is a way out, and the way out is death' (Oates 2011: 247). Being on the edge of things and in a pit of despair, on the one hand Oates dwells upon her past life with her husband, and on the other listens to her internal suicide voices. Only by reminding herself that she has no right to appropriate her husband's death – 'the widow must remember: her husband's death did not happen to her but to her husband' – she is able to question the idea that 'only death can free' her from suffering (Oates 2011: 228). Barnes (2014), when trauma after his wife's death seemed to be without limits, could not see any possible road from his grief other than death. However, he resisted his wish to die because he saw himself as his wife's 'rememberer'. In other words, although he believed his recovery was impossible, he rejected thoughts of suicide because if he killed himself, he would be killing her too.

Although the authors of memoirs feel that with the death of a loved one the life they know ends and they are resigned to it, they still agonize over what would replace the suffering of grief. For Barnes (2011: 132), the only tools of detachment from the pain of loss, from which he does not want to recover, is his appreciation of 'the miraculous trickery of art'. While art's tricks do not bring the lost loved one back, they allow a revisiting of the past to make it present or enable representation of the past in the present. Moreover, Didion and Oates do not want spare themselves the suffering of grief if this can be achieved only at the price of total disconnection from the lost loved one. Didion (2012), familiar with Freud, consciously rejected his argument from *Melancholy and Mourning* that it is only when we are able to acknowledge loss that we can finalize the work of mourning. For Oates (2011), any thought of detachment from her dead husband's memory was initially unacceptable; however, with time passing and as her image of him becomes less immediate and more remote, she realizes that, despite her desire to hold on to the lost one, she is on the road out of grief, which is the road to life. Travelling on this difficult road or 'pilgrimage to life', full of confusing feelings, such as anger, self-pity and guilt, Oates (2011: 345) feels that she betrayed her dead husband when her image of him became less immediate and more remote. For the same reason, Didion (2012: 225), who initially found it very difficult to accept the irreversibility of her husband's death, later started to blame herself for betraying her husband. All these feelings of guilt, responsibility, betrayal, self-pity, anger, agony and fear illustrate the significance of the second theme visible in all memoirs: the tensions underlying the experience of grief.

In the first acute agony of grief, Didion (2012: 63–77) questioned the nature of grief and analysed her feelings and responses to her husband's death and to being left alone. While overwhelmed by anger, she realized that a cause of the anger was 'this feeling of being left alone' (Didion 2012: 161). Moreover, as soon as Didion recognized that anger was simply a good antidote to grief, it was replaced by a feeling of guilt. This new emotion was a result of her belief that her husband did not survive because of her: 'I believed that I should have been able to prevent whatever happened' (Didion 2012: 173). Holding herself responsible, she searched for details of what did in fact happen, investigated hospitals records, reconstructed the whole clinical history of her husband's illness. Didion (2012: 195, 192) knew that in grieving we are left with no further focus than ourselves, and this can be a source of self-pity; for her, this was the main enemy as it can 'derange the mind'. Even when grieving, Didion (2012: 192), who had an aversion to 'dwelling on self-pity' and sentimentality, neither wanted to feel sorry for herself nor to be concerned only with herself.

In the memoirs of grief, there is considerable evidence that the power of grief does not just make people feel stunned, traumatized and lonely, but can also make them incapable of thinking rationally and can change grieving people's attitudes to life. Barnes, in the depths of his grief and solitude, wants to believe that 'the fact that someone is dead may mean that they are not alive, but doesn't mean that they do not exist'(Barnes 2011: 127). Both Didion and Oakes, while on the surface looked like they were acting normally and rationally, were really drowning in suffering and did not care at all about their everyday routines. They did what they were told to do; collected their dead husbands' belongings, arranged for cremations and memorial services, and publicly acknowledged that their husbands were dead (Didion 2012; Oates 2011). Despite that, their thinking remained 'suspiciously fluid', with a continuous focus still being on 'bringing him back' and asking him questions (Didion 2012: 43, 44). For a long time after her husband's death, Oates (2011: 351) did not believe what had happened: 'This is not real, this cannot be happening ... I am talking to him, I almost in wonder.' As any changes in such a connection with the beloved dead tend to be attributed to time passing, we should turn now to the third commonality in the presentations of grief: the role of time.

When discussing the impact of time on the grieving process, the first thing to emphasize is that grieving people most frequently feel that they are living in suspended, empty and void time, as if they are waiting for something to happen (Lewis 1961). Many bereaved people wish they could reverse time, some want time to stop and still others desire its acceleration. But, at some point, all of them feel that they need to learn how to 'kill time'. Moreover, grieving older people, who find it difficult to accept the irreversibility of the death of their spouse, also do not believe that time heals anything; instead, they are convinced that the time of their loss escalates things, they think that time works against them. In the widow world, writes Oates (2011: 143), 'there is most primitive sort of time: what has happened, irremediably, has somehow not-yet-happened'. Although 'the widow knows that time cannot be but turn back and the death cannot be erased, she wants the world-time-to have ended' (Oates 2011: 275). Didion, in contrast, wants to stop time to have a chance to grieve or reflect on her tragic loss. Viewing time as 'fire in which we burn' (from Dalmore Schwartz's poem, quoted in Didion 2012: 198), she wishes for time to stop to give her the time for bereavement (Didion 2012: 197). While finding herself in the empty and void time, Didion (2012: 189), with a piercing sense of detachment from the outside world and with well-established and domestic life rituals and habits (such as setting table and lighting candles) losing their meaning, tries to 'kill time' by engaging herself in various ways and occupying herself with various tasks. In order to 'kill time', Oates too takes on many external appointments, attends meetings with her readers and seminars with students and gives public lectures. Still, these things are often not enough to alleviate the widow's dominant feeling that her 'life has ended;, that all she can know about the grief experience 'is a familiar set of words ... all suffer, and we all die' (Oates 2011: 275, 242).

So the widow must confront her feeling that her 'life is over' (Oates 2011: 172). Even though she is 'shaken to the roots of being', even though losing the husband is like losing a part of herself and being left a 'depleted, broken self', she still searches for a meaning in narratives of her life (Oates 2011: 88). However, the grieving woman's attempts to overcome a loss of meaning by rebuilding a coherent narrative of her life does not mean she has forgotten the dead husband. It is, rather, the evidence of the widow's continuous exploration of her husband's identity in order to place him firmly in her memory. Oates (2011: 248) wonders whether she did know her husband and whether she knows herself: 'We have no personalities unless there are people who know us. Unless there are people, we hope to convince that we deserve to exist.' Slowly, she realized that the presence of friends, family and other people can help her feel closer to the world without losing the connection to the dead beloved.

The maintenance of connections to the dead beloved can be attained internally through memories of the deceased, by being their 'rememberers'. It can also be sustained externally through funerary and mourning rites as well by practice, such as passing on a deceased's name within the family, or engraving the name of deceased on a tombstone, branch or tree. Today, with the increased use of technology, memories are preserved by creating grief blogs or virtual memorials that allow people to share their feelings and memories about the deceased on social media forums. Such ways of maintaining the connection to the dead, by integrating the memory of the dead into outgoing lives and by keeping 'alive' memories of beloved dead through various rituals and practices, are also important means of reducing our own anxieties about our future death. It what follows, we explore how the COVID-19 pandemic, by forcing changes to memorial and funeral services, impacted older bereaved people's abilities to cope with their grief.

The grief in the pandemic

As already mentioned, grief is a historically specific cultural script, structured by social conventions and expectations in all societies. While recalling that, until recently, variations in ways of mourning the loss were a result of changes in the religious realm, demographic growth, legislative actions and technological progress (Houlbrooke 2020), here we explore how the pandemic, which has presented us with the main challenge to our ways of mourning the loss, has impacted the nature of grief. The pandemic has presented us with a major challenge to our ways of mourning loss. Grief in the midst of the pandemic, with its thousands of deaths, was more complex, lonely, vast and traumatic than grief in in non-heath crisis times because of the scale of unexpected suffering, because the pandemic 'deprives of the ambivalence of human grief' (Rose 2020: 43) and because the necessary restrictions imposed in the shadow of the pandemic shrank the space for anything like complex reckoning with life and death. By reducing the room left for grieving, the COVID-19 rules and procedures – which prevented people from being alongside loved ones as they died, or even at their graveside after death – added to bereaved people's loneliness and their sense that their individual grief was unimportant. However, although the pandemic's conditions left many grieving people feeling alone, the COVID-19 tragedy also created a collective experience of grief. In the United Kingdom, with the whole country grieving, the overwhelming and lonely grief of families who lost loved ones to COVID-19 was noticed, and various attempts were made to honour the COVID-19 victims.

The pandemic, by inflicting grief on thousands of people and by imposing new rules on burial rituals, has accelerated the process of change in mourning practices. 'The pandemic has been a crash course in how to create the most traumatic conditions for bereavement' (Clarke 2016:178). The UK, with thousands of people still mourning loved ones lost to COVID or to death from preventable non-COVID conditions, has been presented with the largest peacetime mass trauma event in more than a century. For thousands of elderlies, the pandemic has not only meant the higher individual risk, but also death of partners or close friends, which left them with private, intense and prolong grief and with not many spaces and opportunities for healing. As the official figures suggest, as many as 318,000 people in England and Wales over the age of 65 lost their partners between the first lockdown and May 2021 (Independent Age 2021). This loss of life from COVID has inflicted days of trauma on thousands of older people and their families left bereaved by the coronavirus. While during normal times one in ten of bereaved adults would be expected to develop prolonged grief, which is intense, very and persistent, but 'for COVID grievers, that proportion may be even higher, because the pandemic has ticked off many risk factors' (Yong 2022).

Because of the requirement of the health safety measures and regulations, COVID-19 made grieving people feel profoundly lonely, detached from society and particularly from their support networks. The pandemic has also altered the ways in which people could mourn their private loss because they knew little about their loved one's final days as they were unable to be with them at the moment of their death or could only say goodbye over Skype or Zoom. During the first lockdown, the guidance published by Public Health England, which established social distancing measures and restricted the number of people who could attend funerals, profoundly changed grieving and mourning rituals in Britain. The pandemic also had a big impact on the funeral industry, which – while barley coping with demand during that health crisis – had to meet government guidelines and adjust its services to people opting for simpler funerals as grieving families were not permitted to hold the send-off they had wanted. During the first wave of the pandemic, funeral directors and faith leaders were advised that only members of the deceased person's household or close family members could attend funerals and that all who did attend would need to adhere to social distancing at all times, including when travelling to and from the funeral. New hygiene rules, restricting practices involving close personal contact with the body of a person who had died from or with symptoms of COVID-19, required mourners to wear additional personal protective equipment (PPE) if any contact with the deceased occurred; this further reduced the opportunity of grieving families to take part in any rituals or practices. Hence, the aftermath of a COVID-19 death was lonely as people were unable to celebrate their loved ones' lives.

In the United Kingdom, the COVID-19 procedures and rules were a burden for many communities, religious leaders, undertakers and city councils, and for people who were banned from attendance at funeral ceremonies because of the coronavirus crisis. For example, Bradford, Leeds and Kirklees councils, while reducing their cremation charges, did not permit chapel services at crematoria and instead offered 'direct cremations', in which there was no ceremony and mourners were not present, and 'burial services at gravesides, with a maximum of 10 mourners observing physical distancing guidelines' (Sherwood 2020). During the first year of COVID-19, the new rules for burial services and the new reality of funerals meant that in all religious communities mourners were unable to observe the usual rituals. The Anglican Church banned church funeral services, advising that immediate family only may attend at gravesides, and that burials could be livestreamed to other relatives and friends (Sherwood 2020). During the pandemic, families increasingly decided on cremations, which meant the proportion of direct cremation increased significantly in the United Kingdom: in 2020, one in seven funerals was a direct cremation, compared with one in thirty-three in 2019. Moreover, COVID-19 impacted not only the type of funeral but also attendance, partly as a result of the imposed regulations but also because many families postponed the communal get-together until after the pandemic. Subsequently, compared with 2019, there was an almost five-fold rise in cases where there was no service and no mourners present at the cremation and there were also increasing reports of 'people being buried or cremated with no immediate family present' (Sherwood 2020).

The most painful impact of the pandemic was on the individual mourners, particularly on older persons grieving alone after their partners' death: 'Grief is messy at the best of times, but COVID bereavement is exceptionally complex' (Clarke 2021: 178). During COVID-19, older people's grief was profound, as the reduced funeral and mourning rituals could not bring solace; instead, feelings of isolation, loneliness, anxiety and despondency were increased. The pandemic's simplification of funeral rites destroyed people's familiarity with conventional funerals, while the reduced nature of mourning services did not offer comfort. Hence, older persons' encounters with death presented them with a magnified burden. The COVID-19 restrictions meant that burials were rushed, sparsely attended affairs, where those few family members who did attend could not hug each other or congregate afterwards. 'We were denied every ritual. We hadn't said goodbye, we hadn't been prepared, we didn't see the body' (Clarke 2021: 178). The grief-stricken people, who were not allowed to touch, to see or even to say goodbye to their dying spouses, parents or siblings, were also unable to gather to attend funerals, memorial services or ceremonies afterwards. 'The bereaved must suffer alone, stripped of the rituals and basic comforts of grieving such as congregating with others, swapping stories about the life of the one who has been lost, honouring them with the shared memories and affection' (Clarke 2021: 176).Without the proper mourning and funerary rites, people did not know how to cope and how to handle their feelings, thus the grief process left them with profound wounds. Apart from the disruption to funerary rituals, which left the dying and the bereaved to suffer alone, the subsequent lockdowns inflicted a lot of pain on older people, who were left to mourn in solitude, without the comfort of families and social networks, or even the reassurance of ordinary activities and the sounds of mundane life around them. This new sensitivity and texture of grief during lockdown was probably behind the increased number of calls made by bereaved people to various charities to help them to find a space to tell their story (Clarke 2021; Marsh 2021; Sherwood 2020). The desire to share their grief, prompted by people's need not to feel alone in their grief, helped the bereaved to endure tragedy and situate their individual suffering within a wider frame.

The COVID-19 pandemic revealed the importance of the human presence and touch in brining solace after the loss of a loved one. It also taught us to be adaptable and to adjust the existing technological resources to help people in pain. This adaptability during the pandemic can be illustrated by the emergence of several virtual support networks, the websites of various counselling services or the platforms of end-of-life care charities. The online provisions of bereaved family members with resources, from information portals to professional online bereavement counselling, have been important to their process of grieving and remembering. The yearning to honour the COVID-19 dead with shared memories and offer support to their grief-stricken families led to the creation of virtual mourning networks, such as COVIDSpeakEasy and the COVID-19 Bereaved Families for Justice UK group. During the COVID-19 crisis, the limitations on numbers of people at crematoria and cemeteries compelled funeral houses to digitalize their services and enabled mourners to be in touch via Zoom or WhatsApp. This new development, with funeral homes offering video links so people could say goodbye virtually, with increased numbers of those who had suffered a bereavement going online and with the live video-streaming of funerals, virtual memorials, grief forums and grief blogs, has expanded the space for grieving. As well as online sites, which publish COVID-19 victims' portraits and narratives of their lives, there are also some local sites, such as that launched in May 2020 by St Paul's Cathedral in London, where mourners could submit names, photographs and short messages in honour of their loved ones. By allowing people whose loved ones had died from the virus to tell their stories, these digital resources made their individual grief visible and thus offered cyber-solace in the midst of the pandemic, with its thousands of deaths. Although these electronic practices were framed around traditional funerary rituals, a Zoom call would never replace the intimacy of a face-to-face gathering, physical contacts and the sharing of grief. And although the technological development was of enormous importance in providing online support, including digitalized mourning services, for many older people – especially those less digitally literate, these new encounters with death were rather unsettling. Furthermore, during the COVID-19 pandemic, the public acknowledgement of the importance of honouring the coronavirus dead created a momentum not only for calls for funding for bereavement counselling but also for more space for collective grief.

The urge to validate bereaved people's pain and to create a space for collective grief has been behind the emergence of many online memorials to honour and commemorate the COVID-19 victims as well as behind many voices on social media platforms, in newspapers and books calling for a way to honour the COVID-19 dead and prevent 'global humbling' (Bennett 2020; Marsh 2021; Smith 2020). The importance of collective mourning has been recognized by some institutional actors. As the massive loss of lives inflicted by the pandemic continued, the unions (Unison, the Royal College of Nursing and the Royal College of Midwives) scheduled a minute's silence honouring the health, care and other key workers who had died from coronavirus (Badshah 2020). Moreover, on the day the COVID-19 death toll surpassed 100,000 in the United Kingdom – that is, 26 January 2021 – the Archbishops of Canterbury and York, Justin Welby and Stepan Cottrell, in an open letter to the nation, asked all people to pause and reflect on the enormity of this pandemic. Pointing out that '100,000 isn't just an abstract figure. Each number is a person: someone we loved and someone who loved us', they observed that 'all grief profoundly affects us, but this pandemic grief is so hard. Therefore, we need to support each other. We do this by following the guidelines. But we also do it by reaching out to each with care and kindness' (Welby and Cottrell 2021).

However, the most important appreciation of a need for the public mourning and the drive to provide a space for it was initiated by an English grassroots movement aiming to honour the pandemic victims. The growing acknowledgement of the grief experienced by tens of thousands of people and the realization that the COVID-19 dead did not receive any public recognition resulted in calls for collective grief and for a commitment to memorize the pandemic victims. As a number those of mourning the lost in the pandemic increased, various groups challenged with considering how best to mourn came up with different ideas about how to a memorialize the COVID-19 victims. Among many new ideas to create a powerful tribute to UK pandemic victims, the project that really caught people's imagination was a plan for a national COVID Memorial Wall in London, proposed by the founders of the COVID-19 Bereaved Families for Justice campaign. From March 2021, the Wall – located across the river from the Houses of Parliament – has been daily painted with red hearts, each representing a life lost to COVID-19. By the beginning of 2022, the Wall had been decorated with more than 150,000 red hearts and was recognized as an important place for people to come to reflect, to remember and to heal (Lynskey 2021). The main aim behind the idea of public mourning, as initiated by this initiative of spontaneous memorialization, was to create a collective site of mourning that would make grieving people feel they were not alone, that they were listened to and that their individual grief was not 'insignificant' (Marsh 2021).

While, during times of war, public mourning rituals and ceremonials – usually initiated by the state's action – serve the important purpose of kindling the national spirit, at times of peace, spontaneous memorialization and expressions of grief in public have been rather unusual. As the virus swept the country and the COVID-19 death toll grew, people in the United Kingdom, while facing an 'epidemic of grief' (Marsh 2020), recognized the need for public mourning of COVID-19 victims (Bennett 2020). Such yearning for public mourning was something new, as in the past calls for public mourning were only associated with efforts to honour the war dead, to erect memorials for the unknown soldier and to pay homage to the lives of military people and civilians killed in the two World Wars. While normally national memorials to the victims of war or catastrophes are supported by and negotiated with the authorities, in the case of the COVID-19 memorial, bereaved campaigners and activists, without official permission, achieved something unusual. Not trusting the government with the task of memorialization, the COVID-19 Bereaved Families for Justice proudly claimed that, 'The most important part for me was that it was *us* doing it: a grassroots movement of bereaved families and friends' (Lynskey 2021, italics in original).

The COVID-19 pandemic brought massive suffering and pain to many nations, each of them handling the 'pandemic of grief' in a different way. In the United Kingdom, the Westminster location of the national COVID Memorial Wall is a direct reproach to politicians for their lack of support (Lynskey 2021), in the United States, the plight of the COVID victims was not honoured under Trump's administration. Many grieving Americans felt isolated and lonely, and saw 'that their loved ones immediately became statistics – that their individual tragedy was subsumed by the pandemic's enormity' (Yong 2022). Only with the election of Joe Biden did the victims' families and friends feel they had been heard. On 19 January 2019, in his inaugural speech delivered facing the sea of memorial flags – one national flag for each of the 400,000 Americans who died of COVID-19, President Biden emphasized the unity of the nation and remembered all COVID-19 victims, while New York has started the process of approval for transforming Hart Island, the site of mass burials for victims of COVID, into a large-scale memorial to those lost in the pandemic.

However, in the countries where authorities have censored the topics related to the pandemic, not much has been done to honour those who died of COVID-19. For example, in China, in order to prevent mourning from 'bringing shame on the country', the authorities introduced selective blocking of accounts and censorship of all entries on social media on which people posted their diaries of the COVID-19 pandemic, which were initially read and reshared by millions (Standaret 2021). 'Even mourning is said to shame China,' said bloggers from Wuhan who were repeatedly censored for sharing their suffering from COVID-19 online and who continue to fight for a space for to tell their stories (Standaret 2021).

The death of loved ones during the pandemic left many grieving people without rituals and undertakings that might help them to mourn. With the COVID-19 burial rules restricting funerals and memorial services, and with the lockdown limiting the ability to participate in social life and the accessibility of therapeutic care, many bereaved people suffered alone. However, the coronarius pandemic did not just introduce isolation; it also taught us that although grieving is individual, and even though we grieve differently, in the context of the enormous health crisis, people long for grieving to be less lonely and less restricted, and to have a chance to reach out to one another. By making the bereaved feel very lonely and that their individual grief was insignificant, COVID-19 has increased people's yearning for a collective grief. Together with the huge death toll, this has created 'a shared experience that countered the loneliness of grief' (Yong 2022).

To fully grasp the nature of traumatic conditions of bereavement created by the pandemic, we also need to look at how this health crisis has impacted dying, which will the topic of the following chapters. The public's new familiarity with the death of older people, together with a new rhetoric used by politicians and social media, constructed the view of the death in old age as no longer 'natural' or 'normal', but rather unexpected and unprepared for. It is not just that the United Kingdom has failed to prepare for the pandemic; the nation has also been unprepared to deal with the problems of an ageing population and increased rates of death in old age. Prior to the pandemic, the UK health system already faced many difficulties, such as the nation's declining longevity trends – especially for those living in deprived areas – and the highest death rates of older patients in the Western world (Gregory 2021). Yet, despite these facts, until the pandemic the deaths of aged people were relatively well hidden. It has taken the high mortality rate from COVID-19 to display and exhibit death in old age in much clearer terms.

In conclusion, the pandemic, which disproportionally impacted older people – especially those with pre-existing health conditions – increased the visibility of death in old age. The recent health crisis has also altered the historical trends in the improvement in longevity and has reopened debates about the quality of the end-of-life care. In the next chapter, we will explore who the older people facing the increased risk of COVID-19 might be, and look at their common characteristics and how are they are perceived by society.

CHAPTER 6

Public debates about the value of the end

Discussing the attributes of a good death

In the previous two chapters, we examined older persons' direct and indirect encounters with death and the impacts of both type of encounters with death on people's awareness of mortality. Apart from the encounters with death in the private sphere, we are also frequently confronted with 'the problem of death' in the public sphere: we come across it in public debates, run into it in policy discussions and have been unable to avoid it during the recent pandemic. As today the boundary between private and public life seems to have virtually disappeared (Thompson 2011), and as advances in medical science have 'created a new difficulty for mankind: how to die' (Gawande 2010: 40), the importance of debates about death in the public sphere cannot be overlooked. Since public debates about death and the quality of end-of-life care frame the context in which individuals' views on death are confronted and challenged, we will first analyze the underlying conceptions behind discussions of the idea of a good death. Then, in order to explain the difficulties of enabling a good death, we will explore debates about solutions to overcome the obstacles to a good death. The final section of the chapter will examine the fallout from narratives of COVID-19 on our evaluation of just how realistic the assumptions behind the notion of a good death might be.

Across the centuries, there have been many ideas of a good death, as its definition has changed with shifts in the authority to identify the essence of a good death, from religion to medicine and from medicine to the individual (Walter 2017). In the past, when people shared religious norms about how to die, they perceived death as an inevitable fact of life, knew that death was never far away and were prepared for it. The good death was defined by the authority of religion as one 'where people were aware that death was immanent and therefore they had the opportunity to prepare themselves for it, both spiritually and in terms of their earthly business' (Howarth 2007: 20). Believing in religion's promise of the afterlife and an eternal reunion with the beloved helped to ensure a peaceful death. From the religious perspective, death was seen as an integral feature of life and the good death ensured the prospect could say farewell to their family and prepare to cross the threshold to the afterlife (Aries 1981).

In contrast to this religious view, the twentieth century secular 'medical-rationalist discourse' reduced death to an identifiable disease under the control of medical professionals (Bauman 1992). With the developments in science, technology and medicine, the good death was defined as painless, quick and unconscious, while the medialization and institutionalization of death removed control over dying and death from the family and community (Bauman 1992; Lang 2020). From the middle of the twentieth century, these two processes – the institutionalization and medicalization of death – have been affecting the experience of dying (Howarth 2007; Kellehear 2007; McManus 2013; Walter 2020). But it is the medicalization of death that is seen as particularly responsible for the dehumanization of dying, as excesses of modern medicine are blamed for contributing to viewing death as something that medicine should somehow 'sort out' (O'Mahony 2016: 271). This identification of death as a medical problem orients medicine to fight death and grants medicine's justification for subjecting dying people to a range of technological, often intrusive and futile, interventions in an attempt to keep them alive. The rhetoric that constitutes death as a technical failure, or the perception of death as the failure of the medical profession, coexists with seeing dying as 'a medical event, rather than a natural event in which medicine plays a part' (Walter 2017: 18).

Since the publication of Illich's (1976) *Limits to Medicine*, the medicalization of death has become the subject of criticism from academia, the general public and medical professionals. Illich (1976: 207) exposed the medicalization thesis's arguments and assumptions, questioned many negative consequences of 'the end of epoch of a natural death', criticized modern scientific medicine as a 'monolithic world religion' and asserted that it was the medical professionals who were now in control of where and how death occurs. Yet even before Illich's public stand, critics of the modern way of dying disapproved of the medicalization of dying for being blind to patients' wishes, medicine's excessive spending and patients' unnecessary suffering. The theoretical developments in the field of medical sociology and studies of death concerned with criticizing the medicalization of death pointed out at least three significant problems connected with the medical model of death: medicine's excessive spending, patients' immense suffering and blindness to patients' wishes. For example, Glaser and Strauss (1968), who revealed the dehumanizing consequences of dying in a modern hospital, pointed to a need for lay people to reclaim the experience of dying and to redirect public debates to the issue of death and its significance in life. Elizabeth Kübler-Ross (1969), in her research with people dying in hospitals, criticized medicine for disregarding dying patients' needs and wishes. Viewing death as the final stage of growth, she raised concerns about basic human values in institutional dying and pioneered the 'natural death' or awareness of death approach. All these scholars argued that in Western developed societies, the growing specialization of medicine and the use of medical technology to sustain life artificially have resulted in dehumanization of dying in the modern hospital, as dying people feel both marginalized and feared (Glaser and Strauss 1968; Illich 1976; Kübler-Ross 1969). While exploring the dehumanizing effects of medical interventions on the experience of dying persons, they rejected the medical model of death.

Following the theoretical questioning of the medical model of death, the lay public has raised the importance of the idea of a good death. The death awareness movement, which emerged during the 1970s, has made the public more aware of the consequences of the medicalization of death. By adopting Elizabeth Kübler-Ross's (1969) idea that death is the final stage of growth and therefore something to be embraced, the death awareness movement asserts that, as part of natural processes, death cannot be avoided and therefore must not be denied. Hence, the awareness movement – sometimes also described as 'the happy death movement' (Lofland 1978) – identified the modern 'death taboo' as its enemy. The movement's criticism of the medicalization of death in the context of post-material values, and the culture privileging the authority of the individual, have expanded the contestation of the medical model of dying to a wider public forum. This lay attempt to de-medicalize dying reacted against the power of medical profession and the depersonalization of dying, and called to reclaim the experience of dying and for death to be recognized as the rightful domain of dying people and their families. A more recent effort to encourage openness about death includes the global death café movement, where strangers meet or blog to converse about death. The first death café was set up by the Swiss sociologist Bernard Crettaz in 2004 and involved informal meetings dedicated to 'café, tea and discussion of death'. The idea that it could 'increase awareness of death with the view of helping people make the most of their (finite) lives' has spread around the world and there are now 12059 death cafés in 75 countries, with the first in Britain set up in 2011. According to the official website, during the COVID-19 pandemic, there were no face-to-face meetings, but the virtual death café contacts have been very successful and growing.

The most successful of all attempts to resist the medicalization of dying and to propose the new idea of a good death came from the British hospice and palliative care movements aiming to help dying people by offering them care, easing pain and respecting their preferences. Both these initiatives have their origins in the critique of medicalized dying, pioneer holistic, humanistic end-of-life care and have the aim of increasing people's awareness of death by encouraging them talk about death and enabling individuals to think about where they want to die (Howarth 2007; Lang 2020). Since the opening of St Christopher's Hospice in London in 1967, the hospice movement has aimed to provide 'total care' to both the patient and their family. As a result of Cicely Saunders' insistence on the importance of offering compassion, dignity, consolation, counselling, listening and respect to dying people, and her efforts to introduce effective pain management, people in hospices can expect to be helped 'not only to die peacefully', but to 'live until they die' (Cicely Saunders, quoted in Humphrys and Jarvis 2009: 136). In Britain, palliative care has been a recognized medical specialization since 1987, and since then has developed into a diverse range of professional and non-professional practices, including hospital care. In the United Kingdom, there are now more than 300 hospices, which all offer total care to patients with progressive illness and their families. Despite this diversity and expansion, palliative care remains strongly associated with the idea of a good death (Lloyd 2000: 176). By defining palliative care as 'the highest possible quality of life for the patient and family', this approach's views a good death 'is closely associated with a good quality of life while living with and dying from progressive illness' (Lloyd 2000: 176). With the United Kingdom being widely prized as an international leader in hospice and palliative care, the philosophical and ethical ideas of these movements, together with the death awareness movement's calls for improving dying through open conversations and informed choice, have spread into many other Western countries.

In the United States, where the healthcare and the bioethics movement over the twentieth century developed medical guidelines on the quality of dying, the hospice programs – which began in the early to mid-1970s – have emphasized the need for a more holistic approach to dying people's needs. Today there are about 3000 modern hospices in the country, with the first opened in New Haven, Connecticut in 1974. All hospice initiatives are results of 'many grassroots efforts of communities wishing to develop volunteer homecare services' (Lattanzi-Licht and Connor 1995: 143). By increasing doctors' awareness of a need to rethink how to help their patients achieve a good death, such attempts to de-medicalize dying have reduced the discrepancy between expert medical discourse and an intensely personal sense of loss.

In the United States, debate about standards for end-of-life care in American hospitals only began at the beginning of the 1980s, with a widespread conversation about the problem of death taking place in newspapers, popular magazines and on television and radio:

> Throughout the 1980s and into the 1990s it became increasingly clearer to critics and analysts of the healthcare system that large numbers of people had become critical of the management of dying, the procedures of dying and the institutional circumstances which dying was taking place. (Kaufman 2005: 2)

The changes in US legislation, the gradual sub-specialization of medicine and shifting public expectations, together with America's market-oriented healthcare delivery, the culture of individualism and the modern technological medicine's goal to battle deaths, have led to the prioritization of delivering quick and technologically intensive interventions (Chapple 2010; Erickson 2013; Kaufman 2005). Changes to the quality of dying in hospitals across the country have been illustrated with many cases of medical over-treatment, patients not having control of their own destiny and cases of dying patients needlessly undergoing rescue. The depersonalization of death and lack of coordinated clinical care to meet the particular needs of dying patients and their loved ones at that crucial time are recurring difficulties in US hospitals (Chapple 2010; Erickson 2013; Kaufman 2005).

Although the American healthcare system has adopted the criteria of a successful dying based on law and medical guidelines, and the country's Institute of Medicine developed a definition of a good death, the quality of death has not actually been improved. Despite acceptance that the good death is one that is 'free from avoidable distress and suffering for patient, family, and caregivers, in general accord with the patient's and family's wishes, and reasonably consistent with clinical, cultural, and ethical standards' (Institute of Medicine, quoted in Meier et al. 2016: 262), these conditions are still not always achievable. Even the empowerment of patients – that is, the recognition of the importance of the patient's stated preferences in advance of falling terminally ill – as very crucial if people are to have a good death has not stopped frequent treatments of illness with endless, invasive, not always necessary technological procedures and has not fully secured patients' choice and control over the dying process. Moreover, even if the system requires patients to make choices, in reality it is typically only at certain times and only certain choices are available (Kaufman 2005). Thus, although the American medical system is located within a culture that privileges personal autonomy and assumes that the good death is one where the individual has control, the resources are redistributed unequally and the culture that predominates in the hospital is full of internal ambivalence about death, which is normalized through language of problem-solving and pragmatism: 'Such language ignores or redirect incoherence, anxiety, breakdown, diffuse suffering, and any other expression of affect that lacks rationality' (Kaufman 2005: 17). Thus, although medical professionals accept that, in order to enable a good death, the dying person needs autonomy and the dying process should be the well timed and well organized, the reality is that dying patients' control is often restricted and the whole process is frequently not well coordinated.

In the United Kingdom, public debate about a good death has also gained visibility over the last several decades, with hospices and palliative care services demonstrating what can be done to provide physical, psychological, social and spiritual care for dying people and their families. Before the arrival of the hospice movement, the profile of end-of-life care within the NHS and social care services was relatively low. Over the last couple of decades, many discussions of a good death have taken place in the context of public debates about and consultations on the governmental policy papers, strategies and programmes developed to promote high-quality care for all adults at the end of life. In recent years, new pragmatic and collaborative visions of care have been developed by the NHS and by the voluntary sector to provide a good death to a wider number of patients. The existing models of end-of-life care, from the modern hospice movement, through the NHS End-of-life Care Programme (2004–07) to the Delivering Choice Programme run by Marie Curie Cancer Care, all highlight the benefits of taking an integrated, whole-system approach to the delivery of end-of-life care. The experience and expertise of these organizations, together with the promised government support, have offered an opportunity to establish some bases for dealing with the challenges of providing high-quality end-of-life care.

In contrast to the United States, the British government is the important actor and stakeholder in the debates about a good death. For example, the British government originally founded the Dying Matters Coalition, a programme that was created in 2009 by the Department of Health and is now run by Hospice UK; with a help of a wide range of resources, it cultivates an open culture that talks about death and dying (Hospice UK 2002). Another initiative supported by the government is the Gold Standard Framework programme, which offers people in the last year of life more choice about how and where they die; it helps patients to live out their last days in their own homes if that what they want. It started as a small pilot programme in 2001 and, although getting involved in it is voluntary for doctors, it has been expanding quickly across the

United Kingdom. The Gold Standards Framework Centre, through its many training programmes, provides training for generalist frontline staff in health and social care to enable the provision of 'gold standard' care for all people nearing the end of life (Gold Standards Framework 2022). By 'helping doctors to keep communicating', it aims to improve the coordination and collaboration of medical teams and, through such a collaboration, to give patients the death they want: 'Even though this kind of teamwork may not always succeed in giving patients the death they want, it will never be for want of trying' (Humphrys and Jarvis 2009: 151).

The UK government's attempt to construct the first comprehensive and collaborative framework aiming at improving the quality of care for all people nearing the end of life in line with their preferences resulted in the publication of a White Paper in 2003. This consultation document promised that within next few years people near the end of life would have access to all services they needed to die at home, if that was what they wanted (Humphrys and Jarvis 2009). After the process and public consultations, all Primary Care Trusts in the country were ordered to set up to a working group to establish what services were needed in their particular area. In 2008, the government announced the End-of-Life Care Strategy, which aimed to develop a national coalition to raise the profile of end-of-life care and to change attitudes to death and dying in society. The consultations for this strategy revealed the public's preference for dying at home, seen as the preferred place of death because it offers informal support, compassion, comfort and familiarity (Humphrys and Jarvis 2009: 129). Yet doctors involved in public conversations about the good death, while realizing that 'medicine had totally overreached itself and was shaping up as a social institution intrinsically involved in social control' (McManus 2013: 46), also emphasize that medical interventions oriented towards pain and symptom management are essential. In short, they bring to our attention that 'medicalization does not necessarily contradict a good or natural death' (Lang 2020: 2). Consequently, it is commonly recognize that, even though home death enables appropriate end-of-life care, medical and professional care is also necessary. Hence, the government has been promoting 'homecare programmes through which terminally ill people may be offered a wide range of medical, personal, domestic, spiritual and counselling services to enable them to live and die in their own homes' (Howarth 2007: 130).

Over time, public conversations about a good death in the United States, like the debates that have occurred in the United Kingdom, have also involved more parties and new approaches to this topic. More recently, the debates in both countries have reported that new explorations of what constitutes a good death have identified the good death as one we choose, as being 'my choice' and 'my way' (Walter 2017: 40). Hence, the good death appears 'individualized and with planning and timing death at its centre', and emphasizes the psychological, emotional, spiritual and bodily needs of the dying person (Lang 2020: 2). Numerous calls for individual patients not to be denied choice and control over their deaths, and to be allowed to die 'on their own terms', have created 'a babble of voices proclaiming various good deaths' (Walter 1994: 9). The emergence of the discourse that constructs death as a matter of choice, together with cultural and structural shifts towards individualization with its emphases on choice and control, mean that death is now 'medically and politically malleable and open to endless negation' (Kaufman 2005: 3). In short, 'today we inescapably think of death in terms of control, quality and timeliness' (Kaufman 2005: 326). This is generally confirmed by the existing studies of people's notion of a good death, which show that, apart from being pain free, other commonly agreed upon features of the good death include the fulfilment of the dying person's choices and preferences concerning the conditions of the dying process, spirituality, emotional wellbeing, life completion, quality of life and dignity (Meier et al. 2016: 262).

Although this can been seen as an indication of consistency in perceptions of what constitutes a good death, the scrutiny of thirty-six English-language, peer-reviewed articles published between 1996 and 2015 (Meier et al. 2016) also reveals the existence of complex and contrasting perspectives on the characteristics of a good death. Even though the study discovered that in more than 85% of the articles reviewed, some consensus existed on the notion of a good death, it also found that there were also some divergent perspectives on how to ensure a good death among patients, family and health professionals (Meier et al. 2016: 262). While there was some consensus on the notion of a good death, such as a lack of pain, dying in a full control, as an independent self and being surrounded by loved ones, there were also discrepancies, and one of the main discrepancies was among family members' perspectives and patient perspectives. For example, family members rated quality of life as more important than patients did, while religiosity/spirituality and dying at home were rated higher by patients (Meier et al. 2016: 262). Furthermore, the Western script for good death might not reflect ideas of the good death in different cultural contexts – for example, for Senegal's Wolof people the good death is a death within the community, never abroad (Walter 2017). Moreover, defining the good death as requiring 'us to retrain control, know when and where it will happen, have pain relief and access to good medical care' (Wolpert 2011: 222) might miss some religions' specific requirements for how to die – for instance, British Hindus may wish to follow their traditional rituals and ceremonies (Walter 2017).

Another equally important question concerns the relevance of this model of death for aged persons themselves. In the context of expanded longevity, a culture of individualism and the value of control over the end-of-life process, the aged and frail people are presented with the complexity of choice of interventions and options that maybe extend their longevity, yet they are often without the necessary knowledge and resources to respond, and maybe under an illusion of a common belief that 'death occurring in later life is more likely to be constructed as the good death and that elderly people are ready to accept death as an inevitable and natural event' (Howarth 2007: 134). Moreover, older people who are at threshold of life and death are in a need of comprehensive support that their informal social environment often is incapable of providing, so may feel rather confused. They also do not know what to expect as the rhetoric of choice at the end of life coexists with the narrative about death in old age that still frames death in old age as natural and normal.

Despite a growing awareness of the importance of the end-of-life care death, despite some consensus on the idea of good death and despite the advances that occurred in the medical care of the dying over the last century, the difficulty of ensuring a successful death remains. To overcome this difficulty, the criteria of a good death needs to be negotiated between medical professionals, patients and family members, and getting this kind of dying right also needs to be coordinated by efforts from of these three groups. However, even if the key components of enabling a good death – namely, having patient-focused preferences for the dying process and being pain free – are identified and agreed upon, we will never totally succeed in achieving a good death 'because of the nature of the final illness or because of human nature' (Humphrys and Jarvis 2009: 193). The persistence of such obstacles prompts many to search for alternative or more radical solutions to the problem death.

Disputing the obstacle to the good death

As many critical studies of modern death show, from the middle of the twentieth century the institutionalization and medicalization of death, together with advances in medical technology, have created a new context for dying (Howarth 2007; Kellehear 2007; McManus; Walter 2020). The cumulative effect of these processes on the experience of dying has undermined people's right to choose how and when they die, which are now seen as the main conditions of the good death. Hence, debates about how to remove impediments to the good death cannot avoid the issue of people's preferences and choice of how and when they die. Since the beginning of this century, public discussions of the main obstacle to a good death have increasingly supported the argument that people should not be forced to experience death they find intolerable, but rather should be offered the right to assisted dying, which refers to either euthanasia or assisted suicide (Taylor 2016). In recent public debates, the main obstacle to a good death has frequently been identified as the illegality of assisted dying. These public discussions on the necessity of legal changes to secure a right to the good death, together with a question about how such public debates might contribute to older people's reflexive thinking about the management of their end of life, are our main concern here.

In contemporary developed societies, with the increase in longevity, the prolongation of fatal illness and the enhancement of capacities to artificially sustain life, public debates about the need for legal changes to secure one's right to a good death have been focused on arguments for and against euthanasia (the act of deliberately ending a person's life to relieve suffering, with the act carried out by a doctor) and on arguments for and against assisted suicide (the act of deliberately assisting another person to kill) (both the NHS definitions). The frequency of discussions of assisted dying is linked not only to advances in medical science and technology, but also to broader social changes, including secularization, liberalization and individualization (Howarth 2007; Lang 2020). In other words, the public debates about the idea of a good death are framed by societal values, science, art and politics. For example, only quite recently new images of death in films have started to raise questions about obstacles to a good death. Since media representations of 'real death are permissible when they are used for sacred purposes of defining a good death' (McManus 2013: 225), it can be argued that today's artistic images of death are allowed in the public realm because they offer helpful voices in our debates about a good death. Such reward winning movies as *Amour* (directed by Michael Haneke, 2012), *Happy End* (directed by Michael Haneke, 2017) and *Everything Went Fine* (directed by Francois Ozon, 2021) show older people who have suffered unbearable pain, whose quality of life has diminished and who have either tried to commit suicide or asked for assisted suicide, or were helped to die by their loving partner. These movies' very artistic and unsentimental depictions of older people's difficulties when death is near and their sensitive presentation of the issue of assisted dying neither offer an answer nor suggest an evaluation of the film heroes' decision. The films, while showing stories of assisted dying, ask viewers whether is it worth fighting to the end and to consider what they might opt for or accept in order to be released of pain and the indignity of final suffering. In short, the movies leave the decision of what is a good death to viewers.

Over the last couple of decades, in many Western nations, the debate about assisted dying has gained in importance. Although many of these countries still ban both voluntary active euthanasia and assisted suicide, the proponents of liberalization of the law regarding death have made conversations about assisted dying very visible on various policy forums, in legal courts, during parliamentary debates and on television shows for the last several decades. The expansion of the right-to-die movement, which can be seen as the outgrowth of a decades-long evolution in public attitudes towards how we die, has intensified the battle for the legalization of assisted dying. While criticizing the existing system of managing end-of-life pain and suffering for being unnecessarily prolonged by medical practice and too often causing overwhelming distress, the right-to-die movement has put the issues of euthanasia and assisted suicide on the news and political agendas in many countries. Arguing that the main obstacle to a good death is the lack of right to die without fear of the dying process, it calls for new laws that could give people the right to dignity in death by allowing them to decide when and how to die. The movement, by expanding the concept of human dignity from the sphere of life where the principle of dignity offers recognition of basic intrinsic worth of persons, asserts that all people have the right to be treated with dignity, not only in life but also in death (Jackson 2008; Warnock and Macdonald 2008).

The development of the right-to-die movement has been also helped by criticism of the medicalization of death, as expressed in the literature since the 1970s, and by the death awareness movement (both discussed earlier in this chapter). Furthermore, the right-to-die movement could only begin when the timing of death had started to be considered to be a controllable event, which happened a result of two trends. The first is the effect of advances in clinical intervention, in the medical technology to sustain life artificially and the growing specialization of medicine in affluent societies (Kaufman 2010). For people who are kept alive indefinitely on life support, 'death is no matter of "nature taking its course" but a matter of deliberate decision, not their own' (Warnock and Macdonald 2008: 3). The second relates to the fact that, while in the past an individual doctor was responsible for treatment, relying on their own judgement, now 'it is no longer regarded as proper for doctors to exercise such unquestionable decision-making powers, every decision has to be both transparent and justifiable' (Warnock and Macdonald 2008: 3). Because of the impact of the medicalization of death and because of advances in medical technology, the relationship between one physician and a dying patient is no longer a private matter and, of necessity, it has become

> a team endeavor, so a physician could not quietly increase the dose of morphine, as before. Instead, these sorts of decisions were removed from the bedside, discussed among team members, and became subject to ethical and legal oversight. (Angell 2012: 25)

This new context of dying has brought to people's attention the importance of dying people's right to have control over the manner, conditions and timing of their death; by the same token, it has also provided foundations for the right-to-die movement. Its argument that terminally ill people should not endure unnecessary suffering, but should have right to a successful death goes back to 1976 and the Karen Ann Quinlan case, which revealed the capacities of medical technology to prolong dying processes by artificially sustaining life. Karen Ann Quinlan was a 21-year-old American woman who, after taking some drugs and drinking at a party, lapsed into a persistent vegetative state and was kept alive in a permanently unconscious state with a mechanical ventilator and a feeding tube. After several months, her parents asked doctors to turn off the machines that kept their daughter alive. When the hospital refused to disconnect the ventilator and allow Karen Ann to die, her parents went to court for legal permission to stop all life-sustaining treatment, which was not granted as the act of removing life-sustaining treatment was considered to equate to euthanasia. Karen Ann Quinlan's case and her lingering death in 1985 brought to public attention whether and how to bring about an earlier death in permanently unconscious patients, or in patients who, although conscious, are suffering unbearably at the end of life. Karen Ann Quinlan's story received extensive media coverage and initiated a passionate debate across the United States between those who held that life was sacred and those who supported the principle of the patient's right to a dignified death (Angell 2012; Humphrys and Jarvis 2009).

The issue of the rights of dying person was kept on the US public agenda through the 1990s with publicity about similar cases, but also with the high profile of two legal cases involving doctors accused of assisting in deaths (Jack Kevorkian and Timothy Quill). In the last decade of the twentieth century, some states – namely, Washington and California – unsuccessfully tried to introduce assisted dying under the law. In 1994, physician-assisted suicide became legal in Oregon, where voters narrowly approved a Death with Dignity Act. The Oregon law, the first of this kind anywhere in the world, allows doctors to prescribe lethal drugs to terminally ill people who want to die, but only for people judged to be in the last six months of their lives. It has publicized the importance of a dignified death for patients near the end of their lives and reinforced the difference between assisted suicide, which implies that medical personnel provide patients with the lethal means to kill themselves, and euthanasia, which is the act of directly injecting medication to cause death. The Oregon Death with Dignity Act, which is regarded as having more safeguards built into it than any other legislation in the world, has become the model pursued by campaigners for assisted suicide in other US states and other countries (Angell 2012; Jackson 2004).

Now, after decades of public debates and many failed attempts to legalize it, physician-assisted dying is legal in several US states, including – apart from Oregon – Washington, Colorado, Hawaii, Vermont, Maine, New Jersey and California. Yet the exact circumstances in which assisted suicide is allowed vary, with some jurisdictions – namely Oregon and Vermont – only allowing it in the case of terminal illness. However, euthanasia, the act of directly injecting medication to cause death rather than providing medication for the patient to take if they choose, is banned everywhere in the United States. Although assisted suicide is generally still more widely available across the world than euthanasia (Davis 2019; Lang 2020), the legalization of euthanasia outside the United States in the last several years has been more common. Outside Europe (discussed below), euthanasia is legalized in Colombia, Canada, in five states in Australia and in New Zealand.

Across Europe, the assisted dying legislation is fragmented and differs from country to country. Although public debates have taken place everywhere, and although in this century the public acceptance of euthanasia has increased in many European countries, in some countries, like the United Kingdom, a divisive public controversy still occurs over the moral, ethical and legal issues associated with euthanasia, while in Greece and Poland the topic is still a total taboo (Cohen et al. 2014). Yet, in the last two decades, the liberalization of European public opinion has impacted government policies on euthanasia and achieved some success across the continent (Lang 2020). In 2002, as the first country in Europe to do so, the Netherlands passed a law legalizing euthanasia, including physician-assisted suicide – although under strict conditions. These specific circumstances include that the patients must be enduring 'unbearable and endless suffering' and that at least two doctors agree to the procedure. In the following years, euthanasia policies have also been legalized in Spain, Belgium, Luxembourg and Portugal as well as the Netherlands, while physician-assisted dying, under specific safeguards, is permitted in Belgium, the Netherlands, Luxembourg, Germany, Portugal, Switzerland and Spain. For example, in Switzerland it is an offence to assist a suicide if it is done with selfish motives – in other words, it can only occur if the motive of bringing suffering to an end is 'entirely honourable' (Warnock and Macdonald 2008: 6). Acting under this exemption, many not-for-profit organizations have created clinics in Switzerland, such as Dignitas in Zurich, where people from all over the world can choose to end their lives by means of assisted dying (Davis 2019).

In the last two decades in the United Kingdom, a growing number of people and organizations have been willing to accept that the nation should ensure the experience of the good death and that it may mean helping people to have an assisted death. The evolution of the UK public towards the legitimacy of euthanasia and assisted suicide can be illustrated by the opinion polls, as already in 2008 the UK polls showed that about 80% of Britons were in favour of some form of assisted dying (Humphrys and Jarvis 2009: 224). The change can also be also attributed to the public visibility of the issues of euthanasia and assisted suicide and the publicity gained by several voluntary organizations and charities that believe everybody has the right to a good death, which includes the option of assisted dying for terminally ill, campaigning for euthanasia policies. Among these charities, among the most significant are Dignity in Dying, which is a not-for-profit membership organization supporting changes to the end-of-life care, and its sister charity organization Compassion in Dying. Yet, despite the media attention and the fact that British opinion is increasingly in favour of assisted dying, and despite many civil society initiatives seeking a liberalization of laws, the British policy on assisted dying has remained unchanged. In the United Kingdom, assisted suicide and euthanasia are still criminal offences and, moreover, people who help or accompany terminally ill persons with travel for assisted suicide abroad might be punished (Bowcott 2019; Davis 2019).

However, the illegality of assisted dying in the United Kingdom has not stopped the increasing numbers of Britons willing to undergo assisted suicide in the clinic in Switzerland. Moreover, as a result of the publicity given to their stories and subsequent court cases, these reports from the Swiss clinic have contributed to the further evolution of public opinion and prompted the introduction of Bills to the House of Lords to change the law. Thus, the British public has been exposed to many stories of travelling to the Dignitas clinic and accounts of subsequent court battles and attempts to change the policy. Among cases that were be widely broadcast, and marking core steps in the legal battle to remove the main obstacle to the good death, one of the first was the story of Anne Turner, a GP in her mid-sixties who died in the Dignitas clinic in Zurich in 2006. Anne, who suffered from a progressive and incurable degenerative disease, knew that her death would be prolonged, intolerable and slow, and that she would lose her independence and dignity; thus, after unsuccessful attempts at killing herself, she decided to go to the Dignitas clinic. Anne Turner wished to put an end to the taboo surrounding assisted suicide so she invited a reporter and crew from the BBC to join her in Zurich (Humphrys and Jarvis 2009). However, the first person to be filmed when dying after going through with an assisted suicide was Craig Ewert, who had motor neurone disease and who wanted the world to see the instant at which he was ending his life in the Dignitas clinic. The moment when he committed assisted suicide was shown in 2008 on Sky in the film *Right to Die?* It generated a host of front-page stories in the national press. The documentary was strongly criticized by anti-euthanasia campaigners, including the organization Care Not Killing and the Pro-Life Alliance, yet many people saw it as an important and valuable contribution to the debate about the right to die (Morris and Plunkett 2008).

Another documentary about assisted dying was initiated by Terry Pratchett, the acclaimed fantasy author, and produced by BBC Scotland in 2011 under the title *Terry Pratchett: Choosing to Die*. This film registered the final moments of Peter Smedley, a 71-year-old motor neurone sufferer, who decided to end his life at the Dignitas clinic. The documentary sparked strong controversy and was criticized by Christian and pro-life organizations as 'biased'. All accusations were denied by Terry Pratchett, according to whom 'Peter got what he wanted – a good death' (MacManus 2013: 217). The most recent debate about death on the British television was the documentary *We Need to Talk about Death*, which was aired in January 2019 on BBC2 and posed questions about people's right to a good death and how could it be regulated and arranged. Generally, British broadcasters are urged by political leaders to deal with the issue of assisted death 'sensitively and without sensationalism', but the BBC website sets out the arguments in favour of allowing euthanasia in certain cases (Luft 2008).

In a next step, in addition to the public media and civil society engagement, the British courts and parliament have become involved in this issue, with actions in both institutions being widely reported. The legal battle started with the story of Daniel James, who died in the Dignitas clinic in 2008 and whose parents, because they took their paralyzed son to Switzerland, were faced with a threat of criminal charges for being 'accomplices' in the Dignitas suicide. As this case has brought to public attention the possibility of prosecutions for aiding and abetting a suicide, several people wishing to end their lives asked the High Court either for help to end their lives or ensure some guarantee that their helpers, husbands or wives would not be prosecuted if they helped with the death. Legal challenges to the UK ban on assisted suicide, initiated by Tony Nicklinson, Diane Pretty, Debbie Purdy, Noel Conway and Omid T., did not achieve much; the courts did not in dismiss the ban, but ruled that it was up to parliament to decide on the issue. Subsequently several people who wanted to control the time and manner of their deaths, and after the court did not grant their loved ones any protection from prosecution for helping them to abroad to die, took their cases to the House of Lords, which tended to reject such applications by saying that the right to life did not include a right to die and the right to private life did not include a right to decide when and how to die. However, as a result of Debbie Purdy's application to the House of Lords in 2009, its judicial committee, while stressing that it was not part of its function to change the law in order to decriminalize assisted suicide, as that was a matter for parliament, accepted that its role was to clarify uncertainty in the law and asked the director of public prosecutions (DPP) to issue new guidance about when people would be prosecuted for encouraging or assisting suicide (Jackson 2008). In September 2009, the DPP clarified the uncertainty in the law and in the existing practices by ruling that the decision to prosecute would be based on factors including the nature of the victim's illness; it also ruled that, although assisting suicide would remain illegal, discretion would be used.

With the new ruling reducing the probability of any legal action being taken against people if they assisted the suicide of a friend or relative who had a settled and informed wish to die, and in the context of the declining number of people defending the continued prohibition by euthanasia and physician-assisted suicides, the UK parliament could not afford to overlook the issue (Keown 2009). Subsequently, several Private Members' Bills tried to legalize assistance for those who were terminally ill and likely to die within six months. One of the first unsuccessful attempts to change the assisted suicide law in the British Parliament was Lord Joffe's Bill in 2006, which was based on the Oregon system and sought to permit only assisted suicide, not euthanasia. The last time parliament voted on and rejected assisted suicide was in 2015, and it was followed by a long legislative pause until the introduction to the House of Lords of Baroness Meacher's Private Members' Bill on assisted dying in May 2021. However, it seems that, with around 200 amendments tabled, the Bill aiming to legalize physician assisted suicide for patients with a terminal illness and six months or less to live, was already running out of legislative time at the beginning of January 2022, which means the British Parliament will not have an opportunity to debate the issue of assisted dying any time soon.

All these developments, from TV programmes through court hearings to parliamentary debates about the right to die, have continued to liberate public thinking about euthanasia and assisted suicide. In other words, in the United Kingdom, public support for the idea of doctors ending the lives of terminally ill, mentally competent adults has been growing (Davis 2019). This change is illustrated by a poll conducted by the National Centre for Social Research, which found that 93% of people in the United Kingdom approved of, or wouldn't rule out, doctor-assisted suicide if the person were terminally ill (Bowcott 2019). Yet, because of strong views on the other side of the question of a person's right to die at a time of their choosing, even with more than 90% of the general public and the majority of people of faith, people with disabilities and doctors in the United Kingdom calling for the legalization of assisted dying for terminally ill people, debates about and attempts to change the law on the right to die will still take some time (Bowcott 2019).

In the context of our increased longevity, which together with advances in medical technology and wider social changes have been contributing to the increased public attention given to the topic of assisted dying, there is a need to address how elderly people are placed in this debate. Given that older people's attitudes to death will be discussed in the next chapter, here we consider only how the recurring debates on assisted dying have referred to the elderly and how these indirect encounters with death have effected older people's understanding of how their own individual preferences fit with the interests of society and its law. Nowhere is euthanasia proposed as a choice for the old – that is, it is never allowed to be applied solely on the basis of 'advanced age'. Where assisted dying is legal, older people – like others – can opt for and be considered for assisted dying only because of their terminal illness, assuming other conditions are met. However, together with disabled people, the elderly are singled out as being vulnerable by both the supporters and opponents of the liberalization of laws to allow euthanasia, and both groups are used to reinforce the two parties' respective arguments. The proponents acknowledge that the development of laws to allow assisted dying must be handled carefully and that the system in which euthanasia is an option should be really carefully monitored because in principle it involves the risk of life to older and disabled people. They warn against regarding the old as less worthy but they also suggest that perhaps euthanasia should be allowed for the elderly, who feel they are a burden to others and therefore desperately wish to be allowed to die (Warnock and Macdonald 2008). Yet this argument only reinforces attacks deployed against legalizing any form of assisted dying. The opponents of assisted dying claim that it is the 'the slippery slope' argument, as it could encourage people to feel that they almost have a duty to put an end to their lives if they are burden to their families. This common criticism deployed against legalizing euthanasia predicts that the liberation of the law would put pressure on old and ill people and would make any moral concerns about 'the pulling the plug on granny' invalid. According to this stand, relaxing the existing law would be dangerous in practice, not least for the dying, the old, the disabled and the disadvantaged (Keown 2009;

Lang 2020; Livne 2019). Such arguments against any relaxation of the law prohibiting euthanasia and physician-assisted suicide were explicitly used by Prime Minister Gordon Brown in 2008 when opposing Lord Joffe's Bill. He told MPs in the Commons that he would never support legislation to permit assisted suicide as it might put elderly and sick people under pressure to end their lives:

> I believe that it's necessary to ensure that there is a never a case in the country where a sick or elderly person feels under pressure to agree to an assisted death or somehow feels it is the expected thing to do. That's why I've always opposed legislation for assisted deaths. (Brown, quoted in Luft 2008)

The ongoing debate about legalizing assisted dying, which dominates public discussions around the idea of a good death, could challenge older people to ask themselves what death they want, how much more time they want to have and whether they should plan for their own death. The answers to these questions depend on their country's legal system and their own values, resources, and physical and mental health. Because of the conditions and limits of legal euthanasia and because longevity often means multiple morbidities, frailty and dementia at the end of a long life, these are not simple answers. Even when the national law allows consideration of the timing of death and help to die, assisted dying for older people could mean that they have to decide to die before they are ready to do so – for example, when they are threatened by dementia. The recent considerations given to the issue of the legality of assisted suicide for older persons resulted in changes to Dutch laws on euthanasia in 2016, which allow doctors to administer a fatal drug to a patient with dementia if they signed a euthanasia declaration under the supervision of their family doctor before their condition deteriorated – that is, before they could 'no longer express their will' (Boffey 2018). However, as this new law called into question the ability of aged dementia suffers to consciously and independently evaluate their options, it might lead to doctors being prosecuted. In 2022, the Dutch Supreme Court ruled that doctors who committed euthanasia on dementia patients who had previously given written consent would be no longer prosecuted. The realization that one's death is not one's own has been exposed further in public discussions of COVID-19's impact on the timing and conditions of death.

The fallout from narratives of COVID-19

Until the coronavirus pandemic, the most disruptive global health disaster since the influenza pandemic of 1918, modern Western societies either avoided the subject of death or talked about it in terms of the quality of the end-of-life experience. It was the arrival of the pandemic that put death into the daily news and brought dying closer to home for many. To discover the role of the public narratives of COVID-19 in eroding the culture of silence around death and in challenging us to consider what kind of death is a good death, we will look at two types of narratives of COVID-19: the government rhetoric and the dominant discourse in the mainstream media. To examine how both public narratives of COVID have held up a mirror to the idea of the good death, we will explore the disparities between these two discourses – that is, between the official and media one – in terms of their projected value of the end. By exploring media and official narratives of COVID-19 and by following the conclusion from studies of past crises that during the trauma people tend to focus on what matters most to them, including relationships (Cohen Silver 2011; Tergesen 2020), it can be argued that the main fallout from the public narratives of COVID-19 has been a realization of the importance of the presence of others in tragic situations and the recognition of our mutual interdependence on each other and the role of social institutions in handling any unexpected crisis.

Throughout the pandemic, with daily reporting of COVID-19 cases, it was very difficult to avoid hearing about death. COVID-19 has made many people aware of death and challenged many to come to terms with it. Apart from increasing the visibility of death and weakening the strength of denial of death, the pandemic also introduced us to a rare type of death for modern Western societies: unexpected, untimely, lonely and not too prolonged death. Until the pandemic, in the United Kingdom only one in ten deaths was classified as an incident of sudden death, while modern death in old age tends to be a prolonged dying process from disabling, chronic and degenerative diseases (Walter 2017). During the pandemic, the headlines, reports and discussions of COVID-19 deaths exposed the unpredictability, uncertainty and shock connected with death in the context of the pandemic. The media narrative of coronavirus casualties revealed the disturbing reality of deaths during the pandemic as the quality of the end of life of the virus's main victims – that is, older people – was compromised. It exposed the mismatch between the public's value of a peaceful, good death and the reality of untimely death during the pandemic. Also, owing to media narratives of COVID-19, it became clear that the pandemic led to the replacement of the official concern with a good death with a strategy aiming to prevent death, and that this priority has not always worked in the best interests of the elderly (Trapper 2021). In other words, during the pandemic, the hierarchy of dying was not challenged and the elderly, the disabled and the frail constituted the second tier of low-priority citizens (Clarke 2021).

At the beginning of the crisis, the official rhetoric of COVID-19, dominated by televised press briefings announcing new set of directives, revisions of old policies and numbers of people who had died, were hospitalized and had tested positive sought to minimize the public's panic. Yet, already at the time of the first lockdown, with the realization that it would take far more than calming down the public's anxiety to prevent or lower the number of deaths, there was a need for a new rhetoric or metaphor. From the end of March 2020, alongside medical language of treatments, tests, protection and shielding, politicians frequently resorted to wartime metaphors and images to describe the 'battle' against COVID-19. To stress the gravity of the pandemic threat to the country and its health system, the 'war on the virus' was declared, which promoted the image of hospitals as 'war zones', physicians as 'warriors' and sick people as 'fighters'. Yet, following Susan Sontag's (1978) argument in *Illness as Metaphor*, it can be argued that the most truthful way of thinking about diseases is without recourse to metaphor; therefore, the metaphor of 'war' used during the COVID-19 crisis amounted to a reluctance to see the awful reality of the pandemic, and to remove the responsibility for its handling from the authorities. Moreover, as Sontag (1978) asserts, metaphors intrinsic to medicine such as 'war on cancer'), by blaming, silencing and shaming patients, make sick people feel as if their illness was their own fault. In short, while they may be useful for health officials and leaders, metaphors are not useful for sick people in coping with and forming meaning out of their experiences.

The British official COVID-19 narratives, by promoting the usage of the metaphor of war, projecting image of people as 'fighters' and relying on 'blame the victim' language, came close to misrepresenting the true nature of the health risks connected with the virus. The inadequacy of the war metaphor became especially evident in the language used to comment on the prime minister's treatment in intensive care after he was infected with the virus in April 2020. Several cabinet members, while assuring us that 'the PM will beat the disease because he is a fighter', seemed to suggest that you need to be a fighter to win against the virus, or that 'survival is somehow a test of character' (Clarke 2021: 16). Such comments ignored the truth that if somebody doesn't come through, it doesn't mean they can be shamed for not being a fighter. Moreover, the government's constant use of wartime metaphors disregarded the fact that any talk of war could be frightening, especially for the elderly – not only because the elderly are the most the vulnerable members of society, but also because some of them still remember World War II.

The reliance on the war metaphor during the COVID-19 pandemic was reinforced during the second lockdown. At the peak of the pandemic, Prime Minister Boris Johnson suggested that the country was fighting a second Battle of Britain and praised people for their 'Blitz spirit' – the term War World II authorities used to describe the reality of being bombed and to promote resilience and solidarity in the face of hardship and trauma caused by the war (Overy 2020). In a televised address to the nation, the prime minister announced the first lockdown as 'the moment of national emergency', and urged people to 'beat the coronavirus'. He told the public that the outbreak was the 'biggest threat this country has faced for decades' and that the people of this country would 'rise to that challenge' and we 'will beat it together'. In the context of the pandemic, many British politicians easily invoked the message of danger and stressed that the war had exploded, and that non-stop battles could go on until a final victory over the virus was achieved. As the effectiveness of any political language is contingent on circumstances, such attempts to proclaim an uplifting narrative with the help of the political myths of the 'Blitz spirit' could not match the success of Britain's wartime s propaganda in obscuring the reality of the war.

In other words, reliance on the war metaphor during the COVID-19 pandemic, in the face of unexpected and invisible adversity, was reductive, insufficient, ahistorical, failed to acknowledge reality and aimed to take away accountability for the course of events from the politicians. If we add to it comments written by those who were convinced that COVID-19 was a fake or a conspiracy aimed at curtailing individual liberties, and if we also include voices spreading misinformation about science – all in the context the language of blame and weaponized misinformation – the COVID crisis started to resemble the situation that existed during the Black Death, where various groups, from lepers to witches, were blamed for causing the plague: 'When there's an epidemic of panic, people long for something to blame, because if you can find the thing to blame' (Margaret Atwood, quoted in Flood 2020).

Another metaphor used in the official representation of the COVID-19 pandemic confirms Susan Sontag's (1978) argument about the deceptive and misleading role of metaphor in our thinking about illness. This second government narrative of coronavirus crisis was developed to reflect a more optimistic development ensured by the success of the UK vaccination programme, which from the first months of 2021 enhanced the nation's hopes for overcoming the awful reality of death from the pandemic. At the end of March 2021, with more than 25 million Britons vaccinated with their first dose, the documentary film produced for the UK government constructed a new official metaphor of 'hope'. The film's title, *A Beacon of Hope*, and its message of 'hope' supported the government's anticipation of victory in 'the battle' against the virus. The replacement of a metaphor of 'war' with an image of 'hope' also aimed to redirect public attention from dwelling on the problems of the UK health policy. In contrast to the uplifting political discourse, the dominant narrative of COVID-19 in the mainstream media continued to point to the state's problems in handling the pandemic, such as the high per capita mortality from COVID-19 in the United Kingdom, its lack of preparation and its poor response in the early stages of the pandemic, as well as the failure to implement an effective test and trace programme in the summer of 2020 (Calvert and Arbuthnott 2021; Clarke 2022; Spiegelhalter and Masters 2021). The lifting of all COVID restrictions in England on 21 February 2022 – weeks earlier than expected – was also presented by the prime minster as marking a 'moment of pride', a suggestion that was met with criticism by scientists, health experts and charities for being a premature strategy that could put vulnerable people at risk.

With more information gathered, public narratives of COVID-19, by showing how the virus eroded our control over the timing and conditions of death and how dying became a less manageable process during the pandemic, challenged many people to rethink their attitudes towards dying and death. The pandemic did not just bring to public attention the unexpected deaths of elderly people; the COVID-19 stories also painted the picture of a lonely death, often without any chance of securing intimacy with loved ones, and little opportunity to achieve peace at the end of life. By imposing restrictions on intimacy in death, the pandemic constructed death as dying alone. Newspaper articles with such headlines as 'They Don't Put Loneliness on Death Certificates' showed the trauma and pain of lonely death and made us recognize the importance of human presence as one of the conditions of a good death. Of course, the presence of others, intimacy and physical closeness are reported to be components of a good death in many studies, which all show that patients greatly value maintaining emotional contacts with members of their families during the final phase of their lives (Meier et al. 2016). Even before the COVID-19, people were dying 'not so much in loneliness as in silence' (Elias 1985: 131), and even in normal times, the hospital environment does not always permit intimacy. Yet the pandemic reinforced the value of the presence of others at the end of life – a value that for too long we probably took for granted. In short, the COVID-19 crisis took 'impersonality to an extreme and unprecedented degree' (Clarke 2021: 178). With the media narrative of COVID-19, together with more doctors and nurses speaking about the daily trauma of the intensive care unit, the public realized the horror of lonely death.

During the coronavirus crisis, dying without the presence of loved ones, as reported by media and research accounts, was taking place in hospitals, care facilities and homes (Calvert and Arbuthnott 2021; Clarke 2021; Francis 2021). The awful truth about the drama of COVID-19 death in care homes was reflected by signs on care homes' entrance doors: 'No visitors'. During the pandemic, care homes became no-go areas, places of trauma, best described by one resident, a 113-year-old COVID survivor who said that elderly people 'do not deserve to leave the world this way' (Kassam 2020). In Chapter 9, we look at the drama of COVID-19 deaths in care homes, including the transfer to care homes of more than 6,000 elderly patients discharged from hospitals in order to free hospital beds, with only a third of them being tested (Calvert and Arbuthnott 2021; Spiegelhalter and Masters 2021). This case points to the mutual dependence and links between the heath and care systems, and their reliance on the decisions of authorities.

Moreover, this tragic event suggests that, during the pandemic, not only care homes but also hospitals were not always very safe places. Newspapers reporting that critically ill, very often older patients were denied access to intensive care because resources were inadequate, as well as reports pointing to the rate of COVID-19 infection in hospitals as well as to long waiting lists for treatment at specialist NHS clinic or hospitals, made people unwilling to seek professional help. Subsequently, because of the internal difficulties and problems of hospitals, as well as because of people's unwillingness to enter hospitals, there was a big increase in the number of people who died at home during the pandemic; according to a Marie Curie study, the number of deaths at home in the year after the United Kingdom went into its first lockdown rose by more than a third, and overall during the pandemic there were 40% more deaths at home than usual (Olszowski 2022: 45). Many old people who died at home, sometimes alone but even with family members, did not have the medicine and counselling that would help them to manage pain and secure a peaceful death. As the Marie Curie survey discovered, 76% of people who died at home during the pandemic did not get the support they needed. The study also reported that most of them (64%) did not even get the help they needed to manage pain (Olszowski 2022: 45). The importance of pain management at the end of life, like the significance of the presence of loved ones, has been widely recognized and accepted since the advent of palliative care. The COVID-19 pandemic has reinforced this idea by showing that medical intervention in such cases is essential in the construction of the conditions for a good death. The recent health crisis, apart from strengthening our recognition of the central role of the presence of intimate others and our dependence on professional help, has also demonstrated the importance of a wider institutional context. The United Kingdom's lack of readiness for the pandemic, with the media disclosing that Britain was simply without the required emergency stockpiles of PPE, without the adequate contingency planning and without recently trained key workers for a pandemic, has had painful consequences for many of its citizens (Calvert and Arbuthnott 2021).

The COVID-19 pandemic has made us more aware of some assumptions behind the notion of a good death, such as the importance of others, the essential role of professional help at the end of life and the significance of a broader societal system. Although a comprehensive picture of emotional, health and mental costs in the time of COVID-19 has yet to emerge, there is already some evidence of the toll that the pandemic is taking on emotional wellbeing and the mental health of older people. The coronavirus crisis has confronted people with the changed conditions of death and made them – especially the people at the bottom of the hierarchy of dying, namely the old and infirm – even more vulnerable. The pandemic has not only brought the existing ageism to the surface; it has also accelerated the existing marginalization and vulnerability of older people. The coronavirus epidemic, by changing the parameters of the problems faced by the elderly, has increased the urgency of retaining past gains in end-of-life care and the importance of holding on to the idea of a good death.

PART III

Living towards death

CHAPTER 7

In the shadow of death

Memento mori

This final part explores what happens when aged people grasp the inevitability of death and surveys the heterogeneity of conditions of dying in later life both before and during the COVID-19 pandemic. Its last two chapters examine the various ways of dying and plurality of places where it may take place: home, hospital, hospice or care homes. This chapter looks at what is happening in the context of the *memento mori* (the remembrance of death) and investigates the variety of emotional states and adaptive mechanisms adopted by aged persons 'living in death's shadow', to paraphrase Abel's (2017) book title. The final section of this chapter explores how older people's outlooks on death have been affected by the COVID-19 pandemic, which disrupted any planning and preparation for the last moments of life and inflicted new existential dread.

In modern Western society, in which degenerative and chronic conditions have replaced acute diseases as the major cause of mortality, large numbers of old people live in the proximity of death for many years. Although not everybody retain full cognitive capacity until their last days (these cases will be discussed Chapter 9), many elderly people live with the increased consciousness that they are running out of time. Hence, we are interested in what, if anything, is unique about older people's feelings, actions and preparations associated with the *memento mori* in the period close to death. While the idea that people's awareness of death increases with age was discussed in Chapter 2, here we will explore whether older people's increased awareness of death translates into any attempt to get their affairs in order as preparation for death. Before we examine the planning and preparation for death, we look at common features of the elderly's emotional life associated with their increased consciousness of the shrinking time they have left.

Emotional consequences of the awareness of death at the end of life is not a well-researched and fully explained topic. Several reviews of the social-psychological literature of gerontology show that the topic of awareness of finitude was largely neglected in such studies, and when it was mentioned, it was seen as an invariable orientation related to chronological age (Abel 2017; Marshall 1975, 1980; Tomer Eliason 2013). Although representatives of major paradigms within social gerontology agree that individuals' awareness of finitude leads to various psychological processes, they have never considered the consciousness of death as an intervening variable, but rather as just an age-related factor (Tomer and Eliason 2013; Walter 2020). Hence, the impact of consciousness of death on the elderly's emotional life has not really been fully investigated. Without plausible resolutions of the empirical and theoretical debates within the gerontological literature, we turn to a more reflective philosophical stand concerned with the human experience of the passing time and the temporal dimension of selfhood. Following Ricoeur's (2004) notion of the progression of our lives from birth to death and his idea of self-aware embodied beings, we can identify older people's awareness of finitude as playing the major role in explaining the nature of their orientation to death and to name sadness as the basic emotional response to thinking about death and the brevity of the remining time left in life. However, as one of the main broad feelings experienced by older people in the context of the *memento mori*, sadness can either lead to a person's total withdrawal or prompt them to eagerly engage with the world and others. In other words, people 'whom death has already taken into its shadow' are either passive and resigned or their attention is focused and intensified by the brevity of time that remains (Marcel Proust, quoted in de Beauvoir 1972: 453).

In the first group are people whose abilities to actively engage with life are paralyzed by their awareness of living in the 'collapsing time' – that is, in 'this insane last phase when everything about you goes downhill' (James 2015: 7). This cluster includes older people who, with their increased realization of the end, become indifferent towards reality. Thinking that 'only death can free' us from the cage of old age and illness, and that soon we will have to leave the future to others, can make people feel passive, depressed, full of self-pity and withdrawn from the realities of life (Grumbach 1991: 56). In other words, sadness at the edge of things can facilitate the tendency to disengage with the world, and in turn this can further expand feelings of sadness and refusal to see the relevance of the world around one.

In contrast to the first group, in the second there are people whose ability and willingness to actively overcome sadness caused by their awareness of the impending death lead them to adopt new worldly perspectives, self-examinations and uplifting revisions of contacts with the others. For example, according to Dr Samuel Johnson, the distinguished eighteenth century man of letters, knowing that one soon will die can 'concentrate the mind wonderfully and it can bring wisdom' (quoted in Scarre 2009: 156). Clive James (2017: 4), while contemplating in his poems the experience of being 'old and ill' and living in the 'injured time' or 'collapsing time', states that when one is conscious of one's physical and temporal conditions, such a sad awareness of death focuses one's attention on the world and the people around one. In short, living in the 'injured time' brings sadness, but it also brings unprecedented clarity of insight about oneself and others, and fosters new appreciation of social bonds and relationships. Likewise, one of the protagonists in Muriel Spark's (1972) novel *Memento Mori*, retired detective Henry Mortimer, notes that the remembrance of death, like no other practice, 'intensifies life'. Arguing that thinking about death 'should be part of the full expectancy of life', he states that without 'an ever-present sense of death life is insipid' (Spark 1961: 150). When sadness associated with the death prospect sharpens people's attention and ability to cope with demanding situations, older people – while realizing the impossibility of ignoring death – view it 'as adding "richness and texture" to their lives' (Byrski 2012: 12).

However, sadness evoked in the closest life period to death, when one is old and waits for death to knock and knows that 'death doesn't keep knocking on her door only to be ignored (as men ignore their ageing), but kicks it in to show himself full in the face' (Becker 1973: 215), neither precludes nor facilitates any specific orientation towards the remining life. Furthermore, older people's sadness due to their awareness of mortality and knowledge that their bodies are falling them and their choices are limited, together with their ideas and values they place on life, also translates not into one but various ways in which of relating to death, from fear and denial of death to acceptance of and coming to terms with death (which will be discussed in the following section). Moreover, while recognizing the significance of sadness experienced by older people when they attempt to reckon with the mortality, there is also a need to acknowledge that when elderly people realize the proximity of their end, they often contemplate the ways of preparing for death. As perspectives on death differ in different cultures, and as each historical period supports different views on death, today's preparations and planning for death differ from those in the past societies.

In the past, religion and tradition dictated how to plan and prepare for one's death, while today the elderly are under pressure to formalize their last moments in terms of legal and medical arrangements. In modern societies, with higher levels of secularization and formalization of life generally, and with the medicalization and institutionalization of death, many customs and practices related to death have been disappearing for several decades. One such vanishing tradition is the preparation of outfits and coffins for death, which was a very important part of planning for death in the past. This custom of planning for the final moment, which lasted until quite recently in rural, more religious and poorer parts of Europe, has been studied by Angelia Kuzniak (2020), who over the last 20 years has carried out interviews with many elderly people in small Polish villages. All elderly villagers interviewed (mainly women), while proudly showing their shiny coffins as well as their dresses and shoes prepared for their last trip, beautifully assembled at their houses, talked about how important planning for death was for them, and how ready they felt to go. These old people, taught by a religion that viewed preparation for death as a very serious task, believed that planning for the end was a good way to make peace with death. The old villagers' awareness of death, and their understanding that the time would not stop, helped them to appreciate their remaining time and to value the fact that they were a part of the community life and would be dying at home in the village. Not denying the reality of death, but rather planning for it, was possible because these old people lived in small, stable communities and were very familiar with death as they frequently witnessed it. All these factors, together with the impact of religion, which provided a framework for beliefs and ritual actions that gave meaning to death, tamed the old people's fear of death and created a space where 'death can exist' (Kuzniak 2020: 3). The custom of handling death by making final preparations of this type has now almost totally disappeared, even in these rural communities.

Nonetheless some forms of planning and preparation for death are still very important today in developed Western countries. To illustrate the role of personalized planning for the final ceremony, we can point to Prince Philip's funeral, which took place on 18 April 2021. As all newspapers reported, the Duke of Edinburgh 'was laid to rest in service he planned'. Prince Philip himself arranged, planned and designed the last ceremony and his final journey in details, from songs to the carrier of the coffin (which was his favourite Land Rover Discovery, specially modified to his instructions to become a hearse and repainted in military green). Another interesting example of relatively recent planning of the personalized final service, including designing coffins and selecting the last resting place, is described by Günter Grass (2016) in his final work *Of All That Ends*. Grass depicts how he and his wife imagined their farewell and what steps they took to plan the end of their lives. After months of ill-health, he devoted himself to planning testaments and coffins, and searching for a resting place. Grass wished for a specially designed coffin and for a double grave with his wife in their garden (although burying in private grounds is forbidden by German law). Following many days of discussion of their joint plans, Grass and his wife reached decisions about different woods for their respective coffins (pine for his wife, birch for him) and ways to overcome the country's law against burial on one's own land. Before he died in 2015, aged 87, Günter Grass saw his coffin, in which he would rest on leaves and be covered with leaves (Grass 2016).

Thus, for some people – especially those with the resources for it – the planning of personalized funeral arrangements is a vital part of their preparation for death. Yet today the preparation for death involves much more. Since in contemporary Western societies 'death is characterized by ignorance, a struggle to make sense of things, and anomie – a sense of normlessness and uncertainty as what to do' (Walter 2017: 16), preparation for death focuses on striving to get one's affairs in order. Today, the planning for death or 'taming of time' and 'taming of death' (Christensen and Willerslev 2013) is ensured by taking initiatives to formally regulate emergent problems with a help of various legal arrangements and documents describing preferred medical care and treatment. Modern ways of handling death include attending to practical matters, such as preparing advance statements about medical care, obtaining living wills or establishing a trust or granting a power of attorney. If in the past it was religion and tradition that dictated end-of-life preparations, now the selection of and decisions about preferences are associated with having discussions with family members and professionals (Ai et al. 2006; Clare et al. 2012; Clarke et al. 2012; Garret et al. 2008; Schrader et al. 2009) on the base of information provided by numerous institutions and charities.

In the United Kingdom, many organizations, such as Age Concern, Age UK, Dignity in Dying, Dying Matters and the Natural Death Centre, offer advice on advance decisions and planning for death in a voluntary process of discussion and review concerning future care and treatment. Through social media and printed materials, these charities provide information, forms of relevant documents and advice about how to write a will, where to find additional information and support for planning final steps and for arranging pre-paid funeral plans. For example, Age UK distributes leaflets to homes about how to make a will and informs people how to get a free guide to making a will, which ensures that one's wishes are met and the loved one is looked after. Dying Matters, in its 2013 campaign, invited people to do five things: 'Write a will; record your funeral wishes; plan your future care and support; consider registering as an organ donor; and tell your loved ones your wishes' (Walter 2017: 27).

In England, the single most powerful tool for self-determination at the end is the advance statement, which sets out general preferences to inform best-interest decisions. Whereas this type of advance statement maybe still have no legal force, advance statements about decisions to refuse treatment are legally binding and regulated by the *Mental Capacity Act* (2005), which recommends three ways to prepare for mental incapacity: an Advance Directive (AD) and a Lasting Power of Attorney (LPA) (Walter 2017: 27, 32). Additionally, Age Concern, which has issued 'Instructions for Next of

Kin and Executors upon Death', offers information on a document known as an Advance Decision to Refuse Treatment (ADRT), which can specify treatment that one would always wish to refuse, or specify the circumstances in which this refusal would apply. In the United States, advance care planning has been considered a very important way to help people to plan care and treatment. Since 1990, when the US Congress enacted the Patient Self-Determination Act (PSDAS), all hospitals receiving federal funds have been required to inform patients of their rights to prepare advance directives, to refuse treatment for any reason and to name a proxy to act for them if they have lost the capacity to make such decisions (Kaufman 2005).

From the point of view of the elderly, such advance statements about medical care perform several positive functions. As a study by Clarke et al. (2012) suggests, behind end-of-life healthcare decisions is concern about quality of the life, which older people estimated by their ability to preserve their independence and control over the end of life. Moreover, these decisions make it possible for the elderly to participate in discussions about their care and reduce their concerns about being an inconvenience and problem for their families. Half of all participants in the investigation of the old people's relationships with death stressed the importance of planning for their future demise because they 'don't want to suffer and don't want to be a nuisance' to others (Clarke et al. 2012: 1412). Wishing to maintain independence and not to be a 'burden' to their remaining friends and family members, the old people 'were striving to actively control a largely uncontrollable status passage by making practical plans for their end-of-life' (Clarke et al. 2012: 1414). Older persons' engagement in end-of-life planning is driven by their wish not to be burdensome to their loved ones and by their aspiration to uphold control over their end-of-life healthcare – that is, by the two indicators of quality of life. In short, behind older people's preference to plan for their passage of death is their wish to sustain quality of life at the end of life. Equally importantly, advance care planning can be considered a means to help people die in their preferred place (Seymour et al. 2004).

Yet, although the majority of older people recognize the importance of the end-of-life care strategy, nonetheless only 37% of Americans have advanced care directives for end-of-life care if they become seriously ill or unable to make healthcare decisions, while in the United Kingdom around 54% of adults do not have a will and 5.4 million adults do not know where to begin when it comes to writing a will (Walter 2017, 2020). It raises questions about what barriers prevent the active engagement of elderly people in end-of-life planning and how such obstacles can be removed. To answer this query, we will look at a number of empirical studies of older people's end-of-life planning that seek reasons why so few old people, while approving the worth of the end-of-life planning, actively engage in this type of practice (Clarke et al. 2012; Garrett et al. 2008; Schrader et al. 2009). More specifically, these studies demonstrate that only around half of the older people who declared an interest in planning for the end of life took active steps to organize their affairs, wrote wills or prepared advanced care statements (Clarke et al. 2012; Garrett et al 2008; Schrader et al 2009). Older adults who executed an advance directive and discussed their plans with others tended to have more years of education and greater social support, while their health status and religious affiliations were not positively related to the likelihood of engaging in end-of-life planning (Ai et al. 2006; Clare et al. 2012; Kahana et al. 2004; Schrader et al. 2009). Additionally, a Canadian study of the steps leading to formalizing end-of-life care preferences and factors related to these steps discovered that being female and unmarried predicted planning (Garrett et al, 2008).

Apart from the level of education, gender, religious affiliation, health and family status, other obstacles on the way to formalization of end-of-life preferences include such factors as negative assessments of the effectiveness of the formal procedures, a lack of support from family members and mistrust of professionals (Garret et al. 2008). As the usefulness and effectiveness of some decisions, such as an Advance Decision to Refuse Treatment (ADRT), have come under criticism in both the United Kingdom and the United States (Kaufman 2005; Walter 2017), many questions about the whole idea of planning of the end of life have been raised by all involved parties. Also, some older people believe that at the end they may not necessarily be ready to adhere to an advance statement and 'disengage' from their lives (Seymour et al. 2004). Moreover, apart from having doubts about the effectiveness of the formal steps offered, other obstacles on the way to formalization of end-of-life preferences include the reluctance of families to engage with their elderly members in any discussion of death and preparation for it. Finally, a lack of trust of professionals and lack of support from institutions involved are commonly quoted as barriers to deciding on a specific treatment that one would wish to have or reject at the end of life (Garret et al. 2008).

Hence, it is not surprising that, with so many obstacles in the way of planning for the end of life, aged adults – even those who recognize the importance of the preparation for the end of life – are not often engaged in this practice (Clarke et al. 2012; Kahana et al 2004; Nelson 1979; Seymour et al 2004). More generally, the older people's indecisiveness in terms of planning and preparation for death can be explained partly by the inconclusiveness of the relationships between older people's sense of mortality and their orientations towards death (as discussed in Chapter 2), which translates into the variety and changeability of attitudes towards death.

Attitudes towards death

In the closest life period to death, when old people realize that they are at the end of life, their attitudes towards death vary and can be altered but are not accidental, as they are shaped by cultural and societal contexts and individual circumstances (Clarke et al. 2012; Elias 1985; Latwon 1998). To explore the diversity of and changes in elderly people's attitudes towards death when they know they are at the end of a continuous process that is impossible to stop, we will review the psychological studies of older adults' experiences, feelings and outlooks on death. While acknowledging that the idea of finitude plays a central role in many religious scriptures, and that religion and beliefs in an afterlife often help people to face death, our concern here is with the aged adults in modern Western societies and their attitudes towards death grounded in the frailty and the weariness of their bodies. Hence, while examining the psychological literature on how, at the end of life, the experience of body exhaustion and decline affects old people's attitudes towards death, we will be not considering the impact of religious beliefs on personal attitudes to mortality. Moreover, our focus is not on the fear of abstract death but rather on the situation when, for the aged person, 'death is no longer a general, abstract fate; it is a personal event, an event that is near at hand' (de Beauvoir 1972: 440).

In today's modern, developed society, with the increased longevity that exists, older people live for years confronted by the body weariness and death of family members and friends. Taking into account the diversity and complexity of their individual experiences as well as the heterogeneity of their values, and their cultural and societal contexts, confronting mortality does not translate into one specific and stable attitude towards death. This inconclusiveness of the relationships between older people's sense of mortality and their attitudes to death (as argued in Chapter 2) means that elderly people's attitudes towards death range from being unreconciled with mortality, seeing it natural and not dwelling on it. They pass through stages of denial of death, anxiety and anger to acceptance, waiting for death and finally embracing death (Clarke et al. 2012; Latwon 1998). Because of this diversity, together with a lack of consensual answers to all the major dilemmas raised by death in the philosophical and psychological approaches, the theme of attitudes towards death is too difficult to summarize in any simple way. That is why the main disciplines interested in the topic of death seem to recognize that the subject of attitudes towards death is rather complex and controversial, and comes with many unanswered questions, such as how it is possible to retain the meaning of life in the face of mortality. We will return later to our examination of the importance of sustaining the continuity of purpose when facing up to death, which is the task for philosophers, but first we will check the earlier psychological investigations of older people's attitudes towards death.

The twentieth-century psychological literature and clinical studies of attitudes towards death, because of its lack of concern with older adults' own views, did not shed too much light on the complexity of older persons' attitudes towards death. Until almost the beginning of the twenty-first century, this type of research emphasized fear of death as a negative phenomenon and was concerned with death anxiety across all age categories. The majority of thanatological studies tended to replicate the general conclusion that 'age was negatively correlated with death avoidance, fear and reluctance to interact with the dying' (Nelson 1979: 129). Yet this general negative correlation between age and death fear was never explained; it was only qualified by the finding that the relationship between age and death anxiety may not be linear (Gesser et al. 1987). Despite the importance of the relationship between age and death anxiety, relatively little research was conducted on this topic, and these studies did not contribute much to our understanding the complexity of elderly people's attitudes to death. Their limited outcomes and the narrowness of their perspective can be explained by several factors.

First, the prevailing taboo nature of death and viewing death in old age as 'natural' limited researchers' interest in the experiences of aged and frail people with health issues and a failing body. Second, the predominance of the assumptions that fear of death is 'unavoidable' and that people who are not afraid of death 'are in denial' (Kübler-Ross 1966: 61, 69) narrowed the focus of many psychological and clinical studies on death to a single theme: the fear of death defined as 'an individual psychological coping mechanism' (Zimmermann 2012: 218). Third, the success of thanatological research of older people's attitudes towards death has been challenged by many methodological problems, such as a lack of sound methods for both measuring death anxiety and sampling from the elderly population. Reviewers of the earlier empirical and clinical research concerning the relationship between death anxiety and age also pointed to the difficulties of generalizing from such studies and questioned contrasting conclusions offered by investigations using questionnaires on the one hand, and studies relying structured interview methodologies on the other. All these criticisms of the earlier psychological explorations also showed that that the thanatological studies raised more questions about the nature and extent of death anxiety than they answered, and that they were hindered by definitional problems and a lack of conceptual clarity and simplifications in their comprehension of the notion of fear of death (Clarke et al. 2012; Howarth 1998; Marshall 1986; Neimeyer and van Brunt 1995; Zimmermann 2012).

With the growing understanding that one of the main weaknesses of the psychological studies carried out up to the 1990s was their reliance on an overly simple definition of the term of 'fear of death', more recent investigations have gradually begun to point out that death anxiety may take on various forms. It can present itself as the inability to reconcile to death, or as a feeling of desperation at leaving the future to others, or as the experience of sense of meaninglessness. It may even take the form of a philosophical argument in the favour of the thesis that 'nothing matters'. From the perspective of psychological studies of older people's attitudes towards death, the notion of multidimensionality of fear has increased the research capacity to grasp the various aspects of fear and to differentiate between the fear of ceasing to be, fear of dissolution of the body, fear of the pain of dying, fear of the conditions of dying and fear of affective consequences for survivors (Broom and Cavenaugh 2010; Gott et al 2008; Tomer and Eliason 2013). Yet, while expanding on the complexity of older people's death attitudes, these investigations have still overlooked the dynamic nature of aged persons' relationships with death, while their ill-defined assumptions have limited the scope of their interest and findings. To illustrate these difficulties, we will look at the two main theoretical approaches in the field: the disengagement theory and the terror management theory.

The disengagement theory, which aims to explain how society makes easier for its members to face death in old age, views preparation for death as being achieved through a gradual process of disengagement, seen as being inevitable, universal and triggered by an awareness of proximity to death (Cummings and Henry 1961). It assumes that in later life, bodily restrictions combined with social exclusion render life intolerable and make death an easier experience. Old age, by bringing a greater awareness of the nearness of death, ensures disengagement, which implies acceptance or resignation on the part of elderly people. However, it was soon noticed that being detached from realities of life is not necessarily the only attitude among those who are in death's shadow, and that being on the steep slopes and no longer regarding death from a distance can also lead to a different outlook on the world. In this questioning spirit, many studies demonstrate that for the aged, death is not always about disengagement and resignation (Adams 2020; Clarke et al. 2012; Howarth 1998; Marshall 1980). These critical investigations show how the disengagement theory's assumptions led to overlooking the possibility of alternative developments, such as older people's re-engagement with life in a new manner, and to these studies' lack of the appreciation of cultural and gender differences.

To start with the disengagement theory's first weakness, Howarth (1998: 676), through his interviews with elderly people, established that the majority of people interviewed had not been disengaged from life; on the contrary, most of them 'remained firmly attached to life and spent little time contemplating their own death'. The great diversity of old people's attitudes towards death, from readiness for and acceptance of death to rejection of death, is explained by their quality of life. In other words, 'the more able-bodied and socially active respondents generally reported extensive social contact and had little time for thoughts of death' (Howarth 1998: 676). Moving to the second limitation of the disengagement theory, many critical reviewers observed that, by concentrating on the loss of social roles in later life, this theory failed to acknowledge the role of cultural and gender differences (Arber et al. 2008; Clarke et al. 2012; Hockey 1990; Howarth1998). The disengagement theory, by regarding elderly people as role-limited, ignores the impact of people's professions and interests on their attitude to life and death, overlooks that better off socially and financially more easily continue their engagements and disregard old age as a gendered experience. To some degree, this difference in gendered experience is connected with the fact that, for women, old age is not always accompanied by loss of role engagements or comes with new roles (Hockey 1990; Howarth1998). It is also connected with gendered differences with respect to responses to the loss of quality of life. In contrast to older women, older men were afraid of loss of independence and becoming helpless in the process of increasing physical decline, while emphasizing the importance of being in control of their deaths (Clarke et al. 2012: 1414). Arber et al. (2008), in their interviews with 33 men and 36 women aged from 65 to 93 years, found that in their attitudes towards death and planning for death, older women were 'other-oriented' as they were concerned primarily about not becoming a burden on others, while older men often expressed 'self-oriented ' attitudes as they focused on staying alive for as long as possible, irrespective of the caregiving consequences. Thus, the inattentiveness to the attitudes of older women, negligent of the possibility of the satisfactory living in the present and overlooking of the role of socioeconomic and cultural factors that influenced end-of-life quality, demonstrate many weak points of the disengagement theory.

The limitations of findings by reason of the ill-defined theoretical assumptions also present a weakness in another popular theory that aims to explain people's ways of coming with death: terror management theory. This psychological approach, developed by Greenberg et al. (2004), assumes that fears of death are moulded by a broader system of beliefs about the self, the world and death itself (Tomer and Eliason 2013). The terror management approach assumes that the perception of being close to death may make older adults more prone to be fearful of mortality. As the terror that is associated with an awareness of mortality may cause many negative psychological consequences, the terror management theory emphasizes the necessity of defence against fear of death. Managing the terror produced by the realization that death is inevitable requires the manipulation of the silence, or denial, of death by the construction of feelings of being a valuable and meaningful part of a whole (Tomer and Eliason 2013). Thus, at the core of the theory is the concept of self-esteem, seen as a universal human need that fulfils a protective, buffering function against terror of death. Moreover, the terror management theory de-emphasizes the attitude of acceptance of death not only because its focus on the existential anxiety created by awareness of mortality but also because it assumes that when people are becoming aware of their mortality, they evaluate life as more valuable.

Subsequently, the terror management theory's numerous investigations overlook older people's ability to reconcile themselves with and accept death (Tomer and Eliason 2013). Although, unlike the disengagement theory, the terror management theory recognizes that older people, despite continuing to fear death, are still able to move forward into a manageable relationship with their mortality (Adams 2020), it ignores the attitude of acceptance of death and thus does not shed light on a very diverse social psychological phenomena related to older people's relationship with death (Tomer and Eliason 2013; Walter 2020). Criticisms of the terror management theory have brought to many researchers' attention the need for a theory that will provide a broad integrative framework to illuminate individual differences in orientation to death and the dynamic of older people's attitudes towards death.

In fact, the ancient philosophers had already noted the fluidity and changeability of elderly people's attitudes towards death. For example, Euripides observed that 'the old men complain of their state and say that they long for death: when they are brought to the point they change their minds' (quoted in de Beauvoir 1972: 446). In line with this argument, more recent studies show that changes in attitudes to death are a not uncommon experience in old age and that the aged people's relationships with death are dynamic and learned through situational experiences. By paying increased attention to the dynamic of death attitudes and by demonstrating that some older people fear death, while others are able to reconcile themselves with death, such investigations have developed a more inclusive approach to older people's attitudes towards death. The proposed broader approach offers the opportunity to develop a more comprehensive understanding of the fluidity and diversity of older people's emotions, closely linked with their growing awareness of the brevity of their remaining future (Ardelt 2013; Clarke et al. 2012; Gott et al. 2008; Telnetted and Franklin 2006; Zimmermann 2012).

One such study is Clarke et al.'s (2012) investigation into what happens when older people grasp the inevitability of death and the psychological consequences of this knowledge of finality. To uncover attitudes to death among older people, the authors interviewed 35 people aged 73–91 years with many chronic health problems. (Clarke et al. 2012). Overall, the authors were 'struck by the resilience and selflessness that many of our participants displayed irrespective of their chronic health issues and social and physical losses' (Clarke et al. 2012: 1413). Most participants described how they had begun to confront death on a regular basis as an increasing number of people in their social circles had died. The study showed that older people's awareness of finitude results in various and changeable attitudes towards death. Some of those interviewed perceived death as a welcome, 'if not longed for, end to their suffering and to their being a burden on their spouses and other family members' (Clarke et al. 2012: 1413). Other participants, while stressing the importance of acceptance of death, found that 'the pervasiveness of death in their social circles the inevitability of dying made them grateful for each remaining day they had' (Clarke et al. 2012: 1413). Several of the older people interviewed reported a change in their relationship with death, particularly pointing to a growing fear of a bad death, defined in terms of a loss of autonomy as the result of the failure of their body or mind. The majority of participants were pragmatic about their mortality and emphasized the need to recognize and accept death as inevitable, while appreciating life much more. In contrast to the disengagement theory, the study demonstrated that, despite the physical realities of having multiple chronic conditions and despite their awareness of mortality, older people were not passive or disengaged from living, 'but rather focused their attention and energy on the enjoyment of the present' (Clarke et al. 2012: 1401). Moreover, in contrast to the theory of terror management, the research found that some participants 'viewed death as a welcome release from intolerable suffering and others anticipated their ending as an opportunity to reunite with their spouses in the afterlife or to relieve their still living spouses from the burden of care-giving' (Clarke et al. 2012: 1401).

In a similar vein, while stressing that death does not wear the same face in all societies and cultures, and that the problem of fear of death was traditionally the province of religion, other recent studies confirm the variety of older people's attitudes towards death. They also recognize that attitudes towards death are influenced by the perceived proximity of death, shaped by the individual attitude to life and assert that the end of life is an event that prompts many to ask questions about the meaning of life and to search for spiritual answers. While bringing to our attention the challenge of death to the meaning of life, these investigations emphasize that 'a personal relationship to death in old age is dynamic and capable of many moments of deliberation and multiple shifts in perspective' (Ardelt 2013: 153). The weight of research evidence suggests that, although there is a general tendency for fear of death to diminish with increasing age, neither the absence nor the presence of fear of death in older age is universal and people do not hold only one attitude towards death when 'living in a shadow of death' (Abel 2017; Adams 2020; Ardelt 2013; Zimmermann 2012).

To sum up the psychological studies, older individuals' relations with death are complex, dynamic and difficult to summarize as these attitudes are changeable and not determined in advance, and as everyone adopts them in accordance with their present situation, including their perception of the body weariness, as well as with their former experiences and former choices. The studies convey the combination of engagement and disengagement endured by most of the aged in living their final days, and depict their attitudes to death as ranging from denial, through meditation, to overall meanings, to acceptance of death and offering comfort. If there is any consensus within all psychological studies of older people's attitudes to death, it is the recognition that it is never easy to make a peace with the inevitability of death (Kellehear 2009; Marshall 1980; Walter 2020). As in the psychological studies of attitudes towards death and the philosophical literature, where the problem of death has been central from its beginning, there is no unified, single approach to the relationship between old age and acceptance of death.

Despite its task being 'learning how to die' (Socrates, quoted in Small 2007: 110), philosophy presents us with a diversity of views, with some philosophers arguing that in old life death is more desired than life, while many others reject the view that ageing makes death more tolerable (as discussed in Chapter 2). Even today, the philosophical literature is full of contradictory views on death anxiety. As 'to philosophize is to prepare for death' (Cicero, quoted in Tomer and Eliason 2013: 25), we witness the continuation of philosophical debates over whether death should be conceived as a threat to the meaning of life or as an incentive to deepen its meaning, with some arguing that death gives meaning to life as it sustains our confidence in the importance of what we value (Hägglund 2012), others maintaining that it poses a threat to meaning (Sartre 1965) and yet still more wondering whether the meaning of life could be found in the very act of facing up to death (Camus 2005).

All approaches discussed – both psychological and philosophical – realize that when age and illness cause people to recognize that death will soon interrupt the permanence of life, people are confronted with one of the most difficult moments of their lives. The confrontation with death is even more difficult during not so 'normal' times – that is, during catastrophes or wars or pandemics. Although acceptance of the inevitability of death has never been painless and effortless, reconciling with death during the COVID-19 pandemic was even more challenging, as this health crisis created new challenges for aged people's ability to face up to death.

The pandemic and existential dread

After our examination of the variety of elderly people's attitudes towards death and their ways of preparing for the end of life under normal conditions, in the last part of Chapter 7 we will look at how the pandemic – which has made dying a more unexpected, medical, statistical, lonely and depersonalized event – has impacted older people's outlook on death. Since it is 'not actually death itself that arouses fear and terror but the anticipatory image of death' (Elias 1985: 44), the picture of death associated with the COVID-19 pandemic, which gave prominence to a loss of control, loneliness, uncertainty and risk, could have generated fears and anxieties for many older people. Confronting the end of life in a context of restrictions, shielding, loneliness, limitations and risks connected with the pandemic became an even more difficult, austere and complex procedure than in normal times. In short, during the pandemic, vulnerable elderly people have been facing and experiencing a new level of existential dread.

The coronavirus pandemic, like all pandemics, has preyed on 'fears, both legitimate and illegitimate' and enlarged not only practical and financial hardships but also psychological problems for many people (Baker et al. 2020). The pandemic has increased the visibility of death and has introduced a high level of risk and uncertainty, particularly to the lives of the oldest and most vulnerable people in society. During the COVID-19 health crisis, charities and care specialists encouraged elderly people to talk to loved ones about their wishes if they were to become critically ill with coronavirus, and to 'let people know' their requests in advance (Hospice UK 2002). As a result of being urged to have 'difficult conversations' about the risk connected with COVID-19, more older people than usual attempted to arrange their final matters – for example, many wrote their wills (Smith 2020). These actions were undertaken despite the fact that during the pandemic elderly people did not have many opportunities and possibilities to plan, formally regulate emergent problems and arrange legal documents describing preferred medical care and treatments. Apart from the lack of usual support from local organizations, such as Age UK and other charities, which were not offering any face-to-face services during the pandemic, another barrier faced by the aged in their attempts to arrange their final matters was the fact that the significant proportion of them were unable to go online. More precisely, in the United Kingdom among those aged over 75, two people out of five (40% of 2.2 million) do not use the internet (Age UK 2021). Still the risk connected with coronavirus led larger than usual number of older people to seek contacts, information and help in arranging their affairs via the internet (Age UK 2021). However, while prompting many elderly people to organize Zoom meetings with relatives and write their wills, the COVID-19 crisis also took from many the possibility of designing their last service. Even Prince Philip's funeral did not go as he had planned. Because of the COVID-19 restrictions, the ceremony was attended by only 30 of his family and closest friends, instead of the planned 800 people (Adams 2021). Hence, as COVID-19 overwhelmed and weakened the functioning of many services, including funeral and health systems, not many older people were successful in, or even concerned with, planning arrangements for the end of life.

During the pandemic, fears of the unknown and anxiety about the ambiguities of COVID-19 left many elderly people's psychological need for protection unfulfilled. Normally, people cope with uncertainty by settling on 'narratives' that, by combining certainty and uncertainty, are able to camouflage high levels of uncertainty (Didion 2012). Yet the COVID-19 crisis only produced a story of high uncertainty – that is, a narrative that was incapable of helping people to deal with their fear of death. While in normal times the existential anxiety created by an awareness of mortality maybe reconciled by 'taming of time' and 'taming of death' (Christensen and Willerslev 2013), during the pandemic, elderly people were deprived of narratives that could had provided a buffer against death anxiety enlarged by the new risks. The story around death was no longer a narrative about the need to exercise control to the end, or a wish to plan for death; rather, it was about the new risk of the coronavirus, which disallowed any possibility of undertaking a project of 'good death'. Older people, in addition to a sense of the anguish driven by the puzzlement that 'it takes sixty years of incredible suffering and effort to make such an individual, and then he is good only for dying' (Malraux, quoted in Becker 1973: 269), experienced new existential dread connected with fear that their death could be depersonalized and nothing more than a part of 'the pandemic statistics', thus not of great concern and unimportant, and that their death could exposed their own insignificance. The perception of death as being a less unexpected and more 'impersonal' event and the absence of reassuring narratives may have negatively impacted older people's psychological wellbeing by undermining their feelings of self-esteem or self-regard (Age UK 2022).

The importance of self-esteem, as emphasized by the terror management theory (discussed above), is associated with its buffering function against terror of death. Some philosophers also connect fear of death with the realization of how easily someone can be replaced after their death and view a positive self-evaluation of their life as an important protection against death denial and death anxiety (Kolakowski 2021; Tomer and Eliason Grafton 2013). In normal circumstances, fear of death caused by unsettling questions about one's sense of worth and by anxiety about being overlooked in one's death can be controlled by some protective narratives, yet in the crisis situation people's feeling of desperation at leaving the future to others not only increases fear of death but may lead to rebellion against death, including suicidal thoughts (Amery 1994). Following these ideas, it can be argued that during the COVID-19 pandemic, elderly people experienced increased existential anxiety and fear of death and such mental states and feelings had many negative psychological consequences. During the coronavirus crisis, when people were presented with daily headlines about death, and when thinking about the new risks could not have been avoided, older people often could not avoid feeling that in their death, if it happened, they would be only a part of the bigger statistics of the COVID-19 deceased. In short, the pandemic created an intense environment of anxiety in which the elderly's distress and uncertainty about the future increased significantly.

In terms of the mental health of aged people during COVID-19, even more detrimental than the narrative of self-esteem was loneliness – which even in non-crisis times is often considered to be one of the main problems of older people. However, it is worth remembering that loneliness is not unique to old age and that even during the lockdowns, it also tormented young people who were left at homes to cope with the closure of schools. Nonetheless, older people – who were expected to shield during the COVID-19 crisis, had problems with filling the empty days and experienced the death of friends or family members – suffered profoundly from a lack of contact with others. Although there are some beneficial effects of freely chosen loneliness or solitude, 'solitude imposed by others is a totally different matter' (Storr 1997: 42). The limitations, of the lockdowns, like other solitary restrictions, unleashed a crisis of loneliness, caused some disruptions to normal mental functioning and led to feelings of alienation and anxiety. While there were already 1.4 million chronically lonely older people in England – or around one in twelve people aged 50 and over in England who were often lonely – by September 2021, more than five million older people said they were feeling lonely (Age UK 2021). During the pandemic, all these features of loneliness, such as being without others, suffering anxiety, coping with painful experience of loss of loved ones and the harsh realities of facing bereavement alone, contributed to an increase in older people's feelings of existential despair. The experience of loneliness during the pandemic disproportionately affected people with low incomes and health issues and those from ethnic minorities; as the Age UK (2021) report on loneliness found, around a quarter of Black and South Asian older people experienced an increase in their feelings of loneliness during the pandemic. In short, the pandemic left many older people – especially from ethnic and lower income groups – feeling anxious, depressed and fearful about the future.

The Age UK (2021) research concluded that the pandemic 'is associated with worse physical and mental health in older people'. In other words, older people's loneliness during the coronavirus had a significant impact on their mental health and general wellbeing. Although there is not yet a full picture of the mental costs of the pandemic, the Age UK studies and new figures from the Office of National Statistics (2022) show a dramatic rise in the number of people suffering mental problems since the start of the pandemic. The Office of National Statistics report estimates that about 800,000 more people suffered from mental health problems in 2020–21 than in 2018–19. The findings of other British studies demonstrate that during the pandemic mental health worsened across all social groups and that although pensioners – unlike the people faced with loss of work and income – did not report being in poor mental health because of financial problems, their wellbeing declined because of other factors, such as loneliness, lower levels of medical support and security (Butler 2021). The Age UK 2020–21 Annual Report (Age UK 2022), which looked at the pandemic years, emphasized that for older people living during the unprecedented times caused 'the immense fear and anxiety'. Describing the COVID-19 pandemic as a 'trying time' of immense challenge and change 'catastrophic years', 'deeply traumatic' and a 'difficult time' for elderly people, the report stressed that 'the pandemic continues to cast a long shadow over many people's lives'. This report, while summarizing research into the impact of the pandemic on the elderly, pointed out that elderly people had deteriorated much more quickly than anyone expected and that they struggled with many problems, from practical to mental issues. The older adults talked about living with the risk of the virus and the pain of loneliness; one in four older people said that during the pandemic they lived in more pain, while one in three of the elderlies declared that they were more anxious during the pandemic and observed that they had lost motivation to do the things they enjoyed in the past (Age UK 2022). If we consider the level of social inequality in the United Kingdom, with 2.1 million pensioners living in poverty and with pensioners from ethnic communities being twice as likely to live in poverty, and that the pandemic disproportionately affected people with lower incomes, health issues and from ethnic minorities, it can be concluded that 'these people are unlikely to recover easily from the physical and emotional impacts of the pandemic' (Age UK 2021, 2022).

A survey carried out in the United States, which asked Americans to describe in their own words the pandemic's impact on their lives, did not discover any clear pattern of experiences or any 'typical' experience' (van Kessel et al. 2022). While showing that nine in ten Americans pointed to at least one change for the worse in their lives and 28% of those interviewed implied that their physical or mental health had deteriorated, the study concluded that the pandemic affected ordinary Americans' lives in a variety of ways, and there was no clear overall pattern (van Kessel et al. 2022). However, while remembering that three-quarters of all COVID-19 deaths in the United States were in people aged 65 and older (Zhang 2022), we compare the answers given by younger Americans with those given by their older co-patriots. For example, younger Americans were more likely than older Americans to mention positive developments in their social and intimate relationships: 40% of adults under 50 did so, while just a quarter (25%) of those aged 50 years and older described improvements to their relationships (van Kessel et al. 2022). Some 45% of those aged 65 years and older said the pandemic forced them to remain isolated at home or otherwise unable to enjoy their normal routines in their older years, while only 27% of those aged under 50 described similar difficulties (van Kessel et al. 2022). Another commonality in the Americans' evaluation of the COVID-19 period was their realization that society 'had gone downhill', that the epidemic posed serious challenges for the healthcare system and that it deepened faultlines in the American nation (Morris 2022: 66). The other survey carried out in the United States during the Omicron wave, which was far deadlier there than in other Western nations, also shows that older people were among those groups whose situation was worsened by loneliness, financial problems and difficulties accessing medical services. By February 2022, the United States also lagged behind other countries in terms of its elderly people's overall vaccination and third booster rates, which were 88.5% and 65% respectively (Zhang 2022).

A common theme in all studies of elderly people in the context of COVID-19 is the high level of anxiety suffered by the aged due to the prolonged lockdowns, loneliness and uncertainty about their health status (Khademi et al. 2020). The pandemic's long-term consequences, such as loneliness, depression, loss of control and of meaning, disrupted routines and activities – all factors altering mental health – are also identified as risk factors for suicidal behaviour, which even before the pandemic was not uncommon among older people (Jain et al. 2021). In the years leading to the COVID-19 crisis, the rate of suicide among males aged 75 and over was the highest in nearly all industrialized countries; moreover, among many of these nations, suicide rates increase with age (the website intended for UK healthcare professionals (GP Notebook 2022). In the United Kingdom, the highest number of suicides for many years was among men aged over 70 (Wolpert 2011: 229). Japan has the highest rates of suicide in the world (Jason 2015: 3), while in the United States, where older adults make up 12% of the population, their suicides account for 18% of all suicide deaths. In France over the last decade, an average of around

3000 citizens over the age of 65 took their own life each year, 'a figure not to be neglected insofar as ageing persons make up 20% of the population yet account for 28% of all suicides' (Drouillard 2016: 57). Yet, even though the rate of suicide among older men is high, suicides among the elderly tend to be under-reported, and many 'silent suicides' (such as deaths from overdoses, self-starvation or dehydration) are simply overlooked.

There is little literature on suicide among older adults. On the one hand, some qualitative studies are based on personal interviews with elderly people without any history of suicide attempts; these discovered that for the older adult, suicide was a 'rational, active choice that they intended to exercise when they felt the timing was right, rather than an indicator of suicidal ideation or pervasive depression' (Clarke et al. 2012: 1414). On the other hand, the literature on suicide among older adults that focuses on suicide attempters concludes that suicide risk is correlated with depression, social isolation, loneliness and functional decline (Jain et al. 2021). The same risk factors were very visible during the pandemic, and were shared by many older adults – especially elderly people who were shielding at home, were unable to meet others and often experienced personal loss. Since loneliness, depression and loss of control are themes preceding suicide attempts (Jain et al. 2021), it is not surprising that there are already some evidence of the increased suicide rates among people who were the most affected by the pandemic – for example, in Poland it was reported that there was a significant increase in the suicide rate among two groups – older people and young students – during the pandemic (*Gazeta Wyborcza,* 2 February 2022).

To sum up, the COVID-19 pandemic negatively impacted older people's wellbeing and mental health. In the United Kingdom, from the end of February 2022, with the removal of all main restrictions and with the successful vaccination program – with more than 90% of Britain's elderly population being vaccinated with their third jab or booster (Zhang 2022) – and with new medical treatments, including anti-virals, the situation has improved markedly. Yet, even in mid-2022, with all restrictions lifted, the pandemic has not gone away but continues to be a source of anxiety and fear for many elderly people, especially those with underlying health conditions.

CHAPTER 8

Handling the last stage

Modern death

This chapter will discuss dying when the old person is aware of the impending death and still has a chance to maintain some control and to 'make death proud to take us' (Shakespeare, *Antony and Cleopatra*, quoted in O'Hagan 2020: 158), while Chapter 9 will be concerned with the end of life of older persons who struggle with cognitive disabilities, particularly with dementia and Alzheimer's disease. First, this chapter will examine the fundamental features of modern death, seen as shaped by of the scientization of and technological advances in medicine. After discussing the dilemmas connected with the realities of the medicalization of death, we focus on the impact of the institutionalization of death on elderly people's experience of dying and explore dying within contemporary hospitals, hospices and at home. In the last part of the chapter, we examine what happened to the modern death when COVID-19 governed how people die.

In contemporary Western societies, with the growing influence of medicine in shaping the conditions of death and with the secularization of culture, the main discourse about death is medical and secular (Walter 2020). Although the ways in which people die in old age vary, reflecting a range of physical and mental conditions as well as cultural, gender, educational, economic and race characteristics, there are still some general commonalities in the way modern dying occurs. These are mainly because modern death is controlled and managed through medical institutions and infrastructures (McManus 2013). Because of the prevalence of the biomedical model of death, which ensures medicine's dominance over dying and death, death is seen as a health issue, which medical expertise is needed to address. Still, death differs from person to person, not only because of dying people's characteristics but also because the technological advances in medicine provide individuals at the end of life with new options for medical intervention or additional choices of treatment. Today, with an increasingly large and diverse range of medical professionals managing the dying process and new levels of medical intervention and treatment, we have created a method of modern dying that typically takes place in later life, and that is prolonged, institutionalized, medicalized and sequestered.

The concept of a modern death is well illustrated by Julian Barnes (2009) in his memoir *Nothing to be Frightened Of*, where he depicts the death of his 82 years old father, whose decline had stretched over years. Barnes (2009: 9) observers that his father 'died a modern death, in hospital, without his family, attended in his final minutes by a nurse, months – indeed, years – after medical science had prolonged his life to a point where the terms on which it was being offered were unimpressive'. This description of a modern death brings to our attention the general features of this way of dying, such as the loneliness and medicalization of the hospital death of the elderly person, who is dying of a multiplicity of ailments rather than a single and specific disease, and who usually retains full cognitive capacity until the last day. Before the twentieth century, death was different, not only because dying individuals were younger and because death occurred in people's homes, but also because it was the priest who was called upon to help the dying person, who usually was attended by family members.

Until the twentieth century in the United Kingdom, as in other Western countries, the majority of people died at home; however, by the late 1980s, over 60% of people died in hospital settings (McManus 2013: 44). A more recent study of death in England, where in 2017 almost 70% of all deaths were of people over 75 years of age, confirms the role of hospital in the last year of life of the elderly (Dalrymple et al. 2020). People aged 75 years and older spent more than four weeks in hospital during the last year of life, and their hospital admissions for in the last year of life represented 22.2% of all admissions, despite people aged 75 years and older only representing 8.2% of the population (Dalrymple et al. 2020). Although not all older adults are sick at the end of life and not all are experiencing symptoms of illness, as both general medical and gerontological research tell us, the majority of old people at the end of life suffer physical discomfort, difficulty breathing, weakening of mental capabilities, existential anxiety and growing frailty; they are also increasingly dependent on care (Carr and Luth 2019; Gawande 2015; Hockey 1990). The way modern medicine cares for and treats those who are most vulnerable, and the capacity of today's medicines to relieve pain mean that the most of frail elderly people who die in the hospital 'do so after several days of syringe-driver-induced oblivion' (O'Mahony 2016: 3).

However, over the last several decades, the main features of modern death in old age, although still shaped by the hospital culture's conception of dying as the prerogative of medical experts, have been changing as a result of debates about the medicalization of death and changes in how we determine that somebody is dead. Hence, before we debate the idea a modern death any further, we will look briefly at the transformation of the definition of death and at consequences of the criticism of the medicalization of death. Even though many of us still tend to think, like Shakespeare's King Lear, 'I know death when I see it', we also know that the law requires a more clear-cut definition of death, and that such a definition should be provided by a medical professional. In the past, a mirror was held up to a dying person's mouth and when the mirror ceased to fog, the person was dead. Later, a stethoscope was used to determine cessation of a heartbeat and therefore death. This traditional biological understanding of death, seen as occurring when an individual ceases breathing or when their heart stops beating, was accepted as an adequate conception of death for many decades. For generations, physicians ascertained death after the fact: based on the absence of a heartbeat and breathing and on the basis of the confirmed and persistent absence of these vital signs, the person was to be declared dead (Nelds 1995). More recently, though, new waves of transformations in defining death, brought about by the most fundamental advances in life-sustaining technology and organ transplantations, have led to a revision of the legal definition of death and a review of the main standards or benchmarks of death.

From the last decades of the twentieth century, the irreversible destruction of the brain, which entails the inability to regain consciousness or the capacity to breathe without support, has become the main criterion of death. By 1993, the United States and almost all other nations had adopted a whole-brain definition of death (Troyer 2020; Veatch 1995). Today in the United States and the majority of other countries, in order to be declared legally dead, there must be incontrovertible evidence that the brain has permanently ceased to function. Only some cultures, including Orthodox Jewish, Native American and Japanese, reject this because of a discomfort involved in regarding someone as dead if they are still breathing, whether artificially assisted or not (Wicks 2017). The brain death criteria has been somewhat modified in the United Kingdom, where both the clinical and legal emphasis is on brain stem death. As destruction of the brain stem is irreversible and it is the last part of the brain to be affected by a lack of oxygen, the brain stem is seen as a sign of death rather than dying. 'Brain stem death (BSD) has been accepted by the courts in the United Kingdom as the legal definition of death' (Wicks 2017: 121). Similarly, the NHS website announces that 'brain death (also known as brain stem death) is when a person on an artificial life support machine no longer has any brain functions' and asserts that 'a person who is brain dead is legally confirmed as dead'. In other words, if someone's brain is dead, the damage is irreversible, and thus, according to UK law, the person has died.

The acceptance of the equivalence of brain stem death as the definition of death has been abetted by various practical pressures pushing for this consensus. Two factors are central to these practical considerations: the development of transplant medicine and the cost of intensive care. If someone's brain is dead and, according to UK law, the person has therefore died, the state can lawfully withdrawal life-sustaining treatment in the case of people in a persistent vegetative state. This removal of life-sustaining treatment, after the pronouncement that the brain damage is irreversible, could allow for the transplantation of organs and reduce many costs associated with the prolongation of life. The advancements in medical technology and the development of intensive care medicine, such as the introduction of assisted ventilation, life-sustaining treatment and heart-bypass machines, and transplantation of the heart and other organs, have produced increasing complexity of the understanding of death and have blurred the line between dying and death (Troyer 2020; Wicks 2017).

Even more importantly, the application in hospitals of medical technologies and medical interventions has also shaped 'particular forms of dying' (Kaufman 2005: 9). These developments in medical science and technology have not only postponed dying to older age and made the process of dying more gradual and slower; they have also increased the scope for explicit human decisions about alternative treatments and about the timing of death. Moreover, as these difficult decisions about the treatments and the extent of interventions are made not only by medical professionals but also by patients, the process of dying is undergoing further transformations (Gawande 2015). The medical technologies have put enormous pressure on medical staff to employ the most sophisticated technologies, and on patients and their families to make choices among the available technologies (Kaufman 2005). With many hospitalized old people opting for assertive medical treatments, and with frail old patients 'ending up' in an intensive care unit, hospitals maybe improving their death statistics for days or weeks, but such situations result in confusion about the line 'between some ideal notion of "humane" end-of-life care and aggressive medical intervention that delays death' (Kaufman 2005: 39).

The medicalization of dying, as discussed in Chapter 6, has been questioned since the publication of Illich's (1976) *Limits to Medicine* onwards. The criticism of the medical model of death for dehumanization of dying in the modern hospital, and for the failure of the experiment of making mortality a medical experience, are now commonly accepted. These acknowledged negative evaluations of the medicalization of death point out that many decades of medicine's focus on living longer and 'fighting death' have made death into an affair controlled by medicine, a situation in which dying old people are marginalized and disempowered by the authority of experts (Howarth 2007: 29). This criticism is supported by the growing amount of evidence that the system of technological medical care has failed to meet dying people's needs, and that medical professionals have overlooked the fact that people with serious illness have other priorities besides simply prolonging their lives (Gawande 2015; Howarth 2007; Kaufman 2005). In short, hospital culture that frames death as a 'negative outcome' is criticized for not being well equipped to serve the dying (O'Mahony 2016: xii). The disapproval is especially directed at the failure to care for frail elderly people as a result of seeing death of the aged in hospital 'almost exclusively as the end point of effective medical treatment' (Kaufman 2005: 82).

As studies show, older people dying in hospitals are less likely to be told about their approaching death because the likelihood of reviling a fatal verdict to patients declines with the patient's age and because doctors in their prognosis for the aged tend to be rather evasive about disclosing terminal diagnosis to frail old persons. Physicians therefore navigate the tangled relationship between old age and disease (Howarth 2007). Consequently, for older people, one of the most important dimensions of hospital culture is 'how waiting happens, how it is experienced and how it is both integral to and disruptive of the pathway' (Kaufman 2005: 148). Apart from waiting and suffering, another element of hospital culture that undermines the comfort of the aged at the end of life is a lack of continuity of medical care as a result of too-frequent moves of elderly people from one medical institution to another. For frail elderly patients who value the continuity of care, the fact they are in and out of hospital as one crisis (such as pneumonia) succeeds another (such as a fall) and they experience an average of three 'transitions' from one healthcare setting to another at the end of life, can be very disturbing (Walter 2017: 24). As a result of such movements, the dying moments of many elderly people are spent with 'neither loved ones nor dignity, but instead involve being treated like a package in transit' (Clarke 2020: 124).

As dying in today's hospitals still very often does not come close to the manner of the dying person's choosing, some argue that modern medicine has failed dying people 'so spectacularly that we have reached the point of actively inflicting harm on patients rather than confronting the subject of mortality' (Gawande 2015: 178). However within the critical approach to the medicalization of dying, two points are worth noting. First, within this broad critical perspective, we need to note the actuality of acknowledgement of the complexity and difficulty of the topic of death. The growing realization that the medicalization of death is causing some negative consequences and the continuation of questioning of the impact of the over-interventionist approach to death has led to the recognition that a single approach has no place within frameworks for managing the end of life, given that people die in various ways and that we all need to find our own way to deal with mortality (Carr and Luth 2019; Clarke 2020; O'Mahony 2016). Second, it is important to notice that none of the critics of the medicalization of dying rejects the central role of the physician in pain and symptom management. They all accept the need for medicine when the dying person physically deteriorates and they recognize that dying is firmly placed within the medical framework, as apart from sudden death, dying is managed by health professionals (Walter 2017). As for the majority of people who die aged 80 or older from disabling, chronic and degenerative diseases, the end of life is a 'protracted period of time shaped by the unpredictable trajectories of dying' (Tigge 2020: 2), so they need medical help. During their last month of life, frail elderly people need physical comfort, relief from pain and reduction of suffering as one-half to two-thirds of them experience pain, which is rated by one-third of them as moderate or severe pain (Carr and Luth 2019: 517).

Attempts to eliminate pain and suffering are offered by health professionals to elderly people on the range of trajectories for dying: from a lingering death from common diseases, through intermittent dying, which implies a move onwards followed by slow improvement, before rapidly going down again towards death, to a dwindling dying trajectory that is unpredictable, encompassing accumulated and multiple health problems and implies gradual decline with high but fluctuating disability levels (Nicholson et al. 2012; Samarel 1995). While recognizing the diversity and ambiguity of dying trajectories in old age, or 'the ambiguous dying syndrome' (Bern-Klug 2004), or 'an uncertain and dwindling process of dying' (Nicholson et al. 2012: 1426), health professionals do not propose a return to the pre-modern world when painkillers and other medical assistance were not available. In short, it is not medicalization *per se* that is seen as a negative phenomenon; rather, the problem is 'over-medicalization' (Howarth 2007: 121). By emphasizing that the old age decline is the inevitable ingredient of the human condition that leads to the end of life, the growing visibility of the new life-course stage, which Carr and Luth (2019) label 'the end of life', has brought to public attention the need a for a more holistic system to deal with the end of life.

Although the criticism of the dominant medical discourse of death has led to many attempts to develop such a holistic approach to death, because of the complexity of the ontological, ethical and cultural issues involved, death remains 'not unambiguous' (Wicks 2017: 131). Even though our traditional understanding of death has been altered by debates and developments in medical science and technology, the decline of the importance of religious structures and the culture of individualism, death continues to be seen as a mystifying aspect of human existence. The ongoing ethical debates about death and dying show how law and biomedical ethics are becoming increasingly intertwined, and how blurred the distinctions between life and death, and the ambiguity of where ageing ends and disease begins, have become. With medical advancements allowing individuals to make decisions about the prolongation of life and the timing of death, people are now presented with new dilemmas and questions about death. The growing rate of intensive care unit use in the last month of life is increasing, and there is a need to rethink whether frail elderly people should be subjected to futile and painful medical treatments (Carr and Lutz 2019). We should also search for an answer to the question of whether the lawful withdrawal of life-sustaining treatment is 'ethically appropriate, morally good, and respectful of the human being's rights' (Wicks 2017: 130).

The ambiguity in our thinking about death in old age is still reflected in modern hospital culture's lack of endorsement of taking care of dying patients' needs other than their medical requirements, while at the same time making the prevention of death the main priority of health professional. The realization of this ambiguity in our thinking about death in old age and the imprecision involved in defining the relationship between being old and the end of life may challenge the implicit medical practice of resisting futility. While the medical rhetoric that constitutes death as a technical failure has led some health and care professionals to identify death as 'an enemy to combat', with the new narrative of death as 'a meaningful conclusion' marked by dignity and spirituality, many physicians realize that death in old age is a difficult topic to 'confront honestly and directly' (Carr and Luth 2019: 518).

Hence, as the attempts to de-medicalize the process of dying have prompted more honest and direct engagements with death in old age, an increased number of people in the final stage of life opt for less depersonalized and less medicalized death. Yet the emerging new craft of dying still mainly applies within the palliative and hospice care systems, while at the same time the hospital remains the main place of death for the elderly. Nonetheless, the waves of the institutionalization of death are transforming where people die and the ways in which they experience death. Therefore in what follows we will be discussing their impact, paying special attention to the impact of the last wave of institutionalization of death on the complexity of the modern death dilemma.

Where old people die

By looking at the past and present waves of the institutionalization of dying, seen as 'transfer of the old, ill, and dying to care facilities and hospitals, as the displacement of dying and death from everyday life and as connected to the societal taboo of age, illness, dying, and death' (Lang 2020: 1), we will further develop our understanding of a modern death. After a compact presentation of historical changes in the main places of death for the elderly, we will examine places of dying other than hospital that are available for today's elderly people and discuss the conditions and dilemmas of dying at home and in a hospice.

Over the last two centuries, alongside the economic growth and expansion of medical systems, Western countries have been moving through three stages of the institutionalization of dying (Gawande 2015). During the first stage, which lasted until the twentieth century, with the majority of death taking place in people's homes, dying at home was a normal occurrence. For example, in Canada before the last century, the vast majority of death occurred in people's homes; this was also the case in the United States. In the United Kingdom around 1900, most people also died in their own homes (McManus 2013: 44). In the second stage of institutionalization, which was very visible from the mid-twentieth century, there was a substantial increase in the number of deaths in hospitals. For instance, in Canada the rates of death in hospitals escalated from the 1930s to 1966, reaching a peak in 1994, with 80% of all deaths taking place in hospitals (McManus 2013: 44). In the United States in 1958, 61 percent of Americans died in hospitals and in 1977it was 70% (Nuland 1993: 255). By 1980, just 17% of Americans died at home and in the 1990s, 80% of American deaths occurred in hospitals (Nuland 1993: 255), while in the United Kingdom by the late 1980s, over 60% of people died in hospitals (O'Mahony 2016: x).

The second stage of institutionalization of dying was brought about by several factors, such as developments in medical technology, the process of secularization, the fragmentation and reduction of the size of the family unit and changes in occupational structures (Broom 2015). In this phase, dying people were offered a clear script for dying, as adopting the strictly clinical perspective was perceived as a way of improving access to specialized facilities and personnel, while the cultural symbolism of sequestering the dying was seen as meaningful part of the 'civilizing process' (Elias 1994). In other words, the increase in the institutionalization of death in the second stage occurred not only because so many of the dying required high level of acute care that could be only provided in hospitals, but also because the institutionalization was seen as the essential aspect of progress and as the critical element of the process of expanding of the control of bodily functions, emotions and instincts.

Since the beginning of the twenty-first century, modern Western countries have been moving to the third stage in the institutionalization of dying, which is characterized by a shift away from an institutionalized death and a growing trend towards dying at home, although with support from institutions (Gawande 2015). In this third phase, in many developed European countries, the likelihood of home death has increased; these nations' polices of physician support, hospice and palliative care at home have resulted in 'the fairly high percentage of people dying at home ranging between 20 to 30% and shifts of death from hospitals to retirement homes' (Thonnes and Jakoby 2013: 15). In the United Kingdom, the rate of death at home has also been rising – for instance, in England between 2004 and 2016, the percentage of deaths in homes increased by 0.7% and in 2016 nearly a quarter of all deaths in England (23.5%) occurred in people's own homes, while the percentage of deaths in hospital fell by 11% from 57.9% to 46.9% (Gov UK 2018). In the United States, where a significant majority of Americans negatively evaluate solitary death in hospital, the percentage of people dying in hospitals declined from 32.6% in 2000 to 24.6% in 2009 (Shapiro 2019: 125). As a result of the significant majority of Americans rejecting a view of death as the prerogative of experts and hoping to die at home, by 2010 some 45% of Americans were dying in hospice care at home (Gawande 2015: 193).

The current phase of institutionalization of dying is the result of new developments in medical science and technology, a rise in life expectancy and the emergence of new cultural values, secularization, growing affluence and weakening kinship ties. In the context of these changes, together with the growing expectation and recognition of a need to improve treatment of the dying, Western nations have moved towards a new approach to the medical management of chronic and degenerative diseases and the dying. 'In the third stage of institutionalization as a country's income climbs to the highest levels, people have the means to become concerned about the quality of their lives, even in sickness, and deaths at home actually rise again' (Gawande 2015: 192). In contrast to the second stage, in this last wave of institutionalization of dying, people are presented with more choices, and increased importance is attached to allowing people to die in the place of their choice. There is also an increased likelihood of home death and of dying at home with hospice care. In short, the choices and decisions offered to a dying person are now more plentiful but also less simple (Carr and Luth 2019; Gawande 2015; Lang 2020). In this recent phase, the 'business of deliberating on your options – figuring out your priorities and working with a doctor to match your treatment to them' is considerably more complicated and exhausting (Gawande 2015: 220).

Unlike the previous phases, the third phase of institutionalization does not offer a well-defined and simple script for dying as the choices it provides for dying persons are not without unknowns and ambiguities. In other words, 'this is an unsettled time, we have begun rejecting the institutionalization version of ageing and death, but we have not yet established our new norm' (Gawande 2015: 193). Moreover, this unsettled time has added to the complexities of the modern death not only a set of new ambiguities and a lack of clear script for dying, but also several new features connected with unmet expectations. First, in the recent wave of institutionalization of dying in Western European countries, places of death are not distributed at random but reflect social factors, such as gender, socio-economic status and the degree of urbanization that have shaped people's capacity to choose their place of death (Lang 2020; Thonnes and Jakoby 2013). In the United States, the rates of dying at home also varies by race, with around 40% of Black people, but just 25–30% of White people, dying in institutions (Carr and Luth 2019: 522). In the United Kingdom, dying at home 'has become a kind of middle-class ideal'; hence, it is 'not suitable for everyone' (O'Mahony 2016: 121). Second, in the third stage of institutionalization, death in old age is marked by the fact that the gains achieved by the end-of-life care and hospice movements are often not easily available; they are not only unequally distributed, but there is a shortage of places in hospice or palliative care facilities for the dying in the majority of Western countries (Thonnes and Jakoby 2013). Third, despite the majority of people wishing to die at home, and despite the decline in the percentage of people dying in hospitals in the last few decades, half of older people still die in hospitals. For example, in England around 70% of people would prefer to die at home, yet 42.8% of those aged 85 years and over die in hospital (Tigge 2020: 2).

These three characteristics of today's situation can been seen as an indication that the modern death often does not meet people's wishes. In other words, with unequal distribution and the shortage of hospice and palliative care places, a lack of support for peacefully dying at home and the continuous importance of hospital care oriented to fighting death, modern dying is 'a medical event, rather than a natural event in which medicine plays part' (Walter 2017: 18). The complexities of the third stage of institutionalization of dying bring to our attention the dilemmas of dying at home and in a hospice, and show why dying at home or in a hospice is not always an option for the elderly. Moreover, the nature of this last phase of institutionalization of dying has revealed that dying at home holds significant rhetorical, emotional and cultural value, and that it is hospice care that allows people to die peacefully at home. Hence, to complete a picture of modern death, we will look at the home and the hospice as locations of the death of elderly people.

The choice of home as a place of death is connected with people's belief that a natural death could diminish and perhaps even extinguish their existential anxiety. In contrast to dying isolated in hospital, death at home is perceived as less fearful because intimacy, empathy and interpersonal relationships are viewed as important factors in ensuring that the last moments are calm and peaceful (Samarel 1995). As Nicholson et al.'s (2012) study demonstrates, dying at home is seen by elderly people as a 'normal' life-course process because staying at home provides them with the sense of continuity with the past and control over their limited future. According to the frail elderly people interviewed, they see the slow gradation into death as better at home because dying at home helps them to see death as a natural course, to understand that 'it's all downhill now' or 'it's not going to get better now' and to accept that 'there is no future now' (Lillian, aged 91, quoted in Nicholson et al. 2012: 1429). Although elderly people occupy increasingly less space within their homes as they become more frail, often even limiting their space to a single chair or bed, living at home to the end may help them to 'better release the world when death draws near' (Rowles and Bernard 2013: 17). In other words, the more comfortable and more 'at home' elderly people feel in their smaller places, the more likely it is that they will live out their days with a sense of wellbeing.

At the same time, dying at home may require having informal care, which can be costly. The financial cost of death at home, which can be too high for many families – especially if there is a need to rely on paid home health aides or other helpers – means that dying at home is not accessible for everyone (O'Mahony 2016).The likelihood of securing care increases with demographic factors such as living with a partner and having children nearby, and with economic factors such as having financial resources or a family member who is financially secure enough to be free to provide care (Carr and Luth 2019). Health factors also determine the possibility of dying at home, as receiving informal care from relatives is more likely for older adults with light and mild disability and ill-health (Tigge 2020). In other words, older persons with such diseases as dementia and Alzheimer's disease have high care needs and generally cannot be handled at home by family carers. Hence, taking into account increased in life expectancy and its consequences in terms of the increasing levels of functional disability and ill-health, and the lingering trajectory of death, as well as the fact that now only around 10% of Western Europeans over the age of 80 live with their children and almost half live completely alone (Gawande 2105: 21), dying at home is not always a credible option for all older people. Yet, despite all the financial, demographic and health factors that undermine the likelihood of dying at home, many national economies and cultures are still constructed on the assumption that care for the aged is provided for free by relatives. It is only very recently that the value of and need for home care, in the context of the increasing inability of families to 'absorb the medium-high and very high care needs of older relatives unaided' (Tigge 2020: 5) has been recognized. The growing criticism of over-medicalization of death has now led to the development of homecare programmes in many Western countries.

As a result of the development of new programmes in the United Kingdom, terminally ill people wanting to die at home may be offered some formal support, allowing them to be cared for outside hospital. This help for rapidly declining elderly people includes some medical, personal, domestic and counselling services provided by local authorities, homecare workers, nurses and other social or health service providers (Howarth 2007). In reality, families cannot avoid not to care for their terminally ill old members as the British care system relies on the unpaid labour of an estimated 8.8. million adult carers, with cohabiting spouses delivering almost half of informal aged care (Mosses 2012: 7). However, the provision of mixed care at home, which combines informal care at home with mixed informal and formal care at home and formal care outside the home, is not equally distributed (Tigge 2020). The expanding programme of homecare is not a choice that is equally available to all families: support for increasingly fragile older relatives is clearly differentiated along the axes of class, gender and education (Tigge 2020), yet it has contributed to an increased percentage of deaths in homes. This means that care is provided for old men either for free by female relatives or, in the case of mixed homecare (which is associated with higher levels of education), by low-paid care workers who are predominately women (Tigge 2020: 5).

Furthermore, many elderly people with a strong sense of their proximity to death opt for death in institutions because they do not want to be a 'burden' on their families. Many older people – mainly women – do not want to abuse their families' time, resources and emotional capabilities (Clarke et al. 2012). Moreover, even if they desire to die at home, many older people understand the enormous task that caring for a dying person entails, and decide on a hospital or hospice as they fear that their dying body will offend the sensibilities of the people around them, will be too difficult for family members to handle (Adams 2020). As much of the act of dying 'involves the increasing prominence of unbridled and out-of-control body that can no longer contain its edges', terminally ill old people are concerned about loss of control over their disintegrating bodies, resulting in the decision to choose death in a hospice or hospital (Broom 2015: 145). Thus, dying in hospital is not necessary evidence of an 'erosion of the family', but rather a reflection of dying persons' appreciation of modern medical assistance and their own independence or their negative evaluation of their families' capacity and resources to take care of their needs.

Finally, the desire of elderly people to spend their final days at home and their hope for continuity between long-term care and end-of-life care, and the natural move towards death are often undermined by the need to manage pain and limit suffering. When it comes to actual dying, many elderly people prefer to be cared for by skilled professionals in hospital (Walter 2020). As the end of life is typically marked by spells of pain, increasing fragility, emotional distress and diminishing cognitive capacities, despite how much they want to avoid the medicalization of dying, they need medication for effective treatment of pain and to increase the quality of their remaining days. Beside, as their health conditions deteriorate, there is often no alternative but to call an ambulance. Thus, despite 80% of older Americans with chronic diseases wanting to avoid hospitalization and an intensive care unit at the end of life, many may find themselves being hospitalized and undergoing some treatments (Carr and Luth 2020: 521). In recent years in the United States, the use of intensive care units by terminally ill older people living at home in the last month of life increased from 24% to 30% (Carr and Luth 2019: 520). Hence, dying at home is not always accomplished easily, as at the end of life many people are rushed to hospitals, where they are often 'connected to machines' (Carr and Luth 2019: 520). This could happen despite the fact that some of them have set out their wishes in a legally binding way in an Advanced Care Planning directives (ACP) and declaring whether or not they want resuscitation and a breathing tube. Although only a small proportion of people (for instance, in Britain around 4% and in the United States just 10%), sign relevant documents, and although these wishes are not always heard, still there are some visible consequences of ACP, such as lower rates of hospitalization, intensive care unit admissions and less aggressive treatments (Carr and Luth 2019; Clarke 2020; Kaufman 2005).

Another important feature of the modern death, a distinctive feature of the third wave of institutionalization of dying, is the increased understanding of the importance of caring for the qualities of a person's last day. Hospice care, seen as 'being a kind of hybrid of medicine and domesticity', restores the bonds of hospitality and ensures 'kindness, courage, love, tenderness' (Clarke 2019: 136, 16; Stanworth 2004). New incentives to develop the modern hospice movement, which was started in 1967 with the opening of Cicely Saunders' St Christopher's Hospice in London (see Chapter 7), have been provided by the continuous criticism of inability of the modern hospital to meet the needs of dying patients and to take these patients' wishes into account, together with a growing questioning of the human and financial costs of an interventionist culture. The main principle of the hospice movement is best summarized by Cicely Saunders (quoted in Clarke 2020: 141): 'We will do all we can not only to help you die peacefully, but also to live until you die.'

Since the end of the 1980s, Western countries have witnessed the spread of hospice services, the expansion of specialist palliative care services and the greater penetration of palliative care into the hospital sector. Before palliative care – which developed from hospices – became an accredited medical specialty in its own right in 1987, medicine did not offer specialized treatment for the dying and symptoms control for dying patients 'was haphazard and unstandardized, with many mavericks creating their own set of rules' (O'Mahony 2016: 89). Palliative care has brought guidelines for care and comfort for the dying and recognition of dying patients' wishes for some control of the end of their lives. The rise of palliative care as a medical specialty has increased the role of specialists in palliative medicine, working with an interdisciplinary team to raise the quality of the last months of life of the dying person. The emergence of an entirely new professional field of concern with terminally ill patients has allowed palliative care professionals to focus on quality of life and the minimization of suffering, rather than pursuing life - prolonging treatments. Over the last three decades, the influence of palliative medicine has gradually extended to general medicine; hence, the presence of palliative care within the medical system has been growing (Livne 2019). With death and dying being the major objects of clinical interest of both hospice and palliative care, 'hospice care' and 'palliative care' have tended to be considered synonymous (Lawton 2000: 18). Now, however, as people with terminal illnesses are increasingly choosing hospice care at the end of life, and as the majority of hospice care takes place outside of hospitals (home care or hospice at home, outpatient services and hospice day care), while palliative care increasingly happens within hospital, the difference between these two services has become more pronounced. Although hospice care – like palliative care – provides comprehensive care and support, unlike palliative care, it is provided for a person approaching the end of life. Palliative care – that is, specialized medical care for people living with a serious illness – provides care and support, along with treatment intended to cure a person's serious illness. Nonetheless, both palliative and hospice care, while focusing on the care, comfort and quality of life of a person with a serious illness or who is at the end of life, both provide a pain - free and emotionally supportive transition in the last days.

Moreover, palliative care professionals, who work in settings from hospitals to homes, and who self-consciously see themselves as 'a low-rank medical specialty' (Clarke 2020: 14), reject a single - minded devotion to extending life. Instead, they view their role as being 'to work within, not against the finality of terminal illness' (Clarke 2020: 168). In contrast to the traditional medical model of dying, in which doctors do battle with death and disease, they propose a model of death that accepts the limits of human life, which enables them to focus on helping people with a 'terminal illness live what remains of their lives as fully as possible, and die with dignity and comfort' (Clarke 2020: 14). In other words, palliative and hospice care have paved the way for limits to interventionist medicine to be morally acceptable (Levine 2019). Furthermore, the hospice approach, seen now as standing outside 'rather than within, the medical mainstream' (O'Mahony 2017: 141), has helped to shift attitudes towards favouring quality of life versus length of life, and questioning invasive treatments. Subsequently, in many Western countries over the last few decades, hospice care has become increasingly important and popular.

The new status of hospice care is reflected in the increased use of hospice services at home and in the application of hospice principles to the treatment of patients dying in acute general hospitals. For example, in the United States in 1997, 17% of all American deaths occurred under hospice care, and between 2000 and 2009 the percentage of Americans dying in hospice care doubled (Shapiro 2019: 125); by 2016, this proportion was 48% (Carr and Luth 2019: 523), while many more received palliative care in an institution – usually an inpatient hospice facility for the dying or a nursing home (Gawande 2014: 205). However, the situation is different in the United Kingdom, where 5.7% of all deaths in 2016 occurred in a hospice and where between 2004 and 2016 the percentage of deaths in hospices increased by just 0.1% (Gov UK 2018). In the UK hospices, which mainly provide care for cancer patients, and where people with Parkinson's disease, heart conditions and dementia are unlikely to receive care, old frail and dying people with a non-cancer diagnosis are in the minority. Since hospices are 'more likely to cater for the youngest (50–64 years old) as opposed to the oldest (80+ years old) old adults', it can be said that in Britain hospices 'configure themselves as "shorter term" long term care (LTC) settings specialising in end-of-life care (EOLC) for cancer diagnoses and adults aged 50–64' (Tigge 2020: 5, 8). In 2016 in England, 10.0% of people aged between 65 to 74 years died in hospices compared with 2.1% of people aged 85 years and over (Gov UK 2018). Yet, in recent decades there have been several attempts to make general hospitals 'hospice- friendly' (O'Mahony 2016: 83).

One such programme was the Liverpool Care Pathway for the Dying Patient (LCP), which is a part of the NHS End-of-Life Care Programme. It aimed to apply hospice principles to the care of the dying in acute hospitals, advocated for dying with dignity and created a new understanding of end - of - life care. This programme, as well as the Delivering Choice Programme run by Marie Curie Cancer Care, showed the benefits of taking a whole-system approach to the delivery of end-of-life care. However, the Liverpool Care Pathway was criticized for the introduction of too many bureaucratic forms and protocols, as well as for undermining patients' control at the end of life, while not facilitating a conversation about death with dying patients. Two audits of the Liverpool Care Pathway concluded that 'most of the patients on the Pathway did not know they were dying, and only around half knew details of their diagnosis' (O'Mahony 2016: 87). In the light of further comments on the programme, in terms of older patients' experience in hospice care, the most important issues are the problem of their admission to and their conditions in contemporary hospices as well as the kind of death they can expect in a hospice.

The first problem is critical as while 4% of death occur in hospices (O'Mahony 2016: x), older patients are often sequestered in hospices when their bodily disintegration starts to occur. This marginalization of older patients within hospices is explained by the fact that older people in hospice were described by the staff as 'having already "turned their faces to the wall" and "given up" which in practice meant that they showed no desire to continue living' (Lawton 2000: 154).The interviewed hospice staff observed that they were unable to 'revitalise the elderlies' interest in living' as the aged people were on their road to 'decline' and already accepted their imminent death (Lawton 2000: 154). The elderly patients, facing their dying bodies, with their decay, smells and excretions, 'appeared to actively welcome the prospect of death' (Lawton 2000: 159). Another point about admission to hospices in the United Kingdom is that there is a very low uptake of hospice services by members of the working class, Black people and those from ethnic minorities (Lawton 2000; O'Mahony 2016). Similar inequalities are visible in the United States (Carr and Luth 2019), while Broom's (2015) study of Australian hospices also raises concerns about gender disparities. Moreover, the hospice inpatient unit mainly serves middle class patients and middle-class patients 'were, whenever possible, admitted to the privacy of side rooms, whereas working-class patients invariably found themselves allocated to beds in wards' (Lawton 2000: 170). In the United States, the existence of differences in the level of communication between doctors and highly educated, middle-class, White patients on the one hand, and doctors and less-privileged patients on the other means that guiding patients and families to limit intensive treatments goes most smoothly when patients are from privileged middle-class backgrounds (Levine 2019).

This brings us to the second problem: the question of whether a hospice is a good place to die for the aged and whether the dying elderly patients' needs are met there. Elderly patients know that hospices are stereotyped as 'death houses' or spaces of 'no return', but they value hospices as places where encounters with death are not lonely and where patients receive support, care and kindness from all those involved in the process (Hockey 1990; Lawton 2000). However, elderly people also often realize that the hospice's provision of a dying space comes with specific models of 'dying well'. In other words, dying in a hospice is 'shaped by the presence of normative understandings of the "good death"' (Broom 2015: 138). The prescriptive and normative idea of a 'good death' includes such features as 'being pain free, acceptance, closure, awareness and individuality among other things' (Broom 2015: 60). Yet it is possible that these underlying features of the hospice care model's idea of the 'good death' could differ from older people's own views of a 'good death'.

For instance, one investigation found some components of a 'good death' were in conflict with working-class people's preferences (Lawton 2000), while another study discovered that working-class hospice patients tend to be unwilling to be drawn into conversations about their imminent death (Howarth 2007). More generally, the majority of older hospice patients retrained their class-based preferences and tastes, expressed nostalgia for home and confessed to their inability to perform the expected role of hospice patient (Broom 2015; Lawton 2000). Such data, together with evidence that many terminally-ill elderly people in hospices remained withdrawn and felt either helpless or were in denial of death (Stanworth 2004), suggest the persistence of the silence or inconsequentiality of elderly people's voices. While recognizing autonomy as significant predictor of quality of the end of life and reflecting on the importance of being in hospice as a way of preserving some control, terminally ill older people experiencing in-patient hospice care often expressed anxiety over their lack of control in the last days of life (Broom 2015; Stanworth 2004). Generally, as death can be messy, difficult and chaotic, it is often difficult for elderly hospice patients to be a 'loved patients' (Lawton 2000) and some old people cannot 'rise to the challenge' at the end of life and perform the expected 'dignifying death' (Broom 2015).

Our survey of dying in old age demonstrates the diversity of ways of dying and varieties of places of death. Despite the growing range of trajectories of dying, and improvements in the quality of the end-of-life care, the wishes of elderly people are not always met and they are still too often not offered a chance to speak for themselves or express their concerns, and are dispossessed of control at the end of life. The arrival of the COVID-19 pandemic has brought new threats to the quality of older people's end of life.

When COVID-19 prescribed how people die

In the United Kingdom, the COVID-19 pandemic took the lives of many elderly people, impacted the quality of their end-of-life care and prescribed how they died. During the pandemic, older people were faced with a higher risk of death from the virus than young people, not only because of the weakness of their immune systems and their health problems but also because, as a result of the difficulties experienced by hospitals and of their frailty assessment, they were confronted with the risk of not being prioritized for intensive care. The pandemic exposed the ageism of government COVID-19 policies and the low quality of aged care. Many people touched by COVID-19 deaths, including friends, relatives and members of the COVID-19 Bereaved Families for Justice group, the collectivity that represents more than 6,000 families, shared their encounters with death during the pandemic with a wider public. Likewise, doctors and nurses described how 'COVID necessarily compromises every instinct to deliver humane and compassionate care' (Clarke 2021: 102). Through their stories and media reports, we will explore how the COVID-19 pandemic increased older people's distress and loneliness, limited the space available for their wishes to be followed and reduced the quality of their end-of-life care.

At the beginning of May 2022, more than two years after the World Health Organization (WHO) declared the COVID-19 pandemic, its report estimated that the global actual excess deaths from COVID-19 had reached almost 15 million. This figure is more than twice the official death toll, yet other sources estimate that the global death toll from COVID-19 may be even higher – as many as 18.2 million globally (Campbell 2022). Although there have been many international attempts to estimate the total number of deaths related to COVID-19, the excess mortality measure is recognized as the best means of international comparison and the best model to grasp the ultimate impact of the pandemic on a nation's health and longevity (Murray 2022). Excess deaths – that is, the number of deaths that occurred beyond those expected without the pandemic – is a measure that encompasses both those who died as a result of COVID-19 and those who died indirectly because of the pandemic; it is used as an interpretative tool not only by the WHO, but also by *The Lancet* and *The Economist*. For example, the WHO's report has found that while 53% of the excess deaths occurred in lower- to middle-income countries, only 15% occurred in high-income countries, and 4% in low-income countries, while its complex conclusion points out that geographically isolated and rich nations, with the exception of the United States with its 144 excess deaths per 100,00 people, tended to do better in keeping excess deaths low until the arrival of the vaccines and then achieved high vaccination coverage in elderly people (Balloux 2022: 49). *The Economist*'s (28 March 2022) modelling for the two years of excess deaths due to the COVID-19 pandemic showed that the number of excess deaths due to COVID-19 was greatest in South Asia, North Africa and the Middle East, and Eastern Europe, while the United Kingdom, France and Germany had similar excess death rates, roughly halfway down the global league. Moreover, the excess death model, by helping to account for differences in the age structures of different countries – some of which may have many times more mortality risk than others because their populations are much older – tells us something about the effectiveness of states' policies aimed at protecting the elderly. If we adjust for age, the excess mortality data show that New Zealand, Europe and North America were among the best in the world at preventing deaths among the old, and they were several times better at protecting their elderly – of whom they had many more – than Africa and South Asia. The success of New Zealand's COVID-19 policies and high level of deaths among largely unvaccinated elderly people in Hong Kong (where at the end of March 2022, 65% of those aged over 80 had not been vaccinated, point to the extent to which the ultimate impact of the pandemic is not just a story about COVID-19 but also one about governmental policies and our responses to them (*The Economist*, 28 March 2022).

The United Kingdom recorded over 170,000 deaths linked to the disease and more than 21 million cases of infection. With an estimated 109 excess deaths per 100,00 people, Britain is placed 56th in the global ranking of 'best performing countries' and 15th in the table of European Union countries (Balloux 2022: 49). The excess mortality in Britain at the peak of the pandemic (early April 2020), measured by subtracting the number of deaths during the first year of the COVID pandemic from the number of deaths above the average for the period in the non-pandemic years of 2015–19, stood at 59,000 deaths, with 7,800 of them due to COVID-19 occurring in hospitals, 25,800 in care homes, and 25,200 in people's own homes (Campbell 2020). Deaths surpassed their first-wave peak in January 2021, with daily deaths once again standing at over 1,000. During the first year of the COVID-19 pandemic, up to 8,700 patients died after catching COVID-19 in English hospitals, and the number of deaths from all causes, recorded in private homes among people aged 85 years and over, was 43% above the five-year average in England (Campbell and Bawden 2021). Since the start of the pandemic, in the United Kingdom a third more deaths have occurred at home, while COVID-19 has accounted for a significant proportion of deaths in England and Wales, with 29% of deaths occurring at home, 43% in hospital, 21% in care homes and 7% elsewhere (Scobie and Hutchings 2022). Throughout the whole pandemic, there was also a surge in the number of people dying of often treatable aliments in their own homes because hospitals were unable to accept those who were deemed not sick enough – and even not everyone who required acute care received it. The overwhelmed NHS, lacking resources and forced to rationalize or prioritize treatments, ambulance services and hospital admissions, was unable to offer a bed and treatment to everyone who needed care. This, together, with the high level of the hospital-acquired COVID-19 and high levels of death in care homes, suggests that that some loss of life was potentially avoidable. Although, by May 2022, the number of deaths from COVID-19 had reached a relatively low level, the NHS's long waiting list and its many elderly people who could not be released from hospitals due to the shortage of places in care homes, lead health experts to worry that the next several years will be very difficult.

The United Kingdom does have a high level of vaccination of the older population, with the uptake of two doses of vaccine being above 90% in the oldest age groups and the second booster given to people who are over 75 or clinically extremely vulnerable from mid-March 2022 (ONS 2022). However, even with a successful vaccine program, the overall pattern of those at risk of becoming seriously ill or dying has not changed significantly. Even with the high level of vaccination, many elderly people – especially those with underlying health conditions – continue to feel vulnerable. As they are at far greater risk of death from COVID-19 than younger people, older people with weakened immune systems worry that infections may be receding, but the potential threat of becoming seriously ill remains. Although vaccination has lowered the risk of hospitalization and death – for example, the average age of COVID-19 patients in intensive care during the second wave was 58.8 years, which was only slightly lower compared with 60.4 in the first wave (Spiegelhalter and Masters 2021: 39) – the risk of dying from COVID-19 has remained age-dependent.

This risk has been explained by the role of at least three factors. First, as studies of the disparity in the virus's effect on the old and the young have demonstrated, the immune system in the elderly is less efficient at tackling viruses in the first place, which puts them more at risk of death from the virus than younger people. In other words, 'the elderly were more susceptible to the virus itself, and more likely to be swept away by the storm of the body's late, damaging response to it' (Francis 2021: 82). The new research, which demonstrates that people with COVID-19 and flu – especially older persons – faced a double risk of dying (Swets et al. 2022), further confirms what was true throughout the whole pandemic: that the COVID-19 threat is strongly age associated. Moreover, even when the country removed all restrictions and when its dominant narrative was that the pandemic was over, older adults were not out of danger. At the end of

March 2022, the percentage of people testing positive for COVID-19 in England was increasing, infection levels among the over-seventies were at their highest since estimates began in England in May 2020 and hospitalization with COVID-19 was rising, with admissions of people aged over 65 being 15% higher than their January 2022 peak (ONS 2022).

Second, not only do older people's immune systems increase their risk of death from the virus; the aged are doubly disadvantaged because they are more likely to have underlying health conditions – such as cardiovascular diseases, respiratory diseases and diabetes – which increase the risk of death from COVID-19. For example, during the sixteen weeks between 7 March and 26 June 2020, when 218,354 deaths were registered in England and Wales, the death rate was around 12–13% higher for each year of age, corresponding to doubling for every five to six additional years of age. This is consistent from childhood to old age (Spiegelhalter 2020). During the COVID-19 pandemic, older people with a number of comorbidities were also most likely to have delayed or cancelled medical appointments and planned procedures compared with younger adults. Moreover, as the COVID-19 crisis worsened health inequalities, which were already exacerbated by a decade of spending cuts, vulnerable older people, alongside minority ethnic groups and people in the poorest neighbourhoods, faced the great disruption to medical care, and subsequently increased threats to their lives (Hill 2021; Sample 2021). In general, older people experienced more difficulties with their GPs and hospital care, with 39% more problems reported by those aged 65–75 years than those aged from their mid-forties to mid-fifties (Sample 2021). By the end of 2020, 88% of the all deaths from COVID-19 in the United Kingdom had occurred among residents in care home – those aged over 70 and clinically extremely vulnerable individuals (Spiegelhalter 2020).

Third, as a result of state policies and some form of rationing of treatments in the NHS at the peak of the COVID-19 crisis, not all older people who needed intensive care were prioritized for it. During the first wave, only 2.5% of patients in intensive care were over the age of 80, while in the second wave the average age for admittance to critical care was 61 years. The majority of old people who died of COVID-19 during the first two waves did so on ordinary wards (Calvert and Arbuthnott 2021). These data, together with the fact that the average age of death from COVID-19 at that time was 83 years, suggest that the old were less likely to be sent to critical care (Calvert and Arbuthnott 2021). In other words, the pandemic revealed a lack of resources and health equalities, and also showed that some form of triage was the reality in the NHS. Yet this was not discussed, let alone understood or accepted, by the public.

The reality of pandemic, where 'all people under the age of 75 who needed ICU care got it, but quite a few older people, who would have benefited from it didn't get it and died as a result' (Calvert and Arbuthnott 2021: 37), demonstrates a new level of the complexity of criteria for the allocation of intensive care resources. Not only there was not enough Personal Protective Equipment (PPE), staff or ventilators to go around, there was also a perceived lack of clear principles regarding whether to admit frail older people to hospital and how to determine the allocation of intensive care beds. The NHS guidance document that described how, 'under surge conditions', it might become necessary to allocate treatment to patients that might benefit from them' seems to suggest that the ethic of fairness was replaced by an ethic of benefit (Francis 2021: 149). Although such principles were little discussed during the peak of the pandemic, it was soon suspected that age was one of the underlying criteria for a decision about who should receive life-saving care. This suspicion resulted from some doctors' remarks that, in the first wave, some hospitals 'refused intensive care beds to anyone over 75' (anonymous doctor, quoted in Davies 2021: 13) as well as the media's stories about doctors placing notes 'not to resuscitate' on the beds of elderly patients. The decision to signal the elderly as the most likely group that should not be allocated life-saving treatment, was not only a question of resources, however; it also involved understanding that 'the over-seventies have a very low success rate from ventilation and that the use of ITU (intensive therapy unit) would need to be "optimised"' (Francis 2021: 78). With the survival rate for over-eighties who were admitted to intensive care units being 40% (Calvert and Arbuthnott 2021), it was also possible to argue that to give a ventilator to someone very frail 'could mean bringing unnecessary suffering to patients and raising unnecessary hopes of patients and families' (Francis 2012: 79). Moreover, there were some cases when, even if a hospital did not hesitate to give a ventilator to somebody very old and frail, it could have been in violation of that patient's wishes.

Because hospitals were overwhelmed, understaffed and poorly resourced, their personnel did not have sufficient time, space or opportunity to ask patients whether they had an advance decision in place and subsequently too often patients' preferences or living wills were not considered, so it was very often the role of the family to make sure that wishes of their loved ones were respected (Clancy 2021). Hence, the battles of family members to help their loved ones die a good death in hospital were not always about 'missing out' on a ventilator (Srivastava 2020), but also about making sure that their mothers' and fathers' wishes were heard. As the family members witnessed their loved ones' requests being overlooked, the pandemic exacerbated many families' worries about the capability of hospitals to provide quality end-of-life care for their dying elderly loved ones. Yet the bereaved families members did not

> blame the individual doctors or nurses; they are doing an incredible job in the face of such adversity [rather] chronic underfunding and a bizarre management system allowed significant gaps in their loved one's care to develop. Overall, the government is responsible. (Clanchy 2021)

The grieving families were very critical of the government for taking too many risks with people's health. For example, while they could understand that some very old, very sick people were not candidates for a ventilator, they were furious when an 88-year-old died with COVID-19 after a four-hour wait for an ambulance (Dodd 2021). In addition, more than 40% of 349 bereaved family members surveyed believed their loved ones had contracted COVID-19 in hospital (Kale 2021). According to families, the elderly people who died after acquiring COVID-19 in hospital often seemed to be 'expendable' and 'written off'; they believed old people 'don't count any more' and that the way 'this government speaks, it's like we don't matter' (Bawden 2021; Dodd 2021). The growing understanding of the conditions of hospital deaths from COVID-19 made many frail elderly people feel deeply frightened about finding themselves in hospital and also traumatized their families. One grieving son, at whose mother's inquest the coroner said 'the cancers would have killed her anyway, but the COVID saw her off much quicker than they would have', observed that it was

> not just what I went through that I find so hard to deal with, it's what happened to my mum and all the other old ladies on the ward. Is this how elderly people are treated? As soon as they get COVID, whack them to a COVID factory to die. What chance did Mum have? (Bawden 2021)

The COVID-19 crisis increased overcrowding and raised distress on hospital wards. It also worsened the care of dying patients by not allowing families to be physically present with their loved ones and by replacing human contact with the introduction of PPE and reliance on virtual communication. All rules and restrictions for patients during the pandemic brought hardship to dying patients and their families. It was not just that dying elderly people in hospitals were not allowed to meet family members; they were also in a state of agony and torment by being in a disorientating environment without any unmasked human face around them, seeing rooms full of tubes and machines, people in protective aprons and gloves, and with all communication with hospital staff conducted through the strange and impersonal barriers of PPE (Clarke 2021; Francis 2021). For older patients who were delirious, distressed or suffering from severe dementia, such a situation could be 'intolerably alien' and these disorientated patients were seen to be 'ripping oxygen masks off their faces, cannulas from their veins and even, with the catheter balloon fully inflated, catheters straight out of their bladders' (Clarke 2021: 96). Because of strict visitation rules in hospitals during the COVID-19 crisis, many dying elderly people had no chance to be surrounded on their deathbeds by relatives and friends and their hardship was shared by all parties involved. The findings from UK-wide research into how people coped with the deaths of loved ones during the pandemic show that 70% of people whose loved ones died from COVID-19 had limited contact with them in the last days of life, 85% were unable to say goodbye as they would have liked and these experiences impacted on their grieving and general wellbeing (Booth 2020).

In many hospitals, staff recognized patients' need for human contact and did all they could to alleviate it by organizing virtual communication between patients and their families and by seating themselves at patients' bedsides and offering emotional support. To help patients to communicate with loved ones, and to say goodbye to husbands, wives or children, staff in several hospitals were using any possible means to 'bring humanity back to the spaces the virus has stripped bare' (Clarke 2021:116). Throughout the whole pandemic, doctors, nurses and teams of health workers, for whom the dying patients were not shrunken to numbers of death, tried to elevate the trauma of the patients' loneliness: 'We are making it up as we go along. Phone calls, iPads, knitted hearts, recorded songs, laminated photos of our faces on our plastic gowns' (Clarke 2021: 116). Many patients, before being put on ventilators, had a chance to experience the last call, the last text, the last Facetime or Zoom exchange. Quite often, the last contact that grieving families who were unable to visit their dying loved ones had with their dying father or mother was by text.

Some hospitals, realizing that nothing replaces families, made exceptions to the visitor restrictions and the majority of families were very grateful. However, for many patients and families, the choice was not a simple one and often created new dilemmas. For example, some relatives of dying elderly COVID-19 patients could not come to hospital because they were protecting others or shielding themselves, and some because they obeyed governmental rules; another visited their dying relative but worried about their own safety, as only minimal PPE was provided. For instance, the son of dying older woman who went into hospital without COVID-19, caught it there and was then moved to a COVID-19 hothouse, when he got the phone call informing him that his mother was about to die within the hour and asking him whether he wanted to come to say goodbye, said:

> I felt obligated – I knew it was the wrong thing to do for my safety, but she was my dying mother. The hospital reassured me it was safe, so I sat there while she took her last breath. (Bawden 2021)

In similar way, the COVID-19 rules imposed distressing experiences on dying elderly people, as for them the COVID-19 restrictions on visitors often meant either a painful acceptance of the strict rules or choosing which 'child should visit' them (Kirby 2020). With the COVID-19 restrictions in place, the hospital staff's attempts to organize contacts between patients and families through the innovative usage of mobiles and tablets, and facilitating families' visitations, were not always successful in ensuring healing and making dying a peaceful occasion.

COVID-19 has compromised the ability of hospitals to deliver quality end-of-life care. While the NHS chiefs denied that elderly people were refused care during the pandemic and that many of them contracted COVID-19 infections in hospital, and rejected claims that patients thought unlikely to survive were 'written off', exhausted medical staff kept working very hard to prevent lowering of the standards of the end-of-life care for the COVID-19 victims (Campbell 2020). Health workers, alongside patients and their families, felt the limitations of the COVID-induced conditions, from physical exhaustion caused by working long hours to mental anguish due to facing daily traumas or repeatedly delivering distressing news. The new nature of stress faced by medical staff can be illustrated by a doctor's task of phoning an 80-year-old woman to tell her that her husband was dying, knowing that only several days before she had watched him being loaded into ambulance and was now sitting in her bungalow alone (Calvert and Arbuthnott 2021). Doctors' conversations on the phone with frightened, sick older people shielding at home were also often distressing experiences for both sides. The difficulty of the task doctors faced in reaching and helping elderly people isolating at home can be illustrated by an answer given to a physician by an old sick man who did not want to go to hospital and wished to die quickly and peacefully at home because 'This is no life anyway' (Francis 2021: 78–80). Such exchanges revealed the sadness, unhappiness and isolation endured by vulnerable people in the last days of life during the pandemic.

By introducing new risk and unpredictability to elderly people's lives, the COVID-19 crisis increased their ongoing anguish, misery and fear. Moreover, by enforcing visitor restrictions in overwhelmed and understaffed care homes, and by increasing overcrowding and degrading conditions in poorly resourced hospitals, it also worsened the quality of care of dying patients. In short, not only did many elderly people – particularly those with underlying illnesses – die because of COVID-19; the pandemic also severely compromised the quality of their end-of-life care.

CHAPTER 9

Fate's deception

The *ars moriendi* and the black hole

This chapter explores 'fate's deception', which takes from dying older people their autonomy, control and capacity to plan for their own deaths. After the previous chapter's discussion of dying in full control and as an independent self, here we examine death in old age under the conditions of the decay and dependency, when the mental and physical capabilities to exercise personal control over the dying process are very limited. The first part of this chapter is about death in the fourth age – that is, in the stage when a gradual extinction of self takes place, resulting in 'passing beyond the social world, beyond both its comforts and its contradictions' (Gilleard and Higgs 2010: 125). The following section will expose challenges to caring for older individuals whose physical and mental capacities have deteriorated, and who suffer from dementia and other illnesses in care and nursing homes. The final part of the chapter will draw our attention to the high death rate in UK care homes during the COVID-19 pandemic and will discuss what the health crisis has revealed about the UK government's policies to protect elderly people in residential settings.

The contrast between the manner of death taught by the *ars moriendi*, or the art of dying, and the way of dying achievable in a 'metaphorical black hole' of the fourth age (Gilleard and Higgs 2010:125) is very instructive. The *ars moriendi* was the fifteenth-century religious and spiritual teaching of the craft of 'good dying', which emphasized the importance of including death within people's awareness of living (Gawande 2015: 156). Its explanation for the teaching being as much about 'good living' as about 'good dying' pointed to the fact that to die well means to live a life that is conscious of death. The main idea cultivated in the *ars moriendi* was the concept of 'the beautiful death, truly the correct way to die', with its main element being 'the longed-for ideal of death with dignity' (Nuland 1995: xvii). This idea of death, which created the bases of the myth of a good death, is in total contrast to dying in the fourth age, the stage where people's active agency, cognitive capabilities and physical mobility are undermined by neurodegenerative diseases and other accumulated debilities characteristic of very old age.

Dying in the fourth age, during which agency begins to slip away, does not bear much resemblance to the idea of 'the beautiful death', and it does not meet standards of the script for good death in which open communication enables the dying person to make autonomous choices. In contemporary Western societies, with increased life expectancy, people live long enough to experience various neurodegenerative diseases, such as Alzheimer's disease or other debilitating conditions, all of which render aged people more vulnerable and frail, take away their autonomy and exclude them from decision-making when life is coming to an end. The fate of dementia sufferers, as well as people who are mentally or communicatively incapacitated by stroke or coma, may be depicted as 'a form of living death' (Howarth 2007: 182). Older individuals whose impairment is such that they show very little understanding of what is going on around them may be described as in some ways 'already dead'; hence their dying might be alleged to be 'a blessing' (Sweeting and Gilhooly 1997: 95–96). Yet death in the fourth age is not 'death with dignity', as 'the quest to achieve true dignity fails when our bodies fail' (Nuland 1995: xvii). Moreover, in the case of dementia, when both the corporeal morbidity and the dislocation of body and self are assumed to be prevalent, care is focused on the body rather than the self of the of dying individual (Twigg 2006).

The concept of the fourth age, which encapsulates all 'bleaker aspects of old age', was introduced into modern gerontology by Peter Laslett (1989), while Gilleard and Higgs (2015: 262) linked it to a metaphorical 'black hole' where 'human agency is no longer visible'. Peter Laslett (1989) exposed various indignities of the death in the fourth age, the stage described as a final part of life in which older people are inflicted by functional impairments, disabilities and corporeal limitations. Similarly, Gilleard and Higgs (2010, 2015) depicted the fourth age as the period of ageing characterized by bodily decline and the loss of agency over the body, generally the stage when people's personhoods are unrecognized. The fourth age, in contrast to the third age, which is aligned with a successful ageing, achievements, independence, choice and an active lifestyle, is associated with a decrepit body, problems with cognition and memory, and increased vulnerability, frailty, dependency and loss of autonomy. Hence, apart from being viewed in comparison with the third age, the fourth age should also be considered in terms of its closeness to death (Gilleard and Higgs 2015; Lloyd 2015).

Although all 'death is the ultimate dependency … the ultimate limit of autonomy' (Bauman 1992: 36), this observation is particularly true in the case of death in the fourth age, where people's various needs, deteriorations and deficiencies mean they are reliant on the help and care of others. Even though the fourth age is characterized by a combination of various complex aspects, one of its features is decisive in the identification of people as subjects of the fourth age: it happens when professionals decide that the older individual has lost the capacity for self-care (Gilleard and Higgs 2010; Lloyd 2000). In other words, despite the fact that the fourth age's characteristics 'are not biologically or temporarily determined and vary in how they are interpreted by older people and those around them' (Lloyd 2015: 261), nevertheless the older people's *status* is defined by the imperative of care or the perceived need for institutionalization. 'It is within the power of others – professionals and carers – to determine when an individual has lost the capacity for self-care and management of everyday life and thus makes the transition over the event horizon into the fourth age' (Lloyd at al. 2014: 2). What alerts professionals' concern and leads them to identify the aged as 'ageing without agency' are dementia and frailty, as both these characteristics imply an increased level of dependency (Higgs and Gilleard 2010). In the same vein, the notion of the fourth age draws our attention to the importance of recognizing older people's dependence on care, services and support in all aspect of their lives.

While describing the fourth age as a dark and unknowable place, Gilleard and Higgs (2015: 268) propose viewing this stage of life as 'a feared imaginary of old age', where that fear 'settles on the loss of agency that is associated with frailty, particularly mental frailty and the perceived abjection of an undignified journey towards non-existence'. Behind such a fear of a premature social death is a fear of dementia, which is commonly seen as as 'a recipe for social death in which the body lingers but person is gone' (Walter 2017: 31). Studies confirm that dementia is the most feared diagnosis of older age (Nogrady 2020). People have a deep fear of it because of their anxiety about losing their identity, autonomy and the integrity of their lives. In particular, they are afraid of losing their dignity and cannot 'stand being a vegetable' or 'going gaga' (Clarke 2020: 212). In other words, people fear dementia because they are afraid to become 'so diminished or dissipated or subjugated that you are becomes disconnected from who you are were or who you want to be' (Gawande 2105: 141).

Dementia is a broad concept used to describe a variety of progressive neurological disorders – that is, conditions affecting the brain, memory, thinking, behaviour and ability to perform everyday activities. It is already one of the major causes of disability and dependency among older people. With around 57 million people suffering from dementia globally (a number that is projected to rise to 80 million by 2030 and 153 m million by 2050), this neurological disease presents the world with a moral and social challenge regarding how to deal with the most vulnerable members of our society. There are various forms of dementia, such as vascular dementia, dementia with Lewy bodies, frontotemporal dementia and mixed dementia, yet around 70% of cases are due to Alzheimer's disease (Alzheimer's Society 2022). Having chronic health problems in middle age, such as high blood pressure, diabetes or liver disease, more than doubles the risk of dementia (Gregory 2022b). Yet the greatest risk factor for Alzheimer's disease is age, as the probability of developing this disease '*doubles* every five years after the age of sixty-five. After the age of eighty-five, the likelihood of living with Alzheimer's disease grows to remarkable *1 in 2*' (Erickson 2013: 41, italics in original). The most recent research shows that the age-specific incidence of dementia is declining in several rich countries, and it also increases our hope that a new treatment could become available within the next decade. Nonetheless, for the time being, dementia's overall prevalence increases as societies get older (World Health Organization 2022). Hence, in wealthier countries where people are likely to live longer, deaths from other major causes have decreased significantly but deaths from Alzheimer's disease have increased considerably over the last decade. In short, dementia is the leading cause of dependency, disability and increasingly of death in the majority of rich countries.

Dementia affects around ten million people in Europe (World Health Organization 2022) and is the second leading cause of death in Australia overall, with one in ten Australians aged over 65 suffering from dementia and the numbers increasing (Nogrady 2020: 47). Also in the United States, Alzheimer's disease – the sixth leading cause of death among American older adults – accounts for 60–80% of all dementia (Hovland-Scafe and Kramer 2017: 1920–21). The number of Americans aged 65 or more living a with Alzheimer's disease reached 6.2 million in 2021, which means that one in nine individuals aged 65 years and older has Alzheimer's disease and one in three people aged 65 years and over dies with Alzheimer's disease or another form of dementia (Alzheimer's Association 2022). In Britain, dementia is the country's biggest killer, with around 67,000 people dying from the disease every year (Alzheimer's Society 2022). In the United Kingdom, Alzheimer's and other forms of dementia have overtaken heart disease, strokes and flu at the top the mortality charts (Mannix 2018), and the number of deaths due to dementia for people over 75 years of age have doubled between 2007 and 2017, from 40,253 to 76,199 (Alzheimer's Society 2022). More than 900,000 people are now living with dementia in the United Kingdom, and this number is projected to increase by 75%, to almost 1.6 million by 2050 (Alzheimer's Society 2022).

Despite these big numbers of older people living and dying with dementia, and despite the epidemiologic transition in the causes and timing of death, in the United Kingdom the fourth age is not the basis for policies of care and debates about the quality of the end-of-life care. In the contemporary cultural and policy context, discussions of ageing are concerned with positive ageing associated with 'the third' age and 'good death' at the end of healthy old age. For example, the main focus of England's End-of-Life Care Strategy is on patient choice as a way by which 'good deaths' can be achieved (Borgstrom and Walter 2015: 105). Such narratives and aims overlook the dark side of old age and do not pay sufficient attention to the nature of death and care required for old people with advanced chronic progressive dementia. Yet the increasing prevalence of neurodegenerative diseases, along with the fact that dementia is a driving force behind the need for 24-hour care and that the dying process of individuals with dementia is one of the most widespread forms of dying in many Western countries, including the United Kingdom, means that it is necessary to recognize the reality of dependence and to acknowledge the difficulties and ambiguity of dementia-related death.

Dementia-related conditions make care at home virtually impossible as older individuals living with the later stage of Alzheimer's disease need continuous care and constant supervision to remain safe. Although countries vary regarding where and how care of old people with dementia is organized, everywhere dementia is the single strongest predictor of institutional care (Walter 2020). As dementia is unlikely to be supported at home by informal carers, in the majority of European countries the most likely institutions where over-eighties dementia sufferers are being cared for are either nursing homes or care homes, and sometimes hospitals (Walter 2017). Taking into account that Alzheimer's disease is age related, together with the fact that the average age of entry to a care home is above 80, it is not surprising that older adults with dementia are over-represented in many care homes and nursing homes in the majority of Western countries, including several Scandinavian countries and the United States, where in many nursing homes more than half of all residents may suffer from dementia-related conditions (Erickson 2013; Walter 2017). In the United Kingdom in 2014, according to the Alzheimer's Society (2022), 311,370 people with dementia lived in in a residential setting.

Hence, in many countries the most likely place for death is the care or nursing home. In the United States, despite the fact that 'hospice utilization has steadily increased among patients with diagnoses other than cancer, hospice remains underutilized among those with advanced dementia' (Hovland-Scafe and Kramer 2017: 1920–21). In the United Kingdom, where care home deaths are increasing, 'care homes are becoming the hospices for severely impaired, very old (80+) adults, affected in particular by dementia, Parkinson's disease and stroke, who are thereby more likely to experience dwindling dying over many months or years' (Teggi 2020: 5).

Suffering and dying with dementia come with many risk factors, from a lack of clear prognosis, through a lack of appropriate treatments, to an absence of cure. The process of dying from dementia is difficult for all parties involved. Caregivers and the family often do not know much about treatments and misunderstand the dying process, and they are confused and unprepared for the nature of the death of their loved one. Because of the ways dementia progresses, by first taking away the known person and separating the body from the self, the disease is described as 'dual dying' (Jones and Martinson 1992). Very often when people with dementia die, people say they are 'out of their misery' – that it is 'better for them' (Ernaux 2014: 90). Hence, grief experienced by the family occurs even before physical death, while the increased dependency and decreased agency of the loved one poses additional challenges to family members who are caregivers and impedes the quality of end-of-life care. It is followed by a sense of 'ambiguous loss' when the death takes place and the 'ambiguous dying syndrome' – that is, 'the collection of medical and social uncertainties' connected with dementia (Hovland-Scafe and Kramer 2017) – occurs. Although Alzheimer's disease significantly shortens lives – for instance, in the United States, among people aged 70, 61% of those with Alzheimer's dementia are expected to die before the age of 80 compared with only 30% of people without Alzheimer's disease (Alzheimer's Association 2022) – the likely timing of death is not clear.

Even though the patient's quality of end of life can generally be increased by the appropriate treatments and pain management with the help of morphine or other opioids, in the case of older individuals with dementia, medical decisions regarding the suitability of particular treatments and the management of symptoms are more difficult. Dementia patients are frequently subjected to 'aggressive treatments', which often cause discomfort and have ineffectual results – for example, 25% of patients with dementia in US nursing homes die with a feeding tube compared with only 5% of those dying with cancer (Hovland-Scafe and Kramer 2017: 1925). The older dementia sufferers, due to their high level of malnutrition, fragility and vulnerability, are at increased risk of developing pneumonia. Yet, while suffering from pneumonia, which is the most common cause of dementia-related death, individuals with advanced dementia at the very end if life often receive life-prolonging treatments similar to those without a terminal illness. Dementia sufferers dying from pneumonia have no apparent awareness of the process; they are simply unconscious all the time and their end 'comes without last words' (Gawande 2015: 157).

Even if the fourth age does not necessarily involve social death (Higgs and Gilleard 2015), care home residents with advanced dementia, as a result of the weight of institutionalization and a lack of compassion, are depicted or even treated as an 'uncollected corpse ... which the undertaker has cruelly forgotten to collect', and often placed outside of social relations and condemned to social death (Howarth 2007: 182). Without going into debates about whether we should accept or reject the idea that the old person with dementia has lost their personhood, we should stress the importance of caring and compassion in supporting the continuation of the person's identity:

> Recognising and valuing the social being of the person being cared for in their past sameness and in their present difference can still be caring about the person with dementia – in the sense of protecting and providing for that person. (Gilleard and Higgs 2015: 268–69)

Compassion, which 'becomes increasingly appropriate the more the patient's agency declines', and which ensures caring in memory of a past self that is no longer seemingly present, plays a very important role in caring for dementia suffers (Borgstrom and Walter 2015: 102).

While caring for dying persons with dementia poses a very difficult challenge even in normal circumstances, during the pandemic this task was enlarged. Moreover, not only did older adults with dementia living in UK care homes have the conditions of their care and support altered; they were also over-represented among COVID-19 victims as those living with dementia were disproportionately affected by the coronavirus. Hence, the next section will explore the ability of care homes to deliver quality of end-of-life care before and during the pandemic.

Dementia and death in care homes

First we illustrate the unjust and cruel tricks of fate, or the death that nobody wants, by looking at the care home population with dementia. With 70% of all care home residents having dementia or severe memory problems, the majority of care home occupants require special care (Alzheimer's Society 2022). The COVID-19 pandemic compromised the ability of care homes to deliver quality of end-of-life care as not only were they ravaged by coronavirus, but older people living with dementia are also particularly vulnerable to the virus. For example, dementia was the most common pre-existing condition among those who died from COVID-19 in England and Wales in March and April 2020, with 25% of the deceased diagnosed with dementia (*The Economist* 2020). Here we will explore the main features of care homes and how they contributed to placing residential homes at the centre of the pandemic, while the next section will examine COVID-19 deaths in care homes.

We illustrated some aspects of living in care homes in Chapter 4, without focusing on dementia or seriously impaired geriatric patients, but with the emphasis on the old age as not only full of death, but also full of life. As the cases discussed in Chapter 4 suggest, a residential care home can be a safe place offering relatively independent living where something meaningful can still be expected to happen. However, caring for some residents of care homes – especially older individuals whose physical and mental capacities have deteriorated – poses many challenges. Moreover, despite its name, the care home is 'a space visibly set apart', where all processes lead to a single event: death (Hockey 1990: 93). Hence, even though institutionalization does not necessarily take away one's autonomy and the possibility of pursuing one's interests, nonetheless there is a stigma around care homes. Some residential care might have a bad reputation, as living there might be seen as removing independence, preferred spaces, identity and lifestyles from older people. Predictably, there is a conflict between the care home's preferred image as a place offering compassionate care for the aged and its external image as 'a dying space concerned primarily with the slow process of deterioration' (Hockey 1990: 92). Despite the many years the care home sector has spent trying to spread the message that such facilities are not unfriendly and clinical spaces, and that they offer personal and homely care, members of the general public often view them as 'either sterile and impersonal, or filthy and impersonal' (Shriver 2021l: 13).

In the United Kingdom, only around one-third (288,000) of people with dementia live in residential care settings, while the majority live in their own homes and are often cared for by members of their families (Alzheimer's Society 2022). Because of the often poor reputation of care homes and their high costs, many families – while barely copying with the physical and mental deterioration of their elderly loved ones – feel too guilty or short of resources to place their loved ones in residential care. Still when the condition progresses and full-time care is required, many older people with dementia are moved into care and nursing homes. When a person with dementia becomes very difficult to care for at home, and when families are faced with a need to provide caring environments for their loved ones, there is less hesitation and resistance, and especially if the family's financial situation makes it possible and places are available, to admitting an elderly person with worsening dementia to a nursing home, regardless how heartbreaking it can be for their family. In the United Kingdom, the average prevalence of people living with dementia in care homes is 63% of men and 71% of women (Mong 2020). Hence, the majority of people in UK residential homes are older people with dementia, who tend to die there – although a small proportion of care home residents with dementia die in hospitals, where they are often moved for medical treatments (Walter 2020).

In 2021, the UK care system consisted of 17,598 care homes, including 5,127 nursing homes, and 12,471 residential homes, employed over 700,000 people, with nearly 690,000 of them being care workers. At that stage, the UK care home population was nearly 500,000, with around 70% of all care home residents having some form of dementia (carehome.co.uk 2022). Nursing homes offer a wider range of personal and nursing care than residential homes, although both types of homes care for elderly people with dementia and both offer end-of-life care. In England, where an estimated half a million physically disabled elderly people are living in care homes, more than half (56%) of people newly admitted to a nursing home are expected to die within twelve months and three-quarters will likely die within three years (Pocock et al. 2021: 1638). While in Scotland social care is free, in England the cost of a care home varies, depending on financial circumstances, location and services offered. Currently one needs to pay in full unless one's assets are less than £23,250, although from October 2023 the system will change. More than half of residents in English elderly care homes pay all or some of their fees and around one in seven people pay more than £100,000 (carehome.co.uk 2022). Still, by providing private operators with a subsidy, the state plays an important role in the English care system. Without state support, local authorities – which tend only to pay the full cost of nursing home care once the person's assets have fallen below £14,250 (including the value of their home) – would not have any money even to fund places in care homes for the poorest people. With eligibility criteria for council-funded services being tightened, in most areas only those with very high needs qualify for help, so only around half of care home residents are state-subsidized and also receive support from the local authorities. With around 82% of places being provided by for-profit operators, it is estimated that on an average 'older people spend in a total about £6 billion for care of their own money, and that the net spend by public authorities is similar' (Wolpert 2011: 199).

Over the last few decades, with the increasing number of old people in need of care and with continuous cuts in care funding, the social care system for the aged has been in a very severe crisis. The functioning of care homes, which have often been understaffed, with their employees poorly trained, underpaid and shifting between different homes, has been the subject of many negative evaluations. For example, the Care Quality Commission's annual report for 2018/19 shows that more than one in six care providers are not meeting acceptable standards. Moreover, various analyses of pre-COVID-19 nursing and residential homes show that, in the context of the ageing population in England in recent decades, the rising costs of the social care system and the decline in funding mean the system was on the brink of collapse. This catastrophic malfunctioning of the system, particularly entrenched inequality and uneven quality of provision of services, had many causes. Over the last few decades, care homes have faced many difficulties, from the rising demand for fragmented services and the inability to meet the rapidly growing need for care, through the government's insufficient support and its lack of a long-term plan for the sector, the growing involvement of market forces, staffing shortages, austerity and decreasing support from local authorities. For instance, during the early to mid-2010s, the significant cuts made to adult social care left spending per person in care 7.5% lower in real-terms in 2019–20 than it had been a decade earlier. In short, care homes experienced severe financial uncertainty and structural instability, which left them unable to adequately care for their residents and meet the demands of an ageing population (Age UK 2018; Barker 2014; Howarth 2007; Humphries et al. 2016; Teggi 2020; Twigg 2006; Walker 2021; Wolpert 2011). Many pre-COVID investigations and various commissions' reports on the conditions of care home services, while acknowledging that there is no single simple solution to this disastrous predicament, warned succeeding political leaders that the UK social care system was unsustainable and called for urgent changes. From the Royal Commission on Social Care established by the Blair government in 1999, through Wanless's (2006) report on the need for a long-term strategy, the Dilnot (2011) review of adult social care founding and the Barker Commission report (Barker 2014), all recognized that the existing social care system was inadequate and diagnosed the urgent need for the UK social care system to undergo significant transformation. More specifically, they recommended that the NHS principle should be extended to personal care in older age and offered various ways of funding social care. However, despite successive governments' promises to deliver reforms to the social care system, none of the commissions' recommendations have ever been implemented.

Since the start of the pandemic, the crisis of the care system has become even more severe and. The five-year average of 145,560 deaths of care home residents increased by almost 20% during the pandemic (ONS 2021), and all functions of the care home have been destabilized and challenged. During the pandemic, for the first time in the United Kingdom, people aged 85 years and over were more likely to die in care homes than in hospitals. In 2017, over 111,000 people in England died in a care home, which means that over half of the very old and 37.6% of those aged 85 and over died in a care home (Teggi 2020: 2). The official government data confirmed the increase in the number of people dying from dementia during the pandemic and that dementia was the leading cause of death for female care home residents in both waves. Dementia and Alzheimer's disease were listed in over half of COVID-19 deaths in care home residents in the first wave and just under half of the coronavirus deaths in the second wave (ONS 2021).

Even before the pandemic, relatives of older people with dementia were reluctant to place them in residential settings because of the fear that care homes do not always offer quality care and do not ensure dignity to those nearing the end of life. They were also worried, given that care homes are not available at an affordable price, that a condition such as dementia could lead to the total liquidation of their loved ones' homes and financial assets. Such fears are often reinforced by media reports and reviews of systemic failures in care homes. In the United Kingdom over the last decade, many widely publicized scandals concerned care homes show the failure of care for elders living with the later stage of Alzheimer's disease – especially exposing the absence of compassionate care, which is a very important within palliative care and hospice movements. The numerous scandals have illustrated how 'elderly Britons today die and how they are cared for, or not cared for, in their final months', and bring to our attention an appalling lack of care for, and indignities suffered by, people with cognitive impairment in care homes (Borgstrom and Walter 2015: 105). As the fate of care home residents caught the attention of newspapers, dementia suffers were presented as being 'drugged and robbed' by a system where they have to pay five times their pensions for poor-quality care (Wolpert 2011: 205). A lack of compassion in care or nursing homes is also a problem in many other countries. For example, in Australia nursing homes, the elders are too frequently treated as 'a separate and subhuman class', seen as 'worthless and invisible' (Holland-Batt 2020: 30). Because of this mistreatment of people in aged care and because of the general failure of Australia care standards, the Royal Commission into Aged Care Quality and Safety (RCACQS) was established in 2018 (Holland-Batt 2020). In New Zealand, end-of-life care in care homes is seen to be unsatisfactory and suboptimal (Borgstrom and Walter 2015; Teggi 2020).These failures of in care homes are particularly devastating and disturbing in the context of dementia, as they add – or accelerate – social death to the disappearance of personal agency of dementia sufferers.

Before the pandemic, care homes were not only managing and taking care of the processes of ageing and dying, but also marginalized, isolated and removed death from public view. During the COVID-19 pandemic, the social visibility of death was raised by daily presentations of tragic stories from care homes, interviews with alarmed managers and staff of care homes and the reporting of the daily death toll. All these messages drew to public attention the previously marginalized topic of death of older people in institutional care and drastically worsened the mood of reporting of the tragic fate of care home residents. This alteration of the mood occurred dramatically in early March 2020 when stories emerged of the tragic fate of residents of care homes in Italy, which were deserted by staff fearful of the virus and where residents' dead bodies were found in their beds by the military (Francis 2021). These revelations were followed by articles in British newspapers about the widespread anxieties and shortages of personal protective equipment (PPE) in care homes, while social media compared the fate of residents of care homes to 'lambs going to the slaughter' (Clarke 2021: 92). Additionally, during the first wave of the pandemic, with rumours circulating that older patients had been discharged from hospital to care home without testing, bringing the virus with them, the sudden increase in panic over outbreaks in care homes produced shocking headlines, such as 'Elderly abandoned to worst the virus can do', 'We were the forgotten people', 'Sacrificing the elderly' and 'Callous betrayal of our most vulnerable'. After the peak of hospital admissions in May 2020, as about 15.8% of COVID-19 patients in the United Kingdom contracted COVID-19 after being in hospital for other reasons, all social media reflected on the increasing panic (Grover 2021).

The COVID-19 crisis, by exposing how the care system had been failing older people in the United Kingdom, and by showing the adversities and struggles faced by care homes, revealed the many structural problems in this sector. Among many systemic difficulties faced by care homes are issues connected with poor integration between the care and health systems. Generally, unlike the NHS, the care system is not only costly for users, but the price for its many services cannot readily be justified on ethical grounds. For example, it is difficult to defend the fact that the NHS will treat long-term conditions such as cancer for free, while dementia can cost a sufferer their family home or life savings. During the pandemic, the issue of the relationship between the NHS and the social care system has become disputed territory as the government's prioritization of the NHS over the social care system in its COVID-19 responses has been seen as one cause of the state's failure to prevent the spread of the pandemic to care homes. By creating a much larger task for the already overstretched care system, the pandemic blew social care services further into crisis. By exposing the links between the government's major failures in the provision of a sustainable care system and the care homes' high numbers of deaths from and with COVID-19, it has brought to public attention the government's negligent role in protecting the most vulnerable from the virus. In the middle the pandemic, in June 2020, social care directors said that in English care homes thousands of people lost their lives prematurely because these institutions were 'ill-equipped and under-resourced' to deal with COVID-19 as a result of years of the state under-investing in social care (Butler 2020).

Another problem faced by the care system relates to the fragmentation of care due to frequent transfers of frail, vulnerable elderlies from care homes to hospitals. Such movements are not only often ineffective, leaving the aged person even more vulnerable and frail; they are also traumatic and disorienting experiences for patients and their families. Moreover, these transfers may lead to fragmented care because the old and new care teams engage in limited communication about the patient's health conditions, treatments and personal history (Hovland-Scafe and Kramer 2017). In the United Kingdom, approximately 25% of beds in hospitals are occupied by people who are over 65 years of age and suffering from dementia, who would have been in care homes if not for the care system's shortage of places (Alzheimer's Society 2022). Regular hospitalizations and deaths in hospital of dementia-affected residents of care homes happen in all developed nations, yet there are differences between countries. For example, in Britain only a small proportion of elderly care home residents with dementia who re moved to hospital for treatment die there: only 8% in 2005 and 6% in 2016. In Belgium, though, almost 24% of care home residents die in hospital (Teggi 2020: 6). In the United States, where people aged 65 years and older survive for an average of four to eight years after a diagnosis of Alzheimer's disease, an estimated two-thirds of those who die of dementia do so in nursing homes, compared with roughly 25% of older adults dying in a nursing home from all other conditions (Carr and Luth 2019: 517).

The COVID-19 pandemic also revealed the care system's financial problems and its lack of sufficient numbers of staff, as well as its lack of adequately trained caregivers. For example, in the United Kingdom, only about one-fifth of nurses working with people with dementia in care homes receive any or enough dementia training (Wolpert 2011: 6). All these troubles and difficulties are responsible for the inequalities and precarity in a care process that affects all residents of care homes living with dementia. The lack of resources to pay higher salaries, staff shortages and a lack of trained staff have a very negative impact on the quality of care of Alzheimer's patients in care or nursing homes. Taking into account how demanding, difficult and emotionally and mentally totally exhausting caring can be, and how low carers' salaries are, it is not surprising that there are 100,000 staff vacancies in the care home sector. With a growing need for high-quality care and problems with recruitment and low salaries, the system seems to be unable to solve its staff shortages. The staffing problems, despite the care home sector urgently requesting more staff from the beginning of the pandemic, have been exacerbated by the COVID-19 crisis. Many additional difficulties in retaining staff, recruiting new people, getting visas for them, the state-sponsored employment chaos and states' changing vaccine regulations for care workers have meant that the huge shortage of carers has become even worse. As a result of the pandemic, care homes – quite apart from the staff shortages – have also been affected negatively by the fluctuations in occupancy rates of care homes as many families, worried about the death toll, risk of infection and restricted visiting, have been disinclined to place their loved ones in care homes.

However, the COVID-19 pandemic has not only compromised the ability of care homes to deliver quality end-of-life care, by exposing how the care system has been failing older people in the United Kingdom it has also prompted the government to finalize reforms to stop people facing 'unpredictable and catastrophic costs' of care. In other words, the COVID-19 pandemic has been a catalyst for change in the English health and care system as on 8 September 2021, the government managed to pass through the parliament a long-overdue plan for social care funding. According to this plan, which was not expected to be implemented before 2023, the cost of adult social care will be reduced, while the NHS is getting £36 billion over the next three years 'to tackle the COVID backlogs'. From April 2022, national insurance contributions rates will go up by 1.25% to allow the government to implement a new cap on total care costs, so no individual will have to pay more than £86,000 over their lifetime. From October 2023, anyone in England with assets worth less than £20,000 will have their care costs fully covered by the government, while people with assets between £20,000 and £100,000 will be expected to contribute to the cost of care, but will also be eligible for state means-tested support covering some of the costs. This new social care plan has, however, been criticized for not addressing many essential issues, such as the dysfunctionality of the residential care market, the care system's recruitment crisis, the low pay rates and the lack of training for care workers. Moreover, this plan is far from offering a sustainable funding solution and many of the government's promises – such as the claim that no one will ever have to pay more than £86,000 for care in their lifetime – seem to be unrealistic. It is not only the scope and timing of financial support that are generating criticism; people are also not sure whether the promised extra money will be delivered to the care system or spent tackling NHS waiting times. Moreover, the likelihood of the successful integration of the NHS and social care could be questioned, as the government proposal does not consider any deeper structural changes necessary for the promised integration and does not offer much funding to the care system (Rawnsley 2021).

The pandemic has broken the silence surrounding death in institutional care, exposed many structural problems of the system and provided a new impetus for reforms of the care system. COVID-19, which has been especially dangerous for older people already suffering from dementia and living in care homes, has enhanced the severity and difficulties of care of the elderly and changed care home residents' ways and conditions of dying. Thus, in what follows, we look at the COVID-19 pandemic's impact on the quality of end-of-life care in care homes.

The health crisis at the forgotten frontline

In the 'war' against COVID-19, the UK care system for adults has been on the forgotten frontline. After decades of the government's failure to reform the care system in England, the state's mistakes in handling the coronavirus pandemic have further eroded the social care system's capacity to function effectively, and have prompted a decline in public trust in the state's competence to respond adequately to the health crisis. To date, all discussions and reviews of the UK's failure to protect residents of care homes from COVID-19 point to the complex causes – mainly related to the long-lasting crisis of social care in England and the country's general lack of preparedness for pandemics. As mentioned in the previous part of this chapter, over the last few decades the functioning of care homes, which were often understaffed, with their employees poorly trained, underpaid and shifting between different care homes, was a subject of many negative evaluations. With COVID-19, as with dementia, people may lose the capacity to plan for their own death and, also like dementia, the pandemic has created a much larger task for the already overstretched care system, which has thrown social care services into a deep crisis. By exposing the negligent role of the state in protecting the most vulnerable from COVID-19, the severity of that crisis has forced the government to initiate reforms of the English health and care system, as discussed briefly in the previous section. Here we will examine the links between the government's major failures in the provision of a high-quality and sustainable care system and the state's failure in preventing the spread of the pandemic to care homes.

The fact that around one-third of all deaths with COVID in the United Kingdom have taken place in care homes raises the question of whether meeting obligations towards the most vulnerable people in the society has been the government's priority in the battle against the coronavirus and to what degree the prioritization of the NHS over the social care system in the 'war' against COVID-19 has endangered the lives of elderly people in residential care. Already in the middle of the COVID-19 pandemic, in June 2020, social care directors said that in English care homes thousands of people lost their lives prematurely because these institutions, as a result of years of the state underinvestment in social care, were 'ill-equipped and under-resourced' to deal with the virus (Butler 2020). While a full explanation of the care homes' tragically high level of deaths during the pandemic is likely be delivered by a statutory inquiry into how the United Kingdom dealt with the coronavirus, the existing documents, reports, legal actions and parliamentary reviews of COVID-related policies, such as the All-Party Parliamentary Group on Coronavirus, which published its report in December 2020, allow us to gradually piece together the picture of governmental priorities in its policy to control the virus.

Apart from the government's failures to address a long-standing social care crisis and prepare for the pandemic, some specific governmental decisions increased the risk of infection for care home residents. Among a number of problematic decisions, which ranged from lockdowns called too late to the government's failure to provide adequate PPE or testing to residents of care homes and staff, the most serious and life-threatening mistake was the order made on 17 March 2020 to discharge thousands of people from hospital into care homes without testing them for COVID-19. While other countries – for example, Germany – kept their care home COVID-19 outbreaks to a minimum by not allowing people into care homes from hospitals without a negative COVID-19 test, in the United Kingdom the lives of residents of care homes were put at risk by the decision to place the aged – who were particularly susceptible to catching COVID-19 – back in care homes, where they were most likely to infect other elderly people, without a test. In short, the coronavirus crisis in care homes was exacerbated by the government's order to clear beds in hospitals to guard the NHS's capacity to deal with new COVID-19 patients. The discharge of 25,00 untested hospital patients to care homes took place between 17 March and 15 April 2020 – that is, at the stage when it was already known that people could transfer the virus without having experienced symptoms. Moreover, at this time asymptomatic transmission was not only acknowledged, but hospitals were known sources of COVID-19 infection. So, in order to facilitate the mass discharge, the government had to suspend all regulatory requirements by issuing the rules on discharge to care homes from hospitals, which 'clarified that negative tests were not required before discharge' (Calvert and Arbuthnott 2021: 281).

According to the cross-party public accounts committee (UK Parliament 2020), the decision to return thousands of patients to care homes without knowing whether they had coronavirus was a 'reckless' and 'appalling' policy error, as it contributed to the coronavirus spreading among residents, with devastating consequences. While the public tried to protect the NHS by not burdening it with calls for medical treatment and by postponing visits to hospital, as part of the national effort to 'protect NHS and save lives', the government pushed to vacate NHS beds to prevent hospitals from becoming overwhelmed. In other words, while preserving the good reputation of the NHS was seen as an important aspect of the country's response to the COVID-19 pandemic, the broken social care system was not perceived as an essential part of the government's plans to 'battle' COVID-19.

As the care sector's sufferings became visible on the TV news, in newspapers and on social media platforms, the government tried to calm the public and to assure the care sector that care homes did not need to take precautions to protect their elderly residents. Despite the fact that elderly people constituted the group that was most vulnerable to serious illness from the virus, until April 2020 health officials claimed that care homes did not need to do anything and care workers were advised that they didn't need to use PPE; moreover, for months care homes could not access testing. For example, on 25 February 2020, Public Health England told staff in the care home sector that there was no need for masks, as it was 'very unlikely that anyone receiving care in a care home or the community will become infected', while at the 3 March press conference, Chris Whitty, England's chief medical adviser, explained why care homes did not need to take precautions: 'because if you do that you get no benefit but you get is a social cost' (quoted in Calvert and Arbuthnott 2021: 161). Despite the crisis unfolding, discharging of untested patients from hospitals to care homes continued as the official advice remained that tests were not mandatory. It was only on 15 April 2020, after the death toll peaked and after some enhancement of the testing capacity, that the government ordered testing of all people being discharged from hospitals into care homes (Perraudin 2020).

Yet this decision did not solve all problems, as the government order from mid-March 2020 to vacate hospital beds without testing was also based on the false assumption that there was no need to test discharged patients because COVID-19 sufferers 'can be safely cared for in a care home' (Butler 2020). In reality, the lack of clinical expertise and medical equipment in the care system, as well as the lack of integration between health and social care, meant COVID-19 sufferers in care homes, both those who had been discharged from hospitals with the virus and those who had been infected in care homes, were left without a proper care and often were rejected for admission to hospital, which resulted in even more people dying in care homes than in hospitals. The decision to discharge and the fact and that critically ill care home residents were denied access to hospital, and thus to intensive care, exposed the government's priorities – particularly the importance it attached to the protection of hospital resources at the cost of elderly people's lives. The cross-party Commons Public Accounts Committee agreed that the government's policy was 'slow, inconsistent and at times negligent' (UK Parliament 2020). Instead of the promised 'protective ring round social care', care home residents were being treated as 'collateral damage' (Calvert and Arbuthnott 2021: 284).

Furthermore, the decision to place untested hospital patients in care homes was made without an agreement or consensus from the care providers. In fact, in early March 2020, the major care providers directly asked the government not to go ahead with this practice. As COVID-19 infections in care homes escalated, with staffing stretched by absences and a chronic lack of protective equipment, the providers of care services pleaded with the government not to force them to accept untested patients from hospitals (Savage and Trapper 2021). Pointing to the rapidly increasing number of coronavirus cases in care homes, managers and staff complained about a lack of PPE and testing, non-existent training to care for COVID-19 patients, and the shortage of places in care homes. They particularly stressed that care homes staff did not have access to PPE for months after the pandemic began, and that there was a huge shortage of carers (Savage and Trapper 2021). Despite the Minister for Health's calming rhetoric that England's care homes were well protected, that many homes had experienced no COVID-19 outbreak at all and that COVID-19-negative patients discharged into infected homes faced low risk, the coronavirus crisis was very real in care homes. Because care homes in England lacked the protective equipment, medical support and sufficient numbers of staff to cope with the coronavirus outbreak, large numbers of elderly people died 'prematurely' or suffered from 'unnecessary' serious illnesses. The *Readying the NHS and Social Care for the COVID-19 Peak* (UK Parliament 2020) observed that government support for the front line of the care system was almost non-existent and that, together with the government's lack of both funding and a long-term strategy for the social care system, this had increased the severity of the virus's impact on the care system.

Despite government promises of the testing for discharged hospital patients in mid-April 2020, and despite later promises of testing for all care home residents and staff by June 2020, all testing arrangements remained 'chaotic' and 'fragmented' and were often not delivered. At the end of August 2020, newspapers reported 'UK care homes still denied COVID tests despite Hancock pledge' (Tapper 2020). By May 2020, many operators and staff saw government interference into the aged care system as unsupportive and felt 'completely abandoned' by their local health service: 'The first thing we saw was district nursing teams withdraw – they wanted us to take on dressings and injections. Then GPs stopped coming, and when we got messages it was only about end-of-life care' (Savage and Trapper 2021). And even when GPs did come, their capacity to offer comfort and reassurance to distressed care home residents was reduced by the existence of new rules, protective procedures and requirements to wear masks, gloves and other PPE (Francis 2021).

Although the residents and staff of the majority of care homes across the country were tested regularly by the autumn of 2020, deaths kept increasing in care homes. The steady rise in the death toll in care homes during the last months of 2020 was reflected in the mainstream press, as illustrated by such headlines as 'Two-thirds of residents die in COVID outbreak at Lincolnshire care home', 'COVID kills half of Sussex care home's residents over Christmas', 'COVID-related deaths in care homes in England jump' and 'Data on COVID care home deaths kept secret "to protect" commercial interests'. All these articles drew public attention to the fact that in the second wave of the pandemic, as COVID-19 cases were rising again in care homes, the heath crisis compromised the ability of care homes to deliver the quality of end-of-life care. According to many people working in the social care system, including the managing director of Edendale Lodge, a care home in East Sussex, the new COVID-19 outbreak in care homes was 'horrendous', 'devasting' and 'just unstoppable', and residents were 'sitting ducks', 'written off' and denied any help. For example, in the last month of 2020, thirteen of twenty-seven residents at Edendale Lodge died with confirmed or suspected COVID-19 and more than one-third of the staff tested positive during this outbreak (Marsh and Booth 2021). Also devastated by COVID-19 was the Old Hall at Halton Holegate, a care home where most of those who died were in their nineties; the youngest was 79 and the oldest was 99. Its manager, while telling the press their tragic stories, noted that some of the deaths

> were so sudden staff did not have the chance to administer end-of-life treatment or arrange for loved ones to say goodbye ... a lot of residents did not get to say goodbye to loved ones or receive the normal end-of-life care ... some residents did pass on their own because there was no suggestion anything was going to happen. We went in to do checks and they had gone. (quoted in Booth 2021)

Daily tragic stories and reports were also raising questions about how it was that, despite the governmental talk about its central task being to protect the vulnerable old, care homes were 'given nothing more than a two-day supply of masks apiece, forcing upon staff the impossible choice of abandoning their residents or going to work unprotected' (Clarke 2021: 107).

During the pandemic, the role and image of care homes changed. With many residents in self-isolation for health reasons and with greater shortages of and demands on staff, care homes became less-responsive environments where residents had less communication and were less familiar with staff members. Moreover, due to the visiting restrictions, this loss of relationships with staff in care homes was not compensated for by contact, intimacy and engagement with family members. The changing nature of care homes, which were becoming 'sterile fortresses' or turning 'into prisons' (Francis 2021: 144), was reflected in many devasted families' stories about the lonely and difficult deaths faced by their relatives in care homes and newspaper articles with headlines such as 'Isolated UK care home residents "fading away"', 'A million over-65s "still at risk of loneliness"' and 'Death in the absence of hugs', with were illustrations showing care homes with large 'NO VISITORS' signs and sometime posters of rainbows decorating care homes' windows with the sad faces of residents peering out behind them. Catastrophic media messages were exemplified by dramatic photographs of old, wrinkly hands reaching towards the gloved hands of care workers, with images of elderly, sad faces pressed to windows and videos of old people waving to relatives gathered outside care homes. Even when, in mid-2021, the government guidance permitted every care home resident to have an unlimited number of 'named visitors' who would be able to enter the care home for regular visits after negative tests, residents of some care homes were not allow to see their family members. They therefore felt separated from their loved ones, lonely and locked in a 'fortress'. In protest against some care homes not following the government instructions on facilitating visits and imposing their own stricter rules, 240,000 people signed a petition, 'Please let me hug my family before it's too late!' which demanded a new law ending isolation for care home residents, making visiting a legal right and stopping care homes from deciding on the scope of residents' contacts with the world outside (Booth 2021).

From the first day that vaccinations were available, 8 December 2020, the UK state policy was to get vaccinations to care home residents and staff. Elderly people in residential care and their staff were identified as the highest propriety groups for COVID-19 vaccination. The uptake of the vaccine among care home residents was very high and, since it was launched in winter 2020, the vaccine program has saved the lives of many residents. However, despite the fact that the vaccination of staff of care homes was also considered a priority, the level of vaccination among staff was lower. Moreover, the level of infection among staff was high and increasing, which was seen as increasing the risk of reappearance of coronavirus in care homes. By July 2021, with almost 70% of care home staff double-jabbed, there were 14,660 positive tests among care home staff, three times the 4,552 positive tests recorded in June 2021 (Chaplin 2021).

Subsequently, the government announced that from 11 November 2021, COVID-19 vaccinations would be compulsory for all registered care home staff in England, including anyone entering a care home, such as health workers, inspectors and tradespeople (Campbell 2021). With more than a quarter of UK care home staff not in favour of vaccination, and with high levels of staff fluctuation and exhaustion, many worried that mandatory coronavirus vaccination would not work and would cause more problems and worsen the already serious staffing crisis engulfing the health and care services (Abrahams 2021). To increase willingness to accept the new condition of employment, as the deadlines for care home workers in England were approaching, on 11 November, the government decided that NHS staff would also have to be fully vaccinated against COVID-19 (*BBC News*, 9 November 2021). However, as these compulsory vaccination requirements were widely criticized, on 1 March 2022 the government abandoned mandatory COVID-19 jabs for health and social care workers in England. The decision that social care staff were no longer required to be vaccinated was welcomed by many, who pointed out that by this stage 95% of care home staff had received two doses of a COVID-19 vaccine, so care home employees had been meeting their obligations to frail elderly residents (*BBC News* 2 March 2022). However, for many the reversal of the decision had come too late to repair the damage done to the care sector as many staff had already left care homes because of the previous requirement and were unlikely to return to their jobs. The UK government's policy of vaccination of staff in care homes was rather chaotic and its attempts to balance contradictory values, such as freedom and safety, were criticized for undervaluing care workers' professional responsibility towards their clients.

Many other aspects of the government strategy of handling the spread of infection in care homes and the actions of the operators of care homes – particularly practices in care homes during the COVID-19 crisis relating to experiences of end-of-life care – met with criticism. The cross-party Commons Public Accounts Committee (2020), investigating the government failure to provide adequate PPE and testing to care home staff during the first peak of the crisis, asserted that, 'Our care homes were effectively thrown to the wolves, and the virus has ravaged some of them.' The committee also described the minister's decision to allow elderly residents to be discharged from hospital without being tested as a 'low moment in our national response' (UK Parliament 2020). In a similar critical mood, the

Care Quality Commission, which investigated claims of some care homes that 'a patient's positive COVID-19 status was known to the hospital but not disclosed at the point of discharge', viewed these actions as constituting a potential breach of the *Health and Social Care Act* (Manson 2020). In addition to the criticism from these two bodies and from the care providers, the government was faced with criticism from members of bereaved families, voiced both individually and collectively. For example, the daughter of a man who died in a care home after being inflected with COVID-19 by a resident who was discharged from hospital into that home in June 2020, claimed that the government broke the law by releasing hospital patients into care homes without COVID-19 tests and requested a judicial review of the government's strategy. Arguing that the state policy 'failed to take into account the vulnerability of care home residents and staff to infection and death, the inadequacy of testing and PPE availability', she pointed out that prioritizing the NHS hospital capacity to deal with critically ill COVID-19 patients was 'disproportionate, discriminatory and irrational'. Her case against the government reached the High Court, which ruled that the government's decision to release hospital untested patients into care homes was 'not illegal' (Booth 2020). As the initial applicant, unsatisfied with the verdict, continued to press for the judicial review, she was joined in her legal battle by another woman who had also lost her father to the virus in a care homes after outbreaks of COVID there in spring 2020. These two grieving women argued that the failure to protect care home residents was among the most 'egregious and devastating policy failures in the modern era'. On 27 April 2022, the High Court ruled that the government's policy of discharging patients from hospitals into care homes at the start of the COVID-19 pandemic in 2020 was unlawful because it failed to take into account the risk to elderly and vulnerable residents from non-symptomatic transmission by residents with coronavirus infection (Gillespie 2022).

The government was also under continuous scrutiny by a collective body, the COVID-19 Bereaved Families for Justice group. From the early stage of the pandemic, they asked very important questions, such as why so many residents of care homes died of COVID-19, why 'the protective ring around care homes' promised by the health minister, failed to work and why thousands of people were discharged from hospitals into care homes without being tested. These and other urgent questions, according to this vocal group, demanded an immediate public inquiry into the UK's COVID-19 response. Prime Minister Boris Johnston initially rejected calls from the families of people who had died from COVID-19 for a full public inquiry before announcing one in May 2021. However, as he stipulated the inquiry would not begin its work until Spring 2022, the members of the Bereaved Families for Justice group, who believed that only an instant review could improve policies and protect the most vulnerable lives, rejected the governmental timescale for a statutory inquiry into the country's dealing with the coronavirus as unacceptable. In another change of state policy, in March 2022, ten months after the prime minister promised it to bereaved families, it was announced that there would be a public inquiry. The inquiry, set up to examine the government's strategy of handling the spread of infection in care homes and many others problems connected with deaths in care homes during the pandemic, was also asked by Black, Asian and minority ethnic leaders to address racism and inequalities experienced during the pandemic (Stewart 2022).

By identifying the lessons to be learned from the COVID-19, the statutory public inquiry into the government policies and actions of the operators of care homes, as well as potential further legal claims over the government's handling of the COVID-19 pandemic, might alter our ways of thinking and meeting obligations to frail elderly people, and might contribute to an improvement in the protection and in the quality of end-of-life care of the most vulnerable citizens.

EPILOGUE:

The afterlife of the pandemic

As I write this Epilogue, in the UK COVID-19 death toll is no longer daily news and we all want to believe that the worst of the COVID-19 pandemic is behind us. Hopes for a return to normality are growing as, thanks to vaccinations, innovative treatment and drugs, the chances of becoming seriously ill and not surviving are much lower than they were in earlier waves of the pandemic. Yet COVID-19 is still with us and those with underlying health conditions, including compromised immune systems and older people, are still at risk from coronavirus. Even though many people have built up immunity through vaccinations, boosters and previous coronavirus infections, and there are effective anti-viral treatments for vulnerable groups, there are still plenty of uncertainties as it is not yet clear how COVID-19 will become an endemic disease that we can live with. Despite the fact that COVID-19 is no longer an acute emergency, we cannot assume that the global threat of the pandemic is over: much of the world remains unvaccinated, vaccines have become accessible mainly in wealthy nations and we are still at risk of this pandemic generating a variant that would be more transmissive and more fatal. Moreover people's hope for a return to the world as it was before the pandemic depends both on individual responsibility for their everyday actions and on public health officials' strategies to exit the health crisis.

Thus, given that we have not yet seen a real aftermath of the pandemic, it is rather difficult to tackle its afterlife. However, this book is not really about the pandemic: I have used COVID-19 to discuss the important ethical questions raised by the pandemic. By casting light on the pandemic's impact on societal values and attitudes to death in old age, this volume highlights the moral concerns raised by the recent health crisis. By exploring how the COVID-19 pandemic's age-specific pattern of mortality has challenged our ways of thinking about death and strengthened the relationship between old age and death, a case has been made for the importance of talking about death in later life. By arguing that death in old age in pre-COVID times was invisible, it shows that COVID-19 – which puts immunocompromised people at risk – has forced us all to confront the issue of death in old age. Because the immune system weakens with age, older people's vulnerability to the virus and the subsequent deaths of many elderly people – especially those with other medical conditions – is far greater. COVID-19 has made death in old age visible. The tragedy of the deaths of so many elderly people, together with the realization that with time passing all people's immunity is partly compromised, so being vulnerable is in our future as well, should motivate our reckoning with the issue of mortality and encourage open discussions of death and ways of dying. The topic of death has always been a difficult subject to talk about, but in the next few years, in a post-pandemic climate where we are more familiar with death and many are grieving the loss of loved ones, there needs to be a real effort to discuss the issue.

Although the experiences of elderly people in the pandemic and the emotional legacy of COVID-19 will become clearer in the months and years ahead, we already know the death toll and several dimensions of older people's painful marginalization and loneliness. After demonstrating the tragic fate of elderly people in homes, hospitals and care homes during the recent health crisis, I argue that the COVID-19 pandemic has brought ageism to the surface by exposing that when 'deaths happen to people who are already not valued in a million other ways, it's easier to not value their lives in this additional way' (Yong 2021). This book asserts that one of the most important lessons from the coronavirus crisis is the realization of the need to reject ageism in all its expressions. This means the rejection not only of referrals to elderly people as 'silly old buggers', to use former Australian Prime Minister Bob Hawke's legendary putdown of pensioners, but also the dismissal by some British politicians of COVID-19 as presenting the risk 'only' to very old people. Above all, it means the rejection of the reliance on chronological age as a sole criterion for determining risk or access to medical care, the rejection of a lack of responsibility and obligation of care for the aged and the rejection of a lack of hospice care for the elderly at the end of life. By breaking the silence surrounding death in old age, the recent health crisis has offered an opportunity to discuss how we want to die, to appreciate the value of the end-of-life care and to recognize the need to make hospice care available to all those who need it, at home, in hospitals and in residential care settings.

As the COVID-19 pandemic strained and overburdened the UK health and care systems, subsequently many difficult situations arose where resources were not sufficient for all individuals in need of treatment and care. Hence, for example, while facing many structural problems and struggling to provide basic services, the NHS was faced with the difficulty of prioritizing the provision of treatments, which often resulted in compromising the needs of the aged and concealing the need for end-of-life care (Olszowski 2022). The pandemic has also been a difficult time for hospices, which faced significant disruptions and a decrease in the number of people supported by end-of-life care. Nonetheless, even though there were fewer hospice inpatients during the COVID crisis, hospices still delivered more than one million 'hospice-at-home' services in 2020 and 2021 (Keeble et al. 2022). Generally, the recent health crisis was a time when hospice day services and outpatient settings were facing a decline in the people seen, while more people were dying at home than ever before. Since the start of the pandemic, one-third more deaths have occurred at home and throughout the whole pandemic there have been more than 100,000 extra deaths recorded in a home setting (Keeble et al. 2022). This significant increase in the number of people dying at home in the pandemic's extreme circumstances further reduced the availability of hospice care for elderly people dying at home.

Before COVID-19, only about half of those who needed end-of-life care were getting it, which means the majority of dying older people were neither gaining places in hospices nor receiving care and support in their homes or care homes (Olszewski 2022). With infection cases flowing downwards into society's cracks and with a shortage of hospice care, during the pandemic, increasing numbers of older and poor people at the end of life were not provided with the medical, practical and emotional support they required. Overall, 76% of those who died during COVID-19 did not get the support they needed in managing pain at the end of life, including 64% of people who died at home during the pandemic, which means 40%

more than usual did not get the help they needed (Olszowski 2022: 45). This indicates that the pandemic presented the elderly with the threat of losing 'the gains the end-of-life care and hospice movement have brought about in recent decades' (Age UK 2022). This threat, together with the ageing of the UK population and the number of people dying with multiple and complex conditions, which is projected to increase by 42% by 2040, implies that now is the time to treat hospice care as 'a right, not a luxury' (Olszowski 2022: 45).

Moreover, not only is there an increasing need for end-of-life care, but the needs of patients using hospice services appear to have become increasingly complicated. Confronting many people with death, pain, insecurity and loneliness, the pandemic has increased their need for help and comfort. It has also impelled changes to how hospice care is delivered, with many hospices, as well as providing end-of-life support, also delivering virtual welfare, bereavement and therapy services. As a result of the COVID-19 crisis, there are now greater demands from patients and families for both in-patient end-of-life care and bereavement services (Scobie and Hutchings 2022). Taking into account societal support for easing the exit from life with hospice care as well as growing public support for the right to assisted dying, it is time to discuss not how to delay the inevitable, but rather how to ease the exit and to help dying people individually to decide how they want to end their lives.

It is also worth noting that the increasing support for the right to choose a way of dying and the perception of the end-of-life care as more than a prolongation of the inevitable with expensive drugs are not on the collision course with the new knowledge of how to modify, monitor and even gain control over individuals' ageing processes by adopting an appropriate lifestyle (Levine 2022). Today's advanced research into the biological age – that is, the age at which a person's body is functioning – might help to lower the risk of diseases and chronic illnesses of old age, but it cannot tame death as, 'Against other things it is possible to obtain security, but when it comes to death we human beings all live in a unwalled city' (Hippocrates, quoted in Spinny 2017: 56). Yet this new scientific drive to increase our life expectancy and to make the time of death a controllable event poses new dilemmas about how to bridge the gap between wanting to live and having to die. Such questions, together with COVID-19's urge to make us rethink mortality, can increase our understanding that the acceptance of death is 'a task we must all engage in, and one that we face up to more or less successfully' (Ricoeur 2004: 358). Although we tend not to believe in our own death, as Freud argued, by fostering the recognition that 'in the midst of life we are in death' (Montaigne 1987: 103), the pandemic has educated us about the reality of death.

If, in the coming few years – given the COVID-19 pandemic experience – we attempt to figure out how we want to live the rest of our lives and to seriously address the issue of death in old age, the next decade needs to be a time of change. Yet generally it is wars, not pandemics, that are seen to be able to mobilize people for change. Despite the data showing that since the eighteenth century more lives have been lost to diseases than to battlefield injuries (Spinney 2017), the function of pandemics in the process of social transformation has tended to be overlooked. The role of pandemics in bringing social change is questioned mainly because studies of collective memories suggest that the trauma of pandemics is forgotten by the second generation (Misztal 2003). In other words, despite their regular occurrences, previous pandemics tend not to be remembered or preserved in collective memory, which means we are not learning the required lessons from them. For example, although the global toll of the Spanish flu is estimated to have been between 50 and 100 million (Honigsbaum 2020; Spinney 2017), and despite this death toll being twice higher as for all of World War I (Kucharski 2010: 2), in our popular conception the 1918–19 pandemic 'exists largely as a footnote to World War I' (Spinney 2017: 33). Even though the Spanish flu was 'the greatest human disaster not only of the twentieth century but possibly in all of recorded human history' (Spinney 2017: 66), it has been the forgotten pandemic in practically all affected societies. For instance, the 1918–19 flu pandemic, as Alfred Crosby (1976) argues in his book *America's Forgotten Pandemic*, did not leave an imprint on the American culture because people were quick to forget this health crisis as they needed to trust their future. Moreover, in contrast to the heroism of deaths in war, the tragedy of pandemics feels much more senseless because pandemics, without anybody to blame for their occurrence, lack clear and unifying narratives as well as powerful and mobilizing images. Whereas 'suffering and death inflicted by an unseen virus may be deemed meaningless, hence often forgotten', deaths in war are seen as meaningful sacrifices for a larger cause that should be remembered (Hirst 2020: 251). Until recently, short memories of traumatic past pandemics, together with optimistic assumptions about the power of modern medicine, have led to the dismissal of infectious diseases, general complacency about threats of pandemics and a lack of planning for health crises. As the COVID-19 pandemic has shown, this can costly.

Yet more recent and detailed scrutiny of the history of pandemics seems to reverse the dominant perception of them, and suggests that pandemics can also represent times of change. With the growing evidence that plagues were behind many historical developments, we are slowly becoming aware that pandemics may have been sources of change (Harari 2020). For example, the Black Death – also known as the Bubonic Plague – which struck Europe in the fourteenth century and killed more than 30% of its population was followed by economic collapse and a string of peasant revolts, all of which helped to end the Middle Ages and enabled the progress of the Renaissance. The Great Plague, which hit London in 1665, led to granting a new status to science, as illustrated by the establishment in the United Kingdom of the Royal Society of Science in 1666 (Wright 2020). With the recent interest in the Spanish flu histography, we now know that 'the 1918 pandemic accelerated the pace of change in the first half of the twentieth century and helped shape our modern world' (Spinney 2017: 33). Moreover, the AIDS epidemic enhanced the push for gay rights and impacted many societal practices, ranging from legal decisions through healthcare rules to ways of dealing with human remains (Hirst 2020; Troyer 2020).

This potential of pandemics to bring change in their wake is connected with the fact that, despite always being a threat to the community, such health crises also demonstrate the role of 'the pragmatic utility of solidarity' in ensuring the effectiveness of battles with viruses (Chrisakis 2020: 324). Despite intensifying conflicts and selfishness, pandemics can facilitate solidaristic actions and mutual help. In the history of pandemics, there are examples of both solidarity when people united to save others from deadly pandemic and a decline in community spirit. For instance, in England in 1599, the plague undermined feeling of communal solidarity as social values broke down and households shut their doors to outsiders (Wood 2021). Yet the idea of community and feelings of solidarity have also been defended during pandemics, such as in the famous seventeenth-century case of the English village of Eyam that sealed itself off when infected with the Great Plague of London and by this communal sacrifice prevented the spread of infection to local towns (Wood 2021). In other words, pandemics not only bring out the worst but also the best in people, as there are moments of selflessness and moments of courage.

It seems that when a pandemic becomes a social symbol of unity and solidarity, such a heath crisis can teach people about their responsibility to communities and can induce processes of social change. All examples from the history of pandemics suggest that handling a pandemic requires citizens to accept new rules and restrictions, to help the disadvantaged and support each other, which all necessitate people trusting both themselves and their authorities. On one hand, maintaining public trust and harnessing collective capabilities can be easier in the midst of a big social catastrophe than it is in normal times. For instance, as the Spanish flu erupted during World War I, the US state's high level of social trust helped the authorities to boost social solidarity and acceptance of government interventions and restrictions (Chrisakis 2020). On the other hand, pandemics can also expose countries' failures in cultivating national unity and trust during health crises – for example, the British people's trust in their government fell during the pandemic, from 65% in February 2020 to 37% in January 2021 (Spiegelhalter and Masters 2021: 195). Pandemics, moreover, can strengthen authoritarianism as the COVID-19 pandemic in China has shown (Osnos 2022). Generally, pandemics can reshape the public's views about the governments, while governments' degree of transparency and citizens' trust in the political system are essential factors in successfully cultivating national unity during the pandemic.

The COVID-19 pandemic has been a catalyst for changes in many aspects of life in the United Kingdom and other developed countries. Its attendant social distancing measures have transformed the way many people work and study, and the ways in which health services are delivered. COVID-19 has also changed the law, as questioning of the legality of the many unprecedented interventions of the past two years, ranging from lockdowns and furlough schemes to mask or vaccine mandates, has assumed some significance. The health crisis has provided, as discussed in the last chapter, a new impetus for reforms of the care system in the United Kingdom. Yet, like other pandemics, it has also been a time of insecurity, fear, risk, loss of lives and disruption to societal norms. And, like all heath crises, COVID-19 has inflamed tensions and exposed social divisions, inequalities and hidden problems. In the United Kingdom, the pandemic reduced life expectancy, increased the inequality in longevity, weakened the functioning of many services and has had a devastating impact on healthcare workers. At the same time, it has also been a time of solidarity in many countries. It has heightened people's awareness of common vulnerability, as it has taught us to recognize that in the midst of the pandemic we cannot push the knowledge of death away and also 'demonstrated how interconnected we are all and how the commonwealth is only as well as its weakest member' (Chrisakis 2020: 324). The pandemic has also fostered greater intergenerational solidarity by encouraging personal contact between old and young people. This form of relationship is an important means to overcome intergenerational tensions and the ageism resulting from them. Yet, by posing questions about who should compensate younger generations for lockdowns and disruptions in their education, the pandemic has also exacerbated controversies between old and young people and activated some expressions of ageism whereby older adults have been stereotypically portrayed as members of a homogenous, vulnerable and troubling group.

The full COVID-19 picture will become clear only in the next few years, while debates over which country had 'good' COVID-19 policies will possibly continue for decades. Yet there are already some evaluations of the handling of the pandemic in individual countries and globally. Frequently critical voices blame politicians for their complacency and lack of strategy for inhibiting the virus and limiting death. For example, Sridhar (2022: 21) concludes her global comparison by arguing that 'with the right politics and leadership, much of the suffering and death was largely preventable'. The UK Parliamentary Report (2021) identifies the major deficiencies in the machinery of the UK government – with its lack of openness impairing meaningful communication – as responsible for the inefficiencies of COVID-19 policies. According to the WHO, the best pandemic preparedness depended on 'reducing inequality, improving health and providing a robust social and healthcare system offering' (Balloux 2022: 49). While pointing out that even though the end of the pandemic is not far away, COVID-19 will continue as the virus will keep on mutating and spreading in largely unvaccinated populations of poorer countries. The WHO warns that to stop the spread of COVID-19 globally requires global action now. Only overcoming severe inequities in vaccine availability, speeding up global vaccine delivery and distributing treatments to prevent severe outcomes will enable the world to see the end of COVID-19 in the coming years.

In addition to these various evaluations of handling the pandemic and searches for ways to exit it, there are also already voices proposing that, instead of returning to something like normal life as it was before the pandemic, we should learn from our experience and consider the changes required for the future. For instance, Peter Hennessy (2022) hopes COVID-19, like the post-World War II period when societal solidarity resulted in the establishment of the NHS, may introduce 'a duty of care' for elderly people, to paraphrase the title of his book. On the other hand, Latour (2021: 5) expects that the experience of lockdown during the COVID-19 pandemic may lead to far bigger global changes, which 'would amount to a metamorphosis'. While pointing that the global health crisis is rooted in the global climate crisis, Latour hopes for the pandemic to provide us with better understanding and tackling of the global climate crisis in preparation for the world we will experience in the years to come.

This book also makes a plea to use our experience of the pandemic to think about change – especially change in our relationships with older adults in ways that might be conducive to confronting mortality and discussing ways of dying and the issue of death in old age.

Bibliography

Abel, E. (2017). *Living in Death's Shadow: Family Experiences of Terminal Care and Irreplaceable Loss*. Baltimore, MD: Johns Hopkins University Press.

Abrahams, C. (2021). 'Forcing COVID jabs on England's exhausted care home staff won't work', *The Guardian*, 29 June, <https://www.theguardian.com/commentisfree/2021/jun/29/covid-jab-england-care-home-staff-vaccinations>, accessed 29 June 2021.

Adams, P. J. (2020). *Reflecting on the Inevitable: Mortality at the Crossroads of Psychology, Philosophy and Health*. Oxford: Oxford University Press.

Adams, T. (2021). 'Queen Alone', *The Observer*, 18 April, pp. 1–2.

Age UK (2018). '1.4 Million Older People Aren't Getting the Care and Support They Need', <https://www.ageuk.org.uk/latest-news/articles/2018/july>, accessed 2 September 2021.

Age UK (2019). *Briefing: Health and Care of Older People in England 2019*, <https://www.ageuk.org.uk/globalassets/age-uk/documents/reports-and-publications/reports-and-briefings/health>, accessed 20 January 2022.

Age UK (2020). 'Age UK Research Lays Bare the Drastic Impact of the Pandemic on Our Older Population's Health and Morale', https://www.ageuk.org.uk/latest-press/articles/2020/10/age-uk--research-into-the-effects-of-the-pandemic-on-the-older-populations-health>, accessed 20 January 2022.

Age UK (2021). 'Loneliness and COVID-19', <https://www.ageuk.org.uk/our-impact/policy-research/loneliness-research-and-resources>, accessed 7 March 2022.

Age UK (2022). *2020–21 Annual Report*, <https://www.ageuk.org.uk/globalassets/age-uk/documents/annual-reports-and-reviews/age-uk-annual-report-2021.pdf>, accessed 15 March 2022.

Ai, A. L., Hopp, F. and Shearer, M. (2006). 'Getting Affairs in Order: Influences of Social Support and Religious Coping on End-of-life Planning Among Open Heart Surgery Patients', *Journal of Social Work in End-of-Life & Palliative Care*, 2 (1), 71–94.

Aims, M. (2020). *Inside Story*. London: Vintage Books.

Alzheimer's Association (2022). 2022 *Alzheimer's Disease Facts and Figures*, <https://www.alz.org/media/documents/alzheimers-facts-and-figures.pdf>, accessed 20 January 2022.

Alzheimer's Society (2022). 'Research United: Against Dementia', <https://www.alzheimers.org.uk/research/our-research>, accessed 20 January 2022.

Amery, J. (1994). *On Aging: Revolt and Resignation*, trans. John D. Barlow. Bloomington, IN: Indiana University Press.

Angell, M.(2012). 'May Doctors Help You to Die?', *New York Review of Books*, 11 October, pp. 23–27.

Applewhite, A. (2019). *This Chair Rocks: A Manifesto Against Ageism*. London: Melville House.

Arber, S., Vandrevala, T., Daly, T. and Hampson, S. (2008). 'Understanding Gender Differences in Older People's Attitudes Towards Life-prolonging Medical Technologies', *Journal of Aging Studies*, 22 (4), 366–75.

Ardelt, M. (2013). 'Wisdom, Religiosity, Purpose in Life, and Death Attitudes of Aging Adults'. In A. Tomer et al. (eds), *Existential and Spiritual in Issues in Death Attitude*, pp. 145–59. Mahwah, NJ: Lawrence Erlbaum.

Aries, P. (1981). *Western Attitudes Toward Death: From the Middle Ages to the Present*. Baltimore, MD: Johns Hopkins University Press.

Armstrong, S. (2019). *Borrowed Time*. London: Bloomsbury.

Arnold, C. (2008). *Necropolis: London and Its Dead*. London: Pocket Books.

Ayalon, L., Chasteen, A. and Wahl, H. (2020). 'Aging in Times of the COVID-19 Pandemic: Avoiding Ageism and Fostering Intergenerational Solidarity', *The Journals of Gerontology: Psychological Sciences*, 20, 1–4, <https://www.semanticscholar.org/paper/Aging-in-Times-of-the-COVID-19-Pandemic%3A-Avoiding-Ayalon-Chasteen/e33bfbffecda2e92829760042cb71a72fca2e84f>, accessed 23 September 2020.

Baars, J. (2015). 'Time in Late Modern Ageing'. In J. Twigg and W. Martin (eds), *Routledge Handbook of Cultural Gerontology*, pp. 397–403. London: Routledge.

Badshah, N. (2020). 'Unions Call for Minute's Silence for Key Workers Killed by COVID-19 in UK', *The Guardian*, 20 April, <https://www.theguardian.com/society/2020/apr/20/unions-call-minutes-silence-key-workers-killed-covid-19-uk>, accessed 20 April 2020.

Baker, J. O., Gordon, A. L., Day, E. and Bade, C. D. (2020). 'Pandemics Prey on Fears, Both Legitimate and Illegitimate', *Context*, 29 October <https://contexts.org>, accessed 23 December 2020.

Balloux, F. (2022). 'Sweden? Japan? UK? Debates Over Who had "a Good" COVID Won't End', *The Observer*, 8 May, p. 49.

Baltes, P. B. and Smith, J. (2003) 'New Frontiers in the Future of Ageing', *Gerontology*, 49 (2), 123–35.

Barker, K. (2014). *A New Settlement for Health and Social Care: Final Report*. London: King's Fund, <https://www.kingsfund.org.uk/publications>, accessed 13 December 2021.

Bauman, Z. (1992). *Morality, Immortality and Other Life Strategies*. Cambridge: Polity Press.
Barnes, J. (2009). *Nothing to be Frightened Of.* London: Vintage Books.
Barnes, J. (2011). *The Sense of Ending*. London: Jonathan Cape.
Barnes, J. (2013). *Levels of Life*. New York: Knopf.
Bauman, Z. (2006). *Liquid Fear.* Cambridge: Polity Press.
Bauman, Z. (2011). 'Sociology, Mortality and Solidarity', interview with M. Hviid Jacobsen, *Morality*, 16 (4), 30–39.
Bawden, A. (2021). 'What Chance Did Mum Have? Two Women Who Died with Hospital-Acquired COVID', *The Guardian*, 24 May, <https://www.theguardian.com/world/2021/may/24/what-chance-did-mum-have-two-woman-who-died-with-hospital-acquired-covid>, accessed 24 May 2021.
Beck, U. (1992). *Risk Society. Towards a New Modernity*. London: Sage.
Beck, U. (1996). *Ecological Politics in an Age of Risk*. Cambridge: Polity Press.
Becker, E. (1973). *The Denial of Death*. New York: Free Press.
Bennett, C. (2020). 'Loved and Lost: Grief in the Time of Coronavirus – a Photo Essay', *The Guardian,* 21 August, <https://www.theguardian.com/artanddesign/2020/aug/21/loved-and-lost-simon-bray-photo-essay>, accessed 21 August 2020.
Bennett, G. and Bennett, K. M. (2000). 'The Presence of the Dead: An Empirical Study', *Mortality*, 5 (2), 139–58.
Bennett, K. M. (1997). 'Widowhood in Elderly Women: The Medium- and Long-term Effects on Mental and Physical Health', *Mortality*, 2 (2), 137–48.
Bennett, K. M., Smith, P. T and Hughes, G. M. (2005). 'Coping, Depressive Feelings and Gender Differences in Late Life Widowhood', *Ageing and Mental Health*, 9(4), 348–53.
Bennett, K. M. and Vidal-Hall, S. (2000). 'Narratives of Death: A Qualitative Study of Widowhood in Later Life', *Ageing and Society*, 20, 413–28.
Benoliel, J. and Denger, L. (1995). 'Institutional Dying'. In H. Wass and R. A. Neimeyer (eds), *Dying: Facing the Facts,* pp. 117–42. London: Taylor and Francis.
Berman, J. (2020). *Anti-Vaxxers: How to Challenge a Misinformed Movement*. Cambridge, MA: MIT Press.
Bern-Klug, M. (2004). 'The Ambiguous Dying Syndrome', *Health and Social Work,* 29 (1), 55–65.
Berns, N. (2011). *Closure: The Rush to End Grief and What It Costs Us*. Philadelphia: Temple University Press.
Biswa-Diener, R., Diener, E. and Tamir, M. (2004). 'The Psychology of Subjective Well-being', *Daedalus*, 133 (2), 18–25.
Black, S. (2018). *All That Remains: A Life in Death*. London: Doubleday.

Blackball, M. (2020). 'I Miss People Terrible', *The Guardian*, 17 May, <https://www.theguardian.com/world/2020/may/17/i-miss-people-terribly-the-growing-pain-of-older-peoples-isolation-lockdown>, accessed 17 May 2020.

Blaikie, A. (1999). *Ageing and Popular Culture.* Cambridge: Cambridge University Press.

Blum, A. (2015). 'Death, Happiness and the Meaning of Life', *Journal of Classical Sociology*, 15 (1), 24–38.

Blythe, R. (2005 [1979]). *The View in Winter.* Norwich: Canterbury Press.

Boffey, D. (2018) 'Doctors in Netherlands Asked Family to Hold Down Euthanasia Patient', *The Guardian,* 25 July, <https://www.theguardian.com/world/2018/jul/25/doctor-netherlands-asked-family-hold-down-euthanasia-patient>, accessed 23 May 2022.

Bonsu, S. K. (2007). 'The Presentation of Dead Selves in Everyday Life: Obituaries and Impression Management', *Symbolic Interaction*, 30 (2), 199–219.

Booth, R. (2020). 'Releasing English Hospital Patients into Care Homes "Not Illegal"', *The Guardian*, 21 June, <https://www.theguardian.com/world/2020/jun/21/releasing-english-hospital-patients-into-care-homes-not-illegal>, accessed 23 June 2020.

Booth, R. (2021). 'COVID Kills Half of Sussex Care Home's Residents Over Christmas', *The Guardian*, 7 January, <https://www.theguardian.com/world/2021/jan/07/covid-kills-half-of-sussex-care-homes-residents-over-christmas?te=1&nl=coronavirus-briefing&emc=edit_cb_20210107>, accessed 7 January 2021.

Borgstrom, E. and Walter, T. (2015). 'Choice and Compassion at the End of Life: A Critical Analysis of English Policy Discourse', *Social Science and Medicine*, 136–37 (July), 99–101.

Bowcott, O. (2019). 'Legalise Assisted Dying for Terminally Ill, Say 90% of People in UK', *The Guardian*, 3 March, <https://www.theguardian.com/society/2019/mar/03/legalise-assisted-dying-for-terminally-ill-say-90-per-cent-of-people-in-uk>, accessed 12 April 2022.

Bowley, J. (1969). *Attachment and Loss, Vol. 1.* New York: Basic Books.

Bowley, J. (1981). *Loss, Sadness and Depression.* Harmondsworth: Penguin.

Brennan, Z. (2005). *The Older Women in Recent Fiction.* Jefferson, NC: McFarland.

Bresalier, M. (2020). 'A Spanish Lesson', *The Guardian*, 19 December, <https://www.theguardian.com/world/2020/dec/18/a-christmas-pandemic-like-no-other-they-thought-that-in-1918-influenza-covid>, accessed 3 February 2021.

Bristow, J. (2019). *Stop Mugging Grandma: The 'Generation Wars' and Why Boomer Blaming Won't Solve Anything.* New Haven, CT: Yale University Press.

Britain Thinks (2015). Frailty Language and Perceptions. Age UK, <https://www.ageuk.org.uk/documents/en-gb/for-professionals/policy/health-and-wellbe

ing/report_bgs_frailty_language_and_perceptions.pdf?dtrk=true>, accessed 23 September 2020.

Brombert, V. (2013). *Musing on Mortality; From Tolstoy to Primo Levi.* Chicago: Chicago University Press.

Broom, A. (2015). *Dying: A Social Perspective on the End of Life*. Farnham: Ashgate.

Broom, A. and Cavenaugh, J. (2010). 'Masculinity, Moralities and Being Cared For: An Exploration of Experiences of Living and Dying in Hospice', *Social Science and Medicine*, 71 (5), 869–76.

Brown, R. (1999). *Surviving the Loss of a Loved One: Living Through Grief.* London: Autumn House.

Burch, D. (2020). 'Psychology vs Epidemiology', *Times Literary Supplement,* 16 October, p. 22.

Butler, J. (2020) 'Follow the Science', *London Review of Books*, 16 April, pp. 33–35.

Butler, K. and Bannock, C. (2021). '"A Sacrificed Generation": Psychological Scars of COVID on Young May Have Lasting Impact', *The Guardian*, 2 June, <https://www.theguardian.com/world/2021/jun/02/a-sacrificed-generation-psychological-scars-of-covid-on-young-may-have-lasting-impact>, accessed 1 June 2021.

Butler, P. (2021). 'Lack of Social Care Strategy Left System Weakened When COVID Struck – Report', *The Guardian,* 25 March, <https://www.theguardian.com/society/2021/mar/25/lack-of-social-care-strategy-left-system-weakened-when-covid-struck-report>, accessed 25 March 2021.

Byrski, L. (2012). *Getting On: Some Thoughts on Women and Ageing.* Sydney: Momentum.

Calasanti, T. (2020). 'Brown Slime, the Silver Tsunami, and Apocalyptic Demography: The Importance of Ageism and Age Relations', *Social Currents*, 3 April, <https://doi-org.ezproxy3.lib.le.ac.uk/10.1177/2329496520912736>, accessed 12 December 2021.

Calasanti, T. (2021). 'Ageism, Generational Rhetoric', *Contemporary Sociology*, 50(6), 453–59.

Callahan, D. (1993). *The Troubled Dream of Life: Living with Mortality*. New York: Simon and Schuster.

Calvert, J. and Arbuthnott, G. (2021). *Failures of State: The Inside Story of Britain's Battle with Coronavirus*. London: Mudlark.

Campbell, D. (2020). 'NHS Denies Elderly People Were Refused Care During Early COVID', *The Guardian*, 25 October, <https://www.theguardian.com/society/2020/oct/25/nhs-denies-elderly-people-were-refused-care-during-early-covid>, accessed 25 October 2020.

Campbell, D. (2021). 'Weaknesses That Led to Patients Getting COVID in Hospital Remain', *The Guardian*, 24 May, <https://www.theguardian.com/society/

2021/may/24/weaknesses-that-led-to-patients-getting-covid-in-hospital-remain>, accessed 24 May 2021.

Campbell, D. (2022) 'Global COVID-19 Death Toll "May Be Three Times Higher Than Official Figures", *The Guardian,* 10 March, <https://www.theguardian.com/world/2022/mar/10/global-covid-19-death-toll-may-be-three-times-higher-than-official-figures>, accessed 10 March 2022.

Campbell, D. and Bawden, A. (2021). 'Up to 8,700 Patients Died After Catching COVID in English Hospitals', *The Guardian,* 24 May, <https://www.theguardian.com/world/2021/may/24/up-to-8700-patients-died-after-catching-covid-in-english-hospitals>, accessed 24 May 2021.

Camus, A. (2005 [1945]). *The Myth of Sisyphus.* Harmondsworth: Penguin.

Camus, A. (2020 [1947]). *The Plague.* Trans. Stuart Gilbert. Harmondsworth: Penguin.

Care Quality Commission. (2018). *Annual Report 2018/19,* <https://www.cqc.org.uk/publications/major-report/annual-report-accounts-2018>, accessed 2 March 2022.

carehome.co.uk. (2022). 'Reviews for care homes, residential homes & nursing homes'. <https://www.carehome.co.uk>, accessed 2 March 2022.

Carozza, P. (2008). 'Human Dignity and Judicial Interpretation of Human Rights: A Reply', *The European Journal of International Law*, 19 (5), 931–44.

Carr, D. and Luth, E. A. (2019). 'Well-being at the End of Life', *Annual Review of Sociology*, 45, 515–434.

Case, A. and Deaton, A. (2020). *Death of Despair and the Future of Capitalism.* Princeton, NJ: Princeton University Press.

Caswell, G. and O'Connor, M. (2015). 'Agency in the Context of Social Death: Dying Alone at Home', *Contemporary Social Science*, 10, 249–61.

Chaplin, C. (2021). 'Ministers Accused of Leaving Care Homes "Exposed", *inews,* 13 August, <https://inews.co.uk/news/politics/ministers-accused-of-leaving-care-homes-exposed-as-number-of-covid-19-cases-among-staff-triple-in-july-1150622>, accessed 13 August 2021.

Chapple, H. S. (2010). *No Place for Dying.* Walnut Creek, CA: Left Coast Press.

Chetwynd-Cowieson, A. (2020). 'Don't Blame Young People for Rising COVID Cases', *Huffpost*, 9 September, p. 4.

Chrisakis, N. A. (2020). *Apollo's Arrow: The Profound and Enduring Impact of Coronavirus on the Way We Live.* New York: Little, Brown Spark.

Christensen, D. R. and Willerslev, R. (2013). *Taming Time, Timing Death: Social Technologies and Ritual.* Farnham: Ashgate.

Choron, J. (1963). *Death and Western Thought.* New York: Collier Books.

Chung, S. and Park, H. (2019). 'How Young and Older People Differ in Discriminatory Behaviour Towards Older People?', *Ageing and Society*, 39, 1996–2017.

Cicirelli, V. G. (1998). 'Views of Elderly People Concerning End-of-life Decisions', *Journal of Applied Gerontology*, 17 (2),186–203.

Clanchy, K. (2021). 'Letting Go: My Battle to Help My Parents Die a Good Death', *The Guardian*, 6 April, <https://www.theguardian.com/news/2021/apr/06/letting-go-my-battle-to-help-my-parents-die-a-good-death>, accessed 6 April 2021.

Clarke, L. H., Kortochenko, A. and Budon, A. (2012). '"The Calendar is Just About Up": Older Adults with Multiple Conditions', *Ageing and Society*, 32 (8), 1339–1417.

Clarke, R. (2020). *Dear Life*. London: Little Brown.

Clarke, R. (2021). *Breathtaking Inside of the NHS in a Time of Pandemic*. London: Little Brown.

Clayden, A., Green, T., Hockey, J. and Powell, M. (2015). *Natural Burial: Landscape, Practice and Experience*. London: Routledge.

Coetzee, J. M. (2005). *Slow Man*. London: Secker and Warburg.

Cohen, J., Van Landeghem, P., Carpentier, N. and Deliens, Luc (2014). 'Public Acceptance of Euthanasia in Europe: A Survey Study in 47 Countries', *International Journal of Public Health,* 59 (1), 143–56.

Cohen Silver, R. (2011). 'An Introduction to 9/11: Ten Years Later', *American Psychologist*, 66 (6), 427–28.

Colby, S. L. and Ortman, J. M. (2015). 'Projections of the Size and Composition of the US Population', *Current Population Reports*, March, pp. 25–1143.

Conn, D. and Barr, C. (2021). 'NHS Faces Questions Over COVID Infections Contracted in Hospital', *The Guardian*, 26 February, <https://www.theguardian.com/world/2021/feb/26/nhs-faces-questions-over-covid-infections-contracted-in-hospital>, accessed 26 February 2021.

Cooper, H. and Szreter, S. (2021). *After the Virus: Lessons from the Past for a Better Future.* Cambridge: Cambridge University Press.

Corcoran, S. and Wood, N. (2021). 'Ongoing Pandemic Could Worsen Older People's Mental Health', *Leicester Mercury*, 13 December, <https://www.leicestermercury.co.uk/news>, accessed 13 December 2021.

Courea, E. (2018). 'Pensioner Poverty Rises as Benefits Freeze Bites', *The Guardian*, 9 December, <https://www.theguardian.com/society/2018/dec/09/pensioner-poverty-rises-bnefites-freeze>, accessed 3 March 2021.

Cousins, S. (2020). 'Experts Criticise Australia's Aged Care Failings Over COVID-19', *The Lancet*, <https://www.thelancet.com/journals/lancet/article/PIIS0140-6736%2820%2932206-6/fulltext www.thelancet.com>, accessed 5 May 2021.

Cox, G. (2005). 'Attitudes Toward Dying and Death', *Illness, Crisis and Loss*, 13 (1), 17–29.

Crayford, T., Hooper, R. and Evans, S. (1997). 'Death Rates of Characters in Soap Operas on British Television', *British Medical Journal*, 3165, 16–49.

Crosby, A. (1976). *America's Forgotten Pandemic.* Cambridge: Cambridge University Press.

Cruikshank, M. (2003). *Learning to Be Old.* New York: Rowman &Littlefield.

Cummings, E. and Henry, W. E. (1961). *Growing Old: The Process of Disengagement.* New York: Basic Books.

Dalrymple, U. Makwana, A., Pring, A., Bowtell, N. and Verne, J. (2020). *Older People's Hospital Admissions in the Last Year of Life.* London: UK Government, <https://www.gov.uk/government/publications/older-peoples-hospital-admissions-in-the-last-year-of-life/older-peoples-hospital-admissions-in-the-last-year-of-life>, accessed 5 October 2020.

Danely, J. (2015). *Aging and Loss: Mourning and Maturity in Contemporary Japan.* New Brunswick, NJ: Rutgers University Press.

Davies, D. and Rumble, H. (2012). *Natural Burial: Traditional-Secular Spiritualities and Funeral Innovation*. London: Continuum.

Davies, J. (2017). *Living Before Dying: Imagining and Remembering Home.* Oxford: Berghahn Books.

Davies, W. (2018). 'Nervous States: How Feeling Took Over the World', *The Observer,* 15 March, p. 27.

Davies, W. (2021). 'Short Cut', *London Review of Books*, 17 June, pp. 12–13.

Davis, J. (2020). 'Introduction: Toward an Ethics of Aging'. In J. Davis and P. Scherz (eds), *The Evening of Life: The Challenges of Aging and Dying Well*, pp. 1–16. Notre Dame, IN: Notre Dame University Press.

Davis, L. (2007). *Varieties of Disturbance: The Collected Stories.* New York: Farrar, Straus and Giroux.

Davis, N. (2019). 'Euthanasia and Assisted Dying Rates Soaring', *The Guardian*, 15 July, <https://www.theguardian.com/news/2019/jul/15/euthanasia-and-assisted-dying-rates-are-soaring-but-where-are-they-legal>, accessed 5 February 2021.

Derrida, J. (1992). *The Gift of Death*. Chicago: Chicago University Press.

Dessaix, R. (2020). *The Time of Our Lives: Growing Older Well.* Sydney: Brio.

Didion, J. (2012). *The Year of Magical Thinking*. London: Fourth Estate.

Dilnot, A. (2011). *The Commission Report on Social Care*, London: The King's Fund, <https://www.kingsfund.org.uk/publications>, accessed 12 February 2022.

Diski, J. (2016). *In Gratitude*. London: Bloomsbury.

Dodd, S. (2021). '"We're Expendable": My Father Died with COVID After Four-Hour Wait for Ambulance', *The Guardian*, 27 January, <https://www.theguardian.com/world/2021/jan/27/were-expendable-my-father-died-with-covid-after-four-hour-wait-for-ambulance>, accessed 27 January 2021.

Dodsworth, L. (2021). *A State of Fear: How the UK Government Weaponised Fear During the COVID-19 Pandemic.* London: Pinter and Martin.

Doig, A. (2022). *This Mortal Coil.* London: Bloomsbury.

Donne, J. (2020). *For Whom the Bell Tolls,* <http://www.yourdailypoem.com/listpoem.jsp?poem_id=2118>, accessed 2 December 2020.

Douglas, M. (1986). *How Institutions Think*. London: Routledge.

Draaisma, D. (2001). *Why Life Speeds Up as You Get Older.* Cambridge: Cambridge University Press.

Drouillard, J. (2016). 'Anticipatory Imagination', *Aging Journal of French and Francophone Philosophy*, 24 (3), 56–73.

Duncan, P. and Booth R. (2020). '10,000 More Deaths than Usual Occurred in UK Homes Since June', *The Guardian,* 24 September, <https://www.theguardian.com/world/2020/sep/24/10000-more-deaths-than-usual-occurred-in-uk-homes-since-june>, accessed 24 September 2020.

The Economist. (2020). 'For Those Affected by Dementia, the Pandemic has Been Especially Grim', 3 August, <https://www.economist.com/international/2020/08/03/for-those-affected-by-dementia-the-pandemic-has-been-especially-grim>, accessed 24 September 2020.

Eglot, J. (2020). 'UK Could Have 50,000 COVID Cases a Day by Mid-October', *The Guardian,* 21 October, <https://www.theguardian.com/world/2020/sep/21/uk-could-have-50000-covid-cases-a-day-by-mid-october-says-chief-medical-officer-chris-whitty>, accessed 21 October 2020.

Elias, N. (1985). *The Loneliness of the Dying*. London: Continuum.

Elias, N. (1994). *The Civilizing Process: Sociogenetic and Psychogenetic Investigations*. Oxford: Blackwell.

Ellen, B. (2020). 'Only in Online Cesspits Do the Young Want the Elderly to Sicken and Die', *The Observer,* 15 March, p. 27.

Emanuel, E. J. (2014). 'Why I Hope to Die at 75', *The Atlantic*, <https://www.theatlantic.com/magazine/archive/2014/10/why-i-hope-to-die-at-75/379329>, accessed 25 October 2020.

Engelhart, K. (2022). *The Inevitable: Dispatches on the Right to Die.* New York: Atlantic Books.

Enright, A. (2020). *Actress.* London: Jonathan Cape.

Erickson, K. (2013). *The Way we Die Now: Intimacy and the Work of Dying.* Philadelphia, PA: Philadelphia: University Press.

Ernaux, A. (2014). *A Woman's Story.* London: Quartet Books.

Evans, M. (2020). 'On Being Old and Vulnerable: On the Solidarity and Care During the Covid-19 Pandemic', <https://www.solidarityandcare.org/stories/blog/on-being-old-and-vulnerable>, accessed 17 June 2020.

Feinmann, J. (2006). *How to Have a Good Death: Preparing and Planning with Informed Choices and Practical Advice*. London: Dorling Kindersley.

Ferguson, H. (2009). *Self-Identity and Everyday Life*. London: Routledge.

Fletcher, J. R. (2020). 'COVID-19 and Gerontology's Relationship with Age Categorisation', *Ageing and Society*, 41 (3), 479–92.

Flood, A. (2020). 'Margaret Atwood: COVID-19 Lockdown is Not a Dystopia', *The Guardian*, 16 April, <https://www.theguardian.com/books/2020/apr/16/margaret-atwood-covid-19-lockdown-is-not-a-dystopia-handmaid-s-tale>, accessed 18 April 2020.

Fordham, R. M. (2017). 'Expert Reaction to Paper on Health and Social Care Spending and Excess Deaths in England', Science Media Centre, <http://www.sciencemediacentre.org/expert-reaction-to-paper-on-health-and-social-care-spending-and-excess-deaths-in-england>, accessed 4 July 2021.

Fortnert, B. and Neimeyer, R. A. (1999). 'Death Anxiety in Older Adults: A Quantitative Review', *Death Studies*, 23 (5), 87–411.

Fowler, B. (2007). *The Obituary as Collective Memory*. London: Routledge.

Frailty Prevention (2022). 'What is Frailty?' <https://www.frailtyprevention.co.uk/what-is-frailty.html>, accessed 4 July 2021.

Francis, G. (2021). *Intensive Care: A GP, Community, and COVID-19*. London: Profile.

Fraser, A. (2011). *Must You Go? My Life with Harold Pinter*. London: Phoenix.

Freeman, D., Waite, F., Rosebrock, L. and Petit, A. (2020). 'Coronavirus Conspiracy Beliefs, Mistrust, and Compliance with Government Guidelines in England', *Psychological Medicine*, <https://doi.org/10.1017/S0033291720001890>, accessed 4 December 2020.

Freud, Z. (1915). 'Thoughts for the Times on War and Death', <https://www.panarchy.org/freud/war.1915.html>, accessed 13 June 2020.

Freud, Z. (1953 [1917]). 'Mourning and Melancholia'. In J. Strachey (ed. and trans.), *The Standard Edition of the Complete Psychological Works of Sigmund Freud*, 243–58. London: Hogarth Press.

Frisby, H. (2019). *Traditions of Death and Burial*. Oxford: Shire.

Froggatt, K. (2001). 'Life and Death in English Nursing Homes: Sequestration or Transition?', *Ageing and Society*, 21 (3), 319–32.

Fulton, R. (1995). 'The Contemporary Funeral: Functional or Dysfunctional?'. In H. Wass and R. A. Neimeyer (eds), *Dying: Facing the Fact*, pp. 185–211. London: Taylor and Francis.

Galbraith, J. (2009). *Baby Boomers Face Grief*. London: Trafford.

Galchen, R. (2022). 'Whack-Mole', *London Review of Books*, 27 January, pp. 15–16.

Garrett, D., Tuokko, H., Stajduhar, K. I., Lindsay, J. and Buehler, S. (2008). 'Planning for End-of-life Care: Findings from the Canadian Study of Health and Aging', *Canadian Journal on Aging*, 27 (1), 11–21.

Gawande, A. (2014). *Being Mortal: Illness, Medicine, and What Matters in the End.* London: Wellcome Collection.

Gawande, A. (2010). 'Letting Go: What Should Medicine Do', *New Yorker*, 2 August, pp. 36–49.

Gazeta Wyborcza (2022). 'Efekt pandemii: wzrost liczby samobójstw seniorów i studentów', (BiQdata), 2 February, p. 5.

Geddes, L. (2020). 'Analysis of COVID Search Terms Reveals Britons' Hopes and Fears in 2020', *The Guardian*, 28 December, <https://www.theguardian.com/world/2020/dec/28/analysis-of-covid-search-terms-reveals-britons-hopes-and-fears-in-2020>, accessed 1 January 2021.

Genna, G. (2020). *Reality*. Rome: Scala Italiani.

Gesser, G., Wong, P. T. and Reker, G. T. (1987). 'Death Attitudes Across the Lifespan', *Omega*, 18, 113–28.

Gilleard, C. and Higgs, P.(2010). 'Theorizing the Fourth Age: Ageing Without Agency', *Ageing and Mental Health*, 14(1): 12–128.

Gilleard, C. and Higgs, P. (2015). 'Social Death and the Moral Identity of the Fourth Age', *Contemporary Social Science*, 10(2), 262–71.

Gillespie, T. (2022). 'Hospital Discharge Policy at Start of Pandemic Unlawful', *The Guardian*, 27 April, <https://www.theguardian.com/politics/live/2022/apr/27/boris-johnson-news-pmqs-today-angela-rayner-latest-uk-politics?filterKeyEvents=false&page=with:block-62690e3f8f087151f7bb80a5>, accessed 27 April 2022.

Glaser, B. and Strauss, A. (1965). *Awareness of Dying.* London: Weidenfeld and Nicolson.

Glaser, B. and Strauss, A. (1968). *Time for Dying.* Chicago: Aldine.

Global Aging Research Network (GARN) (2016). *White Book on Frailty*, <https://www.jpn-geriat-soc.or.jp/gakujutsu/pdf/whitebook.pdf>, accessed 27 April 2022.

Gluck, L. (2021). *Poems 1962–2020*. Harmondsworth: Penguin.

Gold Standards Framework (2022). 'About', <https://www.goldstandardsframework.org.uk>, accessed 27 April 2022.

Gorer, G. (1965). *Death, Grief and Mourning in Contemporary Britain.* London: Cresset.

Gorina, Y. and Lentzner, H. (2005). 'Trends of Causes of Death Among Older Persons in the United States', *Aging Trends*, 6 October), pp. 1–12.

Gott, M., Small, Neil, B., Payne, S. and Seamark, D. (2008). 'Older People's Views of a Good Death in Heart Failure: Implications for Palliative Care Provision', *Social Science and Medicine,* 67 (7), 1113–21.

Gov UK (2018). 'Deaths'. <https://www.ons.gov.uk/peoplepopulationandcommunity/birthsdeathsandmarriages/deaths>, accessed 27 April 2022.

Gov UK (2020). 'Older People's Hospital Admissions in the Last Year of Life', <https://www.gov.uk/government/publications/older-peoples-hospital-admissions-in-the-last-year-of-life/older-peoples-hospital-admissions-in-the-last-year-of-life>, accessed 20 January 2022.

GP Notebook (2022). 'Old Age and Death Certificate', <https://gpnotebook.com/simplepage.cfm?ID=x20120623141725030327>, accessed 20 January 2022.

Granek, L. (2010). 'Grief as Pathology: The Evolution of Grief Theory in Psychology', *History of Psychology*, 13 (1), 46–73.

Grant, L. and Scott, A. (2016). *The 100 Life: Living and Working in an Age of Longevity.* New York: Bloomsbury.

Grass, G. (2016). *All of That Ends.* Boston: Houghton Mifflin.

Gregory, A. (2021). 'England has Highest Death Rates of Older Patients in Western World, Study Finds', *The Guardian*, 10 November, <https://www.theguardian.com/society/2021/nov/10/england-has-highest-death-rates-of-older-patients-in-western-world-study-finds>, accessed 20 January 2022.

Gregory, A. (2022a). 'Number of Adults with Dementia to Exceed 150m by 2050, Study Finds', *The Guardian,* 7 January, <https://www.theguardian.com/society/2022/jan/06/number-adults-with-dementia-exceed-150-million-2050-study>, accessed 7 January 2022.

Gregory, A. (2022b). 'Two or More Chronic Health Problems in Middle Age "Doubles Dementia Risk"', *The Guardian*, 3 February, <https://www.theguardian.com/society/2022/feb/02/two-chronic-health-problems-middle-age-double-dementia-risk-multimorbidity-study>, accessed 7 January 2022.

Grenier, A. (2020). 'The Conspicuous Absence of the Social, Emotional and Political Aspects of Frailty: The Example of the White Book on Frailty', *Ageing and Society*, 40 (11), 1–17.

Groen, H. (2017). *The Secret Diary of Hendrick Groen, 83 1/4 years old.* Trans. Hester Velmans, London: Michael Joseph.

Grover, N. (2020). 'COVID has Cut Life Expectancy in England and Wales by a Year', *The Guardian*, 10 December, <https://www.theguardian.com/world/2020/dec/10/covid-life-expectancy-england-wales>, accessed 10 December 2020.

Gross, A. and Cameron-Chileshe, J. (2020). 'Less Than Half UK Population to Receive Coronavirus Vaccine, Says Task Force Head', *Financial Times*, 4 October, p. 4.

Grumbach, D. (1991). *Coming into the End Zone.* New York: W.W. Norton.

The Guardian (2021). 'COVID Statistics', 22 September.

The Guardian (2022). 'COVID Restrictions and Free Mass Testing to End in England', 22 February, <https://www.theguardian.com/world/2022/feb/21/boris-johnson-says-free-covid-tests-in-england-will-end-on-1-april>, accessed 17 November 2022.

Guidance for Doctors Certifying Cause of Death (2020). <https://gpnotebook.com/simplepage.cfm?ID=x20120623141725030327>, accessed 22 September 2020.

Gullette, M. (2015). 'Aged by Culture'. In J. Twigg and W. Martin (eds), *Routledge Handbook of Cultural Gerontology*, pp. 21–18. London: Routledge.

Günter, G. (2017). *All of That Ends.* Trans. Breon Mitchell. London: Vintage Books.

Hägglund, M. (2012). *Dying for Time.* Cambridge, MA: Harvard University Press.

Hägglund, M. (2019). *This Life: Why Mortality Makes Us Free.* New York: Profile Books

Hall, R. (2020). 'Care Home Residents in England Must be Allowed to Live', *The Guardian*, 31 August, <https://www.theguardian.com/society/2020/aug/31/care-home-residents-in-england-must-be-allowed-to-live-not-just-kept-alive-during-covid>, accessed 31 August 2020.

Harari, Y. N. (2020). 'Death shall have no dominion', *The Guardian*, 25 April, <https://www.theguardian.com/books/booksblog/2006/oct/26/deathshallhavenodominion>, accessed 25 April 2020.

Hardt, M. D. (2016). *History of Infectious Disease Pandemics in Urban Societies.* Lanham, MD: Lexington Books.

Hattenstone, S. (2020). 'Michael Rosen on His COVID-19 coma: "It Felt Like a Pre-death, a Nothingness"', *The Guardian*, 30 September, <https://www.theguardian.com/books/2020/sep/30/michael-rosen-on-his-covid-19-coma-it-felt-like-a-pre-death-a-nothingness>, accessed 30 September 2020.

He, D. (2020). Comparing COVID-19 and the 1918–19 influenza pandemics in the United Kingdom, *International Society for Infectious Diseases*, 98, 67–70.

Health Foundation (2022). 'Real Centre', <https://www.health.org.uk/news-and-comment/news/1.5-million-potential-years-of-life-lost-to-covid-19>, accessed 17 March 2022.

Heidegger, M. (1978). *Being and Time.* Trans. J. Macquarie and E. Robinson. London: Willey-Blackwell.

Heidinger, T. and Richter, L. (2020). 'The Effect of COVID-19 on Loneliness in the Elderly. An Empirical Comparison of Pre-and Peri-Pandemic Loneliness in Community-Dwelling Elderly', *Frontiers in Psychology,* 30 September, p. 11.

Heilbrun, C. (1997). *The Last Gift of Time: Life Beyond Sixty.* New York: Dial Press.

Henley, J. and McIntyre, N. (2020). 'Survey Uncovers Widespread Belief in "Dangerous" COVID Conspiracy Theories', *The Guardian*, 26 October,

<https://www.theguardian.com/world/2020/oct/26/survey-uncovers-widespread-belief-dangerous-covid-conspiracy-theories?amp>, accessed 26 October 2020.

Hennessy, P. (2022). *A Duty of Care*. London: Allen Lane.

Hepworth, M. (2000). *Stories of Ageing*. Buckingham: Open University Press.

Herbert, Z. (1995). *Mr Cognito.* Trans. John Carpenter. London: Ecco Press.

Hiam, L., Harrison, D., McKee, M. and Dorling, D. (2018). 'Why is Life Expectancy in England and Wales "Stalling"?' *Journal of Epidemiology and Community Health,* 72(1), 404–08.

Higgs, P. and Gilleard, C. (2015). *Rethinking Old Age*. London: Palgrave.

Hill, A. (2018). 'UK is "Completely and Institutionally Ageist"', *The Guardian,* 26 December, <https://www.theguardian.com/science/2018/dec/26/uk-is-completely-and-institutionally-ageist>, 3 March 2020.

Hill, A. (2021). 'Age No Barrier to Activism: How UK's Young and Old Built Bonds in COVID', *The Guardian,* 17 November, <https://www.theguardian.com/world/2021/nov/17/age-no-barrier-to-activism-how-uks-young-and-old-built-bonds-in-covid>, accessed 17 November 2021.

Hirschman, A. (1993). 'Interview with Carmine Donzelli', School of Social Science Occasional Papers, <https://www.ias.edu/sites/default/files/sss/papers/paper50.pdf>, accessed 23 January 2022.

Hirst, W. (2020). 'Remembering COVID-19', *Social Research*, 87 (2), 251–53.

HM Government (2020). 'Guidance on Social Distancing for Everyone in the UK', <https://www.gov.uk/government/publications/covid-19-guidance-on-social-distancing-and-for-vulnerable-people/guidance-on-social-distancing-for-everyone-in-the-uk-and-protecting-older-people-and-vulnerable-adults>, accessed 23 September 2020.

Hockey, J. (1990). *Experiences of Death*. Edinburgh: Edinburgh University Press.

Hockey, J., Komaromy, C. and Woodthorpe, K. (eds) (1969). *The Matter of Death: Space, Place and Materiality*. Basingstoke: Palgrave Macmillan.

Holland-Batt, S. (2020). 'Magical Thinking and the Aged-care Crisis', *Griffith Review,* 68, 18–33.

Holloway, M. (2007). *Negotiating Death in Contemporary Health and Social Care*. Bristol: Policy Press.

Holmberg, T., Jonsson, A. and Palm, F. (eds) (2019). *Death Matters: Cultural Sociology of Moral Life*. London: Palgrave.

Holstein, M. (2015). *Women in Late Life: Critical Perspective on Gender and Age.* New York: Rowman & Littlefield.

Honigsbaum, M. (2020). *The Pandemic Century: A History of Global Contagion from the Spanish Flu to COVID-19.* New York: Virgin Digital.

Horton, R. (2020). *The COVID-19 Catastrophe: What's Gone Wrong and How to Stop It*. Cambridge: Polity Press.

Hospice UK (2002). 'Dying Matters', < https://www.hospiceuk.org/our-campaigns/dying-matters/join?n=Dying%20Matters>, accessed 8 March 2022.

Houellebecq, M. (2006). *The Possibility of Island*. London: Phoenix.

Howarth, G. (2007). *Death and Dying: A Sociological Introduction*. Cambridge: Polity Press.

Humphries, R. (2016). *Social Care for Older People: Home Truths*. London: The King's Fund, <https://www.kingsfund.org.uk/publications/social-care-older-people>, accessed 2 September 2021.

Humphrys, J. and Jarvis, S. (2009). *The Welcome Visitors: Living Well, Dying Well*. London: Hodder.

Huxley, A. (1932). *Brave New World*. New York: Chatto and Windus.

Ignatieff, M. (2022). *On Consolation: Finding Solace in Dark Times*. New York: Picador.

Illich, I. (1976). *Limits to Medicine*. London: Marion Boyars.

Inman, P. (2021). 'Poverty Rate Among Working Households in UK is Highest Ever', *The Guardian*, 26 May, <https://www.theguardian.com/society/2021/may/26/poverty-rate-among-working-households-in-uk-is-highest-ever>, accessed 25 June 2021.

International Classification of Diseases (ICD) Information Sheet (2020). <https://www.who.int/classifications/icd/en>, accessed 22 September 2020.

Irish, D., Lundquist, K. and Nelsen, V. J. (eds) (1993). *Ethnic Variations in Dying, Death and Grief*. London: Routledge.

Jackson, E. (2004). 'Whose Death is It Anyway', *Current Legal Problems*, 57 (1), 415–42.

Jackson, E. (2008). 'Secularism, Sanctity and the Wrongness of Killing', *BioSocieties*, 3, pp. 125–45.

Jackson, E. and Keown, J. (2011). *Debating Euthanasia*. Oxford: Hart.

Jain, B., Kalesnikava, V., Ibrahim, J. E. and Mezuk, B. (2021). 'Places of Living and Places of Dying', *Age and Society*, 41 (9), 1945–60.

James, C. (2015). *Sentenced to Life*. London: Picador.

James, C. (2017). *Injury Time*. London: Picador.

James, P.D. (1997). *A Certain Justice*. London: Faber and Faber.

Jarvis, B. (2021). 'We've Had Great Success Extending Life: What About Ending It?', *The New Yorker*,10 May, p. 8.

Jasper, K. (1971 [1931]). *Philosophy of Existence*. Philadelphia, PA: University of Pennsylvania Press.

Jong, E. (2015). *Fear of Dying*. New York: St Martin's Press.

Kaczorowska, K. (2020). 'Miliony seniorów zamkniętych w domach rozporządzeniem', *Polityka*, 24 October, pp. 6–7.

Kahana, B., Dan, A., Kahana, E. and Kercher, K. (2004). 'The Personal and Social Context of Planning for End-of-life Care', *Journal of the American Geriatrics Society*, 52 (7), 1163–67.

Kale, S. (2020). 'They were Withering Away', *The Guardian,* 8 September, <https://www.theguardian.com/society/2020/sep/08/they-were-withering-away-why-did-colin-harris-and-nine-others-die-in-a-skye-care-home>, accessed 8 September 2020.

Kassam, A. (2020). '113-year-old COVID Survivor', *The Observer*, 17 May, p. 29.

Katz, J. (2001). 'Introduction'. In J. Hockey, J. Katz and N. Small (eds), *Grief, Mourning and Death Ritual*, pp. 1–17. Buckingham: Open University Press.

Katz, S. (2003). 'New Sex for Old: Lifestyle, Consumerism and Ethic of Ageing Well', *Journal of Ageing Studies*, 17 (1), 3–16.

Katz, S. (2015). 'Ageing, Risk and the Falling Body'. In J. Twigg and W. Martin (eds), *Routledge Handbook of Cultural Gerontology*, pp. 165–73. London: Routledge.

Kaufman, S. (2005). *And a Time to Die*. New York: Lisa Drew.

Kaufman, S. (2010). 'Time, Clinical Technology', *Sociology of Health and Illness,* 32 (2), 225–37.

Keeble, E., Scobie, S. and Hutchings, R. (2022). *Support at the End of Life: The Role of Hospice Services Across the UK.* London: Nuffield Trust, <https://www.nuffieldtrust.org.uk/research/support-at-the-end-of-life>, accessed 20 May 2022.

Keller, M.. L., Leventhal, E. A. and Larson, B. (1989). 'Aging: The Lived Experience', *International Journal of Aging and Human Development*, 29, 67–82.

Kellehear, A. (2002). 'Grief and Loss: Past, Present and Future', *Medical Journal of Australia*, 177 (4), 176–77.

Kellehear, A. (2007). *A Social History of Dying,* Cambridge: Cambridge University Press.

Kellehear, A. (ed.) (2009). *The Study of Dying. From Autonomy to Transformation.* Cambridge: Cambridge University Press.

Kellehear, A. (2014). *The Inner Life of the Dying Person.* New York: Columbia University Press.

Kemp, A. R. (2019). *Death, Dying, and Bereavement in a Changing World.* London: Routledge.

Keneally, T. (2019). *The Book of Science and Antiquities*. London: Sceptre.

Keown, J. (2009). *Euthanasia, Ethics and Public Policy: Argument Against Legalization.* Cambridge: Cambridge University Press.

Kessler, D. (2019). *Finding Meaning: The Sixth Stage of Grief.* New York: Rider.

Khademi, F., Moyedi, S., Golitaleb, M. and Karbalaie, N. (2020). 'The COVID - 19 Pandemic and Death Anxiety in the Elderly', *International Journal of Mental*

Health Nursing, <https://onlinelibrary.wiley.com/doi/10.1111/inm.12824>, accessed 6 February 2021.

Kiernan, S. (2006). *Last Rights: Rescuing the End of Life From Medical System.* New York: St Martin's Press.

King's Fund (2018). 'Home Care in England: Views from Commissioners and Providers', <https://www.kingsfund.org.uk/sites/default/files/2018-12/Home-care-in-England-report.pdf>, accessed 20 January 2022.

Kingston, A., Comas-Herrera, A. and Jagger, C. (2018). 'Projections of Multi-morbidity in the Older Population in England to 2035: Estimates from the Population Ageing and Care Simulation (PACSim) Model', *Age and Ageing* 47, 374–80.

Kitch, C. and Hume, J. (2008). *Journalism in a Culture of Grief.* New York: Routledge.

Klass, D. (1995). 'Spiritual Aspects of the Resolution of Grief'. In H. Wass and R. A. Neimeyer (eds), *Dying: Facing the Facts*, pp. 243–68. London: Taylor and Francis.

Klass, D., Silverman, P. and Nickman, S. (1996). *Continuing Bonds: New Understanding of Grief.* Washington, DC: Taylor and Francis.

Kolakowski, L. (2021). *Smierc Jako Wlasnosc Prywatna*, Krakow: Wydawnictwo Znak.

Kormann, C. (2020). 'What will Cold-and-Flu Season Mean for the Coronavirus Pandemic?', *The New Yorker*, 1 October, p. 12.

Kotter-Gruhn, D., Gruhn D. and Smith, J. (2010). 'Predicting One's Own Death', *European Journal of Ageing*, 7 (4), 293–300.

Krastev, I. (2020). *Is It Tomorrow Yet?* Harmondsworth: Penguin.

Kucharski, A. (2020). *Rules of Contagion: Why Things Spread.* London: Wellcome Collection.

Kuzniak, A. (2020). *Soroczka.* Warsaw: Wydawnictwo Literackie.

Kundera, M. (1991). *Immortality.* London: Faber and Faber.

Kübler-Ross, E. (2011 [1969]). *On Death and Dying.* New York. Simon and Schuster.

Kübler-Ross, E. and Kessler, D. (2004). *On Grief and Grieving.* New York: Simon and Schuster.

Lamb, S. (2015). 'Beyond the View of the West'. In J. Twigg and W. Martin (eds), *Routledge Handbook of Cultural Gerontology*, pp. 37–44. London: Routledge.

Lanchester, J. (2021). 'As the Lock Rattles', *London Review of Books*, 16 December, pp. 13–16.

Landrman, G. (2003). *Rest in Peace: A Cultural History of Death and the Funeral Home in Twentieth-century America.* Oxford: Oxford University Press.

Lang, A. (2020). 'The Good Death and the Institutionalisation of Dying: An Interpretive Analysis of the Austrian Discourse', *Social Science Medicine*, 245, 1–8.

Larkin, P. (1977). *Collected Poems.* London: Faber and Faber.

Laqueur, T. (2015). *The Work of the Dead: The Cultural History of Mortal Remains.* Princeton, NJ: Princeton University Press.

Laslett, P. (1969). 'Size and Structure of Household in England Over Three Centuries', *Population Studies*, 1 (23), 199–223.

Laslett, P. (1989). *A Fresh Map of Life: The Emergence of the Third Age*. London: Palgrave.

Lattanzi-Licht, M. and Connor, S. (1995). 'Care of the Dying'. In H. Wass and R. A. Neimeyer (eds), *Dying: Facing the Facts*, pp. 143–62. London: Taylor and Francis.

Latour, B. (2021). *After Lockdown: A Metamorphosis.* Trans. Julie Rose. Cambridge: Polity Press.

Lawrence, J. (2011). 'Why an Ageing Population is the Greatest Threat to Society', *The Independent*, 17 September, p. 7.

Lawton, J. (2000). *The Dying Process: Patients' Experiences of Palliative Care.* London: Routledge.

Lay, K. (2021). 'COVID Drove British Life Expectancy to Lowest in a Decade', *The Times and The Sunday Times*, 10 November, p. 13

Lee, S. (2020). 'Coronavirus Anxiety Scale: A Brief Mental Health Screener for COVID-19 Related Anxiety', *Death Studies*, 44 (7), 393–401.

Lefebvre, H. (1984). *Everyday Life in the Modern World.* New Brunswick, NJ: Transaction.

Lessing, D. [pseudonym Jane Somers] (1984). *The Diary of a Good Neighbour.* New York: Alfred A. Knopf.

Levin, A. T., Cochran, K. B. and Walsh, S. P. (2020). 'Assessing the Age Specificity of Infection Fatality Rates for COVID-19: Meta-Analysis & Public Policy Implications', <https://doi.org/10.1101/2020.07.23.20160895>, accessed 5 October 2020.

Levine, M. (2022). *True Age*. London: Yellow Kite.

Levy, B., Slade, M., Kunkel, S. and Kasl, S. (2009). 'Longevity Increased by Positive Self-Perceptions of Aging', *Journal of Personality and Social Psychology*, 83 (2), 261–70.

Lewis C.S (2020 [1961]). *A Grief Observed*. New York: Faber and Faber.

Lindemann, E. (1944). 'Symptomatology and Management of Acute Grief', *American Journal of Psychiatry*, 101 (7), 141–48.

Liou, L., Joe, W., Kumar, A. and Subramanian, S. V. (2020). 'Inequalities in Life Expectancy: An Analysis of 201 Countries, 1950–2015', *Social Science & Medicine*, 25 (112964), 1–8.

Littlewood, J. (2001). 'Just an Old Fashioned Song or a "Harlequin Romance". Some Experience of Widowhood'. In J. Hockey, J. Katz and N. Small (eds), *Grief, Mourning and Death Ritual*, pp. 82–94. Buckingham: Open University Press.

Lively, P. (2014). *Ammonites and Leaping Fish: A Life in Time*. Harmondsworth: Penguin.

Livne, R. (2019). *Values at the End of Life. The Logic of Palliative Care*. Cambridge, MA: Harvard University Press.

Lloyd, L. (2000). 'Dying in Old Age: Promoting Wellbeing at the End of Life', *Mortality*, 5 (2), 171–88.

Lloyd, L. (2004). 'Mortality and Morality: Ageing and the Ethics of Care', *Ageing and Society*, 24 (2), 235–56.

Lloyd, L. (2015). 'The Fourth Age'. In J. Twigg and W. Martin (eds), *Routledge Handbook of Cultural Gerontology*, pp.261-269. London: Routledge.

Lloyd, L., Calnan, M., Cameron, A., Seymour, J. and Smith, R. (2014). 'Identity in the Fourth Age: Perseverance, Adaptation and Maintaining Dignity', *Ageing and Society*, 34 (1), 1–19.

Lofland, L. H. (1978). *The Craft of Dying*. Thousand Oaks, CA: Sage.

Lofland, L. H. (1985). 'The Social Shaping of Emotion: The Case of Grief', *Symbolic Interaction*, 8 (2): 171–90.

Luft, O. (2008). 'Gordon Brown Urges "Sensitivity" Over Assisted Suicide Broadcast', *The Guardian*, 10 December, <https://www.theguardian.com/media/2008/dec/10/craig-ewert-assisted-suicide-gordon-brown>, accessed 2May 2021.

Lynskey, D. (2021). 'Wall of Love: The Incredible Story Behind the National COVID Memorial', *The Guardian*, 18 July, <https://www.theguardian.com/world/2021/jul/18/wall-of-love-the-incredible-story-behind-the-national-covid-memorial-led-by-donkeys>, accessed 30 August 2021.

Lyons, A. and Winter, L. (2021). *We All Know How This Ends*. London: Green Tee.

MacIntyre, A. (1985). *After Virtue*. London: Gerald Duckworth.

Mahon, M. (2011). 'Death in the Lives of Children'. In V. Talwar, H. Harris and M. Schleifer (eds), *Children's Understanding of Death*, pp. 65–78. Cambridge: Cambridge University Press.

Mal, N. (2020). 'More Than 400 Deaths Involving COVID-19 Occurred Each Day in UK Care homes', *Plymouth Herald*, 4 September, <https://www.plymouthherald.co.uk/news/uk-world-news/more-400-deaths-involving-covid-4483313>, accessed 4 September 2020.

Malik, N. (2020). 'A Nation Mourns Its COVID-19 Dead. But for Boris Johnson It's a Time for Triumphalism', *The Guardian*, 3 August, <https://www.theguardian.com/commentisfree/2020/aug/03/nation-mourns-covid-19-dead-boris-johnson-triumphalism>, accessed 3 August 2020.

Mannix, K. (2018). *With the End in Mind: How to Live and Die Well*. London: William Collins.

Manson, R. (2020). 'Ministers Accused of Abandoning Care Homes to Coronavirus', *The Guardian*, 14 May, <https://www.theguardian.com/world/2020/may/14/ministers-abandoned-care-homes-to-coronavirus>, accessed 14 May 2020.

Mannheim, K. (1973). *Essays on the Sociological Knowledge*. New York: Harvest HBJ.

Marsh, S. (2021). 'Epidemic of Grief', *The Guardian*, 13 January, <https://www.theguardian.com/world/2021/jan/13/epidemic-of-grief-the-challenge-of-the-uks-massive-loss-of-life>, accessed 13 January 2021.

Marsh, S. and Booth, R. (2021). 'Two-thirds of Residents Die in COVID Outbreak at Lincolnshire Care Home', *The Guardian*, 19 January, <https://www.theguardian.com/world/2021/jan/19/two-thirds-of-residents-die-in-covid-outbreak-at-lincolnshire-care-home>, accessed 19 January 2021.

Marsh, S. and McIntyre, B. (2020). 'Six in 10 UK Health Workers Killed by COVID-19 are BAME'. *The Guardian*, 26 May, <https://www.theguardian.com/world/2020/may/25/six-in-10-uk-health-workers-killed-by-covid-19-are-bame>, accessed 16 November 2022.

Marshall, B. (2015). 'Anti-ageing and Identities'. In J. Twigg and W. Martin (eds), *Routledge Handbook of Cultural Gerontology*, pp. 210–17. London: Routledge.

Marshall, V. W. (1975). 'Age and Awareness of Finitude in Developmental Gerontology', *Omega*, 6 (2), 113–28.

Marshall, V. W. (1980). *Last Chapters: A Sociology of Aging and Dying*. Monterey, CA: Brooks Cole.

Marshall, V. W. (1986). 'A Sociological Perspective on Aging and Dying'. In V. W. Marshall (ed.), *Later Life: The Social Psychology of Aging*, 125–46. Thousand Oaks, CA: Sage.

Martin, P. and de Saille, S. (eds) (2022). *Being Human During Covid-19*. Bristol: Bristol University Press.

May, V. (2018). 'Belonging Across the Lifetime: Time and Self in Mass Observation Accounts', *British Journal of Sociology*, 69 (2), 306–22.

McCurry, J. (2022). 'World's Oldest Person Celebrates 119th Birthday in Japan Nursing Home'. *The Guardian*, 3 January.

McEwan, I. (1998). *Amsterdam*. London: Jonathan Cape.

McManus, R. (2013). *Death in a Global Age*. London: Palgrave.

Meier, E A., Gallegos, J. V., Montross, T. L., Depp, C. A. and Irwin, A. A. (2016). 'Defining a Good Death (Successful Dying): Literature Review and a Call for Research and Public Dialogue', *The American Journal of Geriatric Psychiatry*, 24 (4), 261–71.

Miller, J. (2010). *Crazy Age: Thoughts on Being Old*. London: Little Brown.

Misztal, B. (2003). *Social Theories of Remembering*. Maidenhead: Open University Press.

Misztal, B. (2020). *Later Life: Exploring the Experience of Ageing Through Literature.* London: Routledge.

Mitford, J. (1963). *The American Way of Death.* New York: Simon and Schuster.

Moddy. H. (1992). 'Bioethics and Ageing'. In T. Cole, D. van Tassel and R. Kastenbaum (eds), *Handbook of the Humanities and Aging*, pp. 395–425. New York: Springer.

Mong, S. (2020). *Taking Care of Our Own: When Family Caregivers Do Medical Work.* Ithaca, NY: Cornell University Press.

Montaigne, M. (1987). *The Complete Essays.* Translated by M. A. Screech. Harmondsworth: Penguin.

Morris, A. (2022). 'Fault Lines in American Society Got Deeper', *Scientific American*, 326 (3), 66–69.

Morris, S. and Plunkett, J. (2008). 'Death on TV: Assisted Suicide to Be Screened', *The Guardian*, 10 December, <https://www.theguardian.com/society/2008/dec/10/society-email-briefing>, accessed 23 April 2021.

Mosse, K. (2021). *An Extra Pair of Hands: A Story of Caring, Ageing and Everyday Acts of Love.* London: Wellcome Collection.

Mulpagano, D. (2017). *Surviving Death: How to Overcome the Loss of a Loved One.* Kelly, NC: Toplink.

Murphy, M. (2009). 'The "Golden Generations" in Historical Context', *British Actuarial Journal*, 15(Supp.), 151–84.

Murphy, M., Luy, M. and Torrisa, O. (2019). *Stalling of Mortality in the United Kingdom and Europe.* London: London School of Economics and Political Science.

Murray, C. (2022). 'COVID-19 will Continue but the End of the Pandemic is Near', *Lancet,* 29 January, <https://www.thelancet.com/pdfs/journals/lancet/PIIS0140-6736(22)00100-3.pdf>, accessed 29 March 2022.

Murray, L. (2013). 'Corniche'. In *Subhman Redneck Poems* (pp. 22–23). Sydney: Duffy and Snellgrove.

Neimeyer, R. A. (2000). 'Searching for the Meaning of Meaning: Grief Therapy and the Process of Reconstruction', *Death Studies*, 24, 541–58.

Neimeyer, R. A. and van Brunt, D. (1995). 'Death Anxiety'. In H. Wass and R. A. Neimeyer (eds), *Dying: Facing the Facts*, pp. 49–88. New York: Routledge.

Nelds, S. (1995). 'The Dying Process'. In H. Wass and R. A. Neimeyer (eds), *Dying: Facing the Facts*, pp. 89–116. New York: Routledge.

Nelson, L. D. (1979). 'Structural Conduciveness, Personality Characteristics and Death Anxiety', *Omega*, 10, 123–33.

NICE (2017). 'Multimorbidity: Clinical Assessment and Management – Context', <www.nice.org.uk/guidance/ng56/chapter/Context>, accessed 20 January 2022.

Nichelson, C., Meyer, J., Flatley, M., Homan, C. and Lowton, K. (2012). 'Living on the Margin: Understanding the Experience of Living and Dying with Frailty in Old Age', *Social Science and Medicine*, 75, 1426–32.

Nogrady, B. (2020). 'Longevity, Quality and Turning Back the Clock', *Griffith Review*, 68, 41–52.

Nuland, S. B. (1993). *How We Die.* New York: Vintage Books.

O'Mahony, S. (2016). *The Way We Die Now*. London: Head of Zeus.

Oates, J. C. (2011). *A Widow's Story*. New York: HarperCollins

Office for National Statistics (ONS) (2015). 'National Life Tables, UK: 2012 to 2014', <https://www.ons.gov.uk/peoplepopulationandcommunity/birthsdeathsandmarriages/lifeexpectancies/bulletins/nationallifetablesunitedkingdom/2015-09-23#toc>, accessed 12 October 2020.

Office for National Statistics (ONS) (2018). *Living Longer: How Our Population is Changing and Why It Matters*, <https://www.ons.gov.uk/peoplepopulationandcommunity/birthsdeathsandmarriages/ageing/articles/livinglongerhowourpopulationischangingandwhyitmatters/2018-08-13>, accessed 17 September 2020.

Office for National Statistics (ONS) (2019). *Quarterly Mortality Report, England: October to December 2018 and Year-end Review*, <https://www.ons.gov.uk/peoplepopulationandcommunity/birthsdeathsandmarriages/deaths/articles/quarterlymortalityreports/octobertodecember2018andyearendreview>, accessed 2 May 2020.

Office for National Statistics (ONS) (2020). 'Health State Life Expectancies, UK: 2016 to 2018', <https://www.ons.gov.uk/peoplepopulationandcommunity/healthandsocialcare/healthandlifeexpectancies/bulletins/healthstatelifeexpectanciesuk/2016to2018>, accessed 17 September 2020.

Office for National Statistics (ONS) (2021). 'Deaths Involving COVID-19 in the Care Sector, England and Wales: Deaths Registered Between Week Ending 20 March 2020 and Week Ending 2 April 2021', https://www.ons.gov.uk/peoplepopulationandcommunity/birthsdeathsandmarriages/deaths/articles/deathsinvolvingcovid19inthecaresectorenglandandwales/latest>, accessed 12 March 2022.

Office for National Statistics (ONS) (2022). 'Coronavirus (COVID-19) Latest Insights: Hospitals', <https://www.ons.gov.uk/peoplepopulationandcommunity/healthandsocialcare/conditionsanddiseases/articles/coronaviruscovid19latestinsights/hospitals>, accessed 12 May 2022.

Oliver, D. (2018). 'Why Did They Put Her on a Geriatric Ward?', *British Medical Journal*, 362, <https://www.bmj.com/content/362/bmj.k3701>, accessed 21 January 2022.

Olszowski, S. (2022). 'Hospice Care is a Right, Not a Luxury'. *The Observer*, 20 February, p. 45.

Osborne, H. (2020). 'UK State Pension Age Increases to 66 – and is Set to Rise Further', *The Guardian*, 6 October, <https://www.theguardian.com/money/2020/oct/06/uk-state-pension-age-66-rise-men-women>, accessed 3 March 2021.

Osnos, E. (2022). 'How COVID Strengthened Authoritarianism in China', *The New Yorker*, 13 May, <https://www.newyorker.com/podcast/politics-and-more/how-covid-strengthened-authoritarianism-in-china>, accessed 13 May 2022.

Overy, R. (2020). 'Why the Cruel Myth of the "Blitz Spirit" is No Model for How to Fight Coronavirus', *The Guardian*, 19 March, <https://www.theguardian.com/commentisfree/2020/mar/19/myth-blitz-spirit-model-coronavirus>, accessed 19 March 2020.

Owen, D. (2021). 'Falling Life Expectancy Could Mean Pension Age Rethink, Say Experts', *Leicester Mercury*, 25 October, <https://www.leicestermercury.co.uk/news/leicester-news/falling-life-expectancy-could-mean-6077202>, 25 October 2021.

Owen, P. (2020). 'Frail People Like Me Should Not Be Denied Lifesaving COVID Care', *The Guardian*, 29 September, <https://www.theguardian.com/world/2020/sep/29/frail-people-like-me-should-not-be-denied-lifesaving-covid-careSept>, accessed 29 September 2020.

Oz, A. (1972). *Touch the Water, Touch the Wind.* London: Vintage Books.

Parkes, C. M. (1972). *Bereavement: Studies of Grief in Later Life.* London: Tavistock.

Parkes, C. M. (2010). 'Grief: Lessons from the Past, Visions for the Future', *Psychologica Begica*, 50 (1 & 2), 7–26.

Parkes, C. M., Laungani, P. and Young W. (2015). *Death and Bereavement Across Cultures*. London: Routledge.

Parsons, B. (2018). *The Evolution of the British Funeral Industry*. Bingley: Emerald.

Parveen, N. (2020). 'Family Plead for Change to Care Home Rules after Daughter's Arrest', *The Guardian*, 5 November, <https://www.theguardian.com/society/2020/nov/05/family-plead-for-change-to-care-home-rules-after-daughters-arrest>, accessed 5 November 2020.

Perraudin, F. (2020). 'All Care Home Staff and Residents in England to Be Tested for Coronavirus', *Plymouth Herald*, 15 May, <https://www.plymouthherald.co.uk/news/uk-world-news/care-home-residents-staff-england-4138209>, accessed 15 May 2020.

Perrow, C. (2008). 'Disastrous Evermore? Reducing our Vulnerability to Natural, Industrial and Terrorists Disasters', *Social Research*, 75 (3), 733–52.

Perrow, C. (2007). *The Best Catastrophe: Reducing our Vulnerabilities to Natural, Industrial and Terrorist Disasters.* Princeton, NJ: Princeton University Press.

Phillipson, C. (2015). 'Global and Local Ties and the Reconstruction of Later Life'. In J. Twigg and W. Martin (eds), *Routledge Handbook of Cultural Gerontology*, pp. 389–96. London: Routledge.
Phillips, J. B. (2007). 'The Changing Presentation of Death in the Obituary, 1899–1999', *Omega: Journal of Death and Dying*, 55 (4), 325–46.
Pocock, L., MacKichan, F., Deibel, F., Mills, A. and Wye, L. (2021). 'Stories from the Fourth Age: Autonomy and Lives of Older Care Home Residents', *Ageing and Society*, 41 (7), 1637–50.
Pyali, C. (2017). *The Customary Practice of Senicide, with Special Reference to India*. Munich: GRIN Verlag, <https://www.grin.com/document/372138>, accessed 2 November 2020.
Raleigh, V. (2019). 'What is Happening to Life Expectancy in the UK?', <https://www.kingsfund.org.uk/about-us/whos-who/veena-raleigh>, accessed 17 September 2020.
Ralph, E. (2020). 'Here's How the Pandemic Finally Ends', *Politico Magazine*, 25 September, <https://www.politico.com/section/magazine>, accessed 23 March 2021.
Rando, T. (1995). 'Grief and Mourning: Accommodating Loss', in H. Wass and R. A. Neimeyer (eds), *Dying: Facing the Facts*, pp. 211–42. London: Routledge.
Raphael, B. (1984). *The Anatomy of Bereavement*. London: Hutchinson.
Ray Karpen, R. (2017). 'The Reflection on Women's Retirement', *The Gerontologist*, 57 (1), 103–09.
Ray Karpen, R. (2019). 'Home Place: Introduction. In A. Waytt-Brown, *The Big Move: Life Between the Turning Points*, pp. 1–13. Bloomington, IN: Indiana University Press.
Rawnsley, A. (2021).' Boris Johnson's Generation Game: The Young and Poor Pay for the Old and Rich', *The Observer*, 12 September, p. 7.
Reisz, M. (2020). 'Why Ethicists are Needed to Help Societies Cope with "New Normal"', *Times Higher Education Supplement*, 5 June, p. 3.
Richite, H. and Roser, M. (2019). 'Age Structure', *Our World in Data*, <https://ourworldindata.org/age-structure>, accessed 15 September 2020.
Ricoeur, P. (2004). *Memory, History, Forgetting*. Trans. Trans K. Blamey and D. Pellauer. Chicago: Chicago University Press.
Ridley, M. (2020). 'A New Approach to COVID-19', *The Times*, 10 October, p. 5.
Rieff, D. (2008). *Swimming in a Sea of Death*. New York: Simon & Schuster.
Roe, G. (2017). *Shattered: Surviving the Loss of a Child*. New York: Healing Resources.
Roe, G. (2019). *Comfort for the Grieving Spouse's Heart: Hope and Healing After Losing Your Partner*. New York: Bowker.

Rose, J. (2020). 'To Die One's Own Death', *London Review of Books*, 19 November, pp. 39–43.
Roth, P. (2006). *Everyman*. New York: Houghton Mifflin.
Rowles, G. and Bernard, M. (eds) (2013). *Environmental Gerontology: Making Meaningful Places in Old Age*. New York: Springer.
Roxby, P. (2020). 'Are COVID Patients Getting Younger?', *BBC News*, 22 December, <https://www.bbc.co.uk/news/health-55586994>, accessed 22 December.
Sage, M., Inman, P. and McKie, R. (2020). 'Johnson's U-turn Puts Country Under Tough New Lockdown', *The Observer*, 1 November, pp. 1–7.
Samarel, N. (1995). 'The Dying Process'. In H. Wass and R. A. Neimeyer (eds), *Dying: Facing the Facts*, pp. 89–116. New York: Routledge.
Sample, I. (2021). 'UK Health Inequalities Made Worse by COVID Crisis, Study Suggests', *The Guardian*, 14 June, <https://www.theguardian.com/world/2021/jun/14/uk-health-inequalities-made-worse-by-covid-crisis-study-sugge sts>, accessed 14 June 2021.
Samuel, J. (2017). *Grief Works: Stories of Life, Death and Surviving*. Harmondsworth: Penguin.
Sartre, J.-P. (1965). *Nausea*. Harmondsworth: Penguin.
Savage, M. and Trapper, J. (2021). 'Patients were Sent Back to Care Homes Without COVID Test Despite Bosses' Plea', *The Observer*, 29 May, p. 7.
Scarre, G. (2009). 'Dying and Philosophy'. In A. Kellehear (ed.), *The Study of Dying. From Autonomy to Transformation*, pp. 147–54. Cambridge: Cambridge University Press.
Schrader, S. L., Nelson, M. A. and Eidsness, L. M. (2009). 'Dying to Know: A Community Survey About Dying and End-of-life Care'. *Omega*, 60 (1), 33–50.
Schumacher, B. M. (2010). *Death and Mortality in Contemporary Philosophy*. Cambridge: Cambridge University Press.
Scobie, S. and Hutchings, R. (2022). *End of Life Explained*. London: Nuffield Trust, <https://www.nuffieldtrust.org.uk/resource/end-of-life-care-explained-what-is-it-how-is-it-provided-and-what-are-the-challenges>, accessed 20 May 2022.
Segal, L. (2012). *Out of Time: The Pleasures and Perlis of Ageing*. London: Verso.
Seymour, J., Gott, M., Bellamy, G., Ahmedzai, S. H. and Clark, D. (2004). 'Planning for End of Life: The Views of Older People About Advanced Care Statements', *Social Science and Medicine*, 59 (1), 75–86.
Shapiro, S. (2019). *Speaking for Dying*. Chicago: University of Chicago Press.
Sherwood, H. (2020). 'UK Councils Begin to ban funeral ceremonies due to coronavirus, *The Guardian*, 4 April,< https://www.theguardian.com/world/2020/apr/04/uk-councils-begin-to-ban-funeral-ceremonies-due-to-coronavi rus, >accessed 4 April 2020.

Sherwood, H. and Pidd, H. (2020). 'My rabbi's tools now include a phone: UK Jewish burials changed by Covid-19', *The Guardian*, May 14,< https://www.theguardian.com/world/2020/may/14/my-rabbis-tools-now-include-a-phone-uk-jewish-burials-changed-by-covid-19, > accessed 14 May 2020.

Shriver, L. (2021). *Should We Stay or Should We Go?* London: Borough Press.

Siddell, M. (1995). *Health in old Age: Myth, Mystery and Management.* Buckingham: Open University.

Simmel, G. (2007 [1910]). 'Metaphysics of death', *Theory, Culture and Society*, vol. 24 (7–8), 72–77.

Sloane, D. C. (2018). *Is the Cemetery Dead.* Chicago: University of Chicago Press.

Small, H. (2007). *The Long Life.* Oxford: Oxford University Press.

Smith, C. (2020). 'The structural vulnerability of healthcare workers during COVID-19:Observations on the social context of risk and the equitable distribution of resources', *Social Science and Medicine,* 258, 1-4.

Smith, V. D. (2020). *Arts of Dying: Literature and finitude in Medieval England.* Chicago: Chicago University Press.

Sofka, C. J., Gibson, A. and Silberm, D. R. (2017). 'Digital Immortality or Digital Death?'. In M. Hviid Jacobson (ed.), *Postmortal Society*, pp. 97–121. London: Routledge.

Sontag, S. (1978). *Illness as Metaphor.* London: Picador.

Spark, M. (1972) *Memento Mori.* Harmondsworth: Penguin.

Spiegehalter, D. (2020). 'How Much 'Normal' Risk Does COVID Represent?' Winton Centre', Cambridge University, <https://medium.com/wintoncentre/how-much-normal-risk-does-covid-represent-4539118e1196>, accessed 1 October 2020.

Spiegelhalter, D. and Masters, A. (2021). 'Why Most People Who Now Die with COVID in England have Been Vaccinated', *The Guardian,* 27 June, <https://www.theguardian.com/theobserver/commentisfree/2021/jun/27/why-most-people-who-now-die-with-covid-have-been-vaccinated>, accessed 27 June 2021.

Spinney, L. (2017). *Pale Rider: The Spanish Flu of1918 and How it Changed the World.* New York: Vintage Books.

Spinney, L. (2021). 'How Elimination Versus Suppression Became COVID's Cold War', *The Guardian*, 3 March, <https://www.theguardian.com/commentisfree/2021/mar/03/covid-19-elimination-versus-suppression>, accessed 3 March 2021.

Sridhar, D. (2022). *Preventable: How a Pandemic Changed the World and How to Stop the Next One.* London: Viking.

Srivastava, R. (2020). 'Instead of Prolonging Life, a Dying Patient's Final Wish is an Antidote for Our Times', *The Guardian*, 1 September, <https://www.theguard

ian.com/commentisfree/2020/sep/02/instead-of-prolonging-life-a-dying-patients-final-wish-is-an-antidote-for-our-times>, accessed 1 September 2020.

Stanworth, R. (2004). *Recognizing Spiritual Needs in People Who are Dying.* Oxford: Oxford University Press.

Starck, N. (2007). 'Revelation, Intrusion, and Questions of Taste: The Ethical Change for Obituary Editors', *Journalism Practice*, 1 (3), 373–82.

Standaret, M. (2021). 'Even Mourning is Said to Shame China', *The Observer*, 10 January, p. 30.

Stark, A. (2016). *The Consolations of Mortality: Making Sense of Death.* New Haven, CT: Yale University Press.

Steffen, E. and Coyle, A. (2010). 'Can "Sense of Presence" Experiences in Bereavement Be Conceptualised as Spiritual Phenomena?', *Mental Health, Religion and Culture,* 13 (3), 273–91.

Stevernik, N., Westerhof, G. J., Bode, C. and Ditmann-Kohli, F. (2001). 'The Personal Experience of Aging, Individual Resources, and Subjective Well-Being', *The Journals of Gerontology: Series B*, 56 (6), 364–73.

Stewart, H. (2022). 'Johnson Announces Terms of Reference for COVID Inquiry', *The Guardian*, 10 March, <https://www.theguardian.com/world/2022/mar/10/cabinet-office-announces-terms-of-reference-for-covid-inquiry>, accessed 10 March 2022.

Stillion, J. (1995). 'Death in the Lives of Adults'. In H. Wass and R. A. Neimeyer (eds), *Dying: Facing the Facts,* pp. 303–22. London: Routledge.

Storr, A. (1997). *Solitude*. London: HarperCollins.

Stroebe, M. and Schut, H. (1991). 'Does "Grief Work" Work?', *Journal of Consulting and Clinical Psychology*, 59, 479–82.

Stroebe, M. and Schut, H. (1999). 'The Dual Process Model of Coping with Bereavement', *Death Studies*, 23, 197–224.

Strout, E. (2008). *Olive Kitteridge*. New York: Random House.

Sweeting, H. and Gilhooly, M. (1997). 'Dementia and the Phenomenon of Social Death', *Sociology of Health & Illness*, 19(1), 93–117.

Swets, M. C., Russell, C. D., Harrison, E. M., Docherty, A. and Girvan, M. (2022). 'SARS-CoV-2 co-infection with influenza viruses, respiratory syncytial virus, or adenoviruses', *The Lancet*, 25 March, <https://doi.org/10.1016/S0140-6736(22)00383-X>, accessed 18 March 2022.

Tapper, J. (2020).'UK Care Homes Still Denied COVID Tests Despite Hancock Pledge, Officials Warn', *The Guardian*, 29 August, <https://www.theguardian.com/society/2020/aug/29/uk-care-homes-still-denied-covid-tests-despite-hancock-pledge-officials-warn>, accessed 29 August 2020.

Taylor, C. (2016). *Dying.* Sydney: Canongate Books.

Teggi, D. (2020). 'Care Homes as Hospices for the Prevalent Form of Dying: An Analysis of Long Term Care Provision Towards the End of Life in England', *Social Science & Medicine*, 260, 1–15.

Tergesen, A. (2020). 'How COVID-19 will Change Ageing and Reinterment', *The Wall Street Journal*, 15 November, p. 7.

Ternestedt, B. M. and Franklin, L. L. (2006). 'Ways of Relating to Death: Views of Older People Resident in Nursing Homes', *International Journal of Palliative Nursing*, 12 (7), 334–40.

Thomas, R. (2022). 'COVID Rule Changes Leave Clinically Vulnerable as "Collateral Damage", Charities Warn', *Independent*, 21 January, p. 5.

Thompson, J. B. (2011). 'Shifting Boundaries of Public and Private Life', *Theory, Culture & Society*, 28 (4), 49–70.

Thonnes, M. and Jakoby, N. (2013). 'Where People Die: A Critical Review', *Medical Sociology Online,* 7 (1): 8–19.

Tomer, A. and Eliason, G. (2013). 'Existentialism and Death Attitudes. In A. Tomer, G. Eliason and P. Wong (eds), *Existential and Spiritual in Issues in Death Attitudes,* pp. 25–47. Mahwah, NJ: Lawrence Erlbaum.

Toolis, K. (2017). *My Father's Wake: How the Irish Teach Us to Live, Love and Die.* London: Weidenfeld and Nicolson.

Tooze, A. (2021). *Shutdown: How COVID Shook the World's Economy.* London: Allen Lane.

Townsend, P. (1979). *Poverty in the United Kingdom.* London: Allen Lane.

Trapper, J. (2020) 'They Don't Put Loneliness on Death Certificates', *The Observer*, 8 November, p. 20.

Trapper, J. (2021). 'Intensive Care Staff Tell of Being Overwhelmed by COVID Traumas', *The Observer,* 14 March, p. 12.

Troyer, J. (2020). *Technologies of the Human Corpse.* Cambridge, MA: MIT Press.

Tulle, E. (2015). 'Theorizing Embodiment and Ageing'. In J. Twigg and W. Martin (eds), *Routledge Handbook of Cultural Gerontology*, pp. 125–32. London: Routledge.

Tyler, A. (1995). *Ladders of Years.* New York: Knopf.

Twigg, J. (2006). *The Body in Health and Social Care*. London: Palgrave.

UK Government (2021). *Health Profile for England: 2021*, <https://fingertips.phe.org.uk/static-reports/health-profile-for-england/hpfe_report.html>, accessed 2 May 2022.

UK Parliament (2020). *Readying the NHS and Social Care for the Covid-19 Peak*, <repohttps://publications.parliament.uk/pa/cm5801/cmselect/cmpubacc/405/40505.htmrt>, accessed 12 May 2021.

UK Parliament (2021). *Coronavirus: Lessons Learned to Date*. London: UK Government.

Updike, J. (2009). *My Father's Tears.* New York: Knopf.

Uscinski, J. and Enders, A. (2020). 'The Coronavirus Conspiracy Boom', *The Atlantic*, 30 April, <https://www.theatlantic.com/health/archive/2020/04/what-can-coronavirus-tell-us-about-conspiracy-theories/610894>, accessed 14 December 2020.

van Kessel, P., Baranovski, C., Scheller, A. and Smith, A. (2022). *In Their Own Words, Americans Describe the Struggles and Silver Linings of the COVID-19 Pandemic*, Pew Research Center, <https://www.pewresearch.org/2021/03/05/in-their-own-words-americans-describe-the-struggles-and-silver-linings-of-the-covid-19-pandemic>, accessed 6 March 2022.

Veatch, R. (1995). 'The Definition of Death'. In H. Wass and R. A. Neimeyer (eds), *Dying: Facing the Facts*, pp. 406–43. London: Routledge.

Vulliamy, E. (2020). 'Will COVID Change Italy?', *New York Review of Books*, 24 September, pp. 82–85.

Walker, A. (2018). 'Why the UK Needs a Social Policy on Ageing', *Journal of Social Policy*, 47 (2), 253–73.

Walker, C. C. (2021). 'Predatory Financial Tactics are Putting the Very Survival of the UK Care System at Risk', *The Guardian*,10 August, <https://www.theguardian.com/commentisfree/2021/aug/10/predatory-financial-tactics-survival-uk-care-system-at-risk>, accessed 10August 2021.

Walker, P. (2020). 'No 10 Denies Claim Dominic Cummings Argued to "Let Old People Die"', *The Observer,* 22 March, p. 9.

Walter, T. (1994). *The Revival of Death.* London: Routledge.

Walter, T. (1996). 'A New Model of Grief: Bereavement and Biography', *Mortality*, 1(1), 7–25.

Walter, T. (2017). *What Death Means Now.* Bristol: Policy Press.

Walter, T. (2020). *Death in the Modern World.* London. London: Sage.

Wanless, D. (2006). *Securing Good Care for Older People.* London. The King's Fund, <https://www.kingsfund.org.uk/publications>, accessed 25 May 2021.

Warner, A. (2018). *Grief Day by Day: Simple Practices and Daily Guidance for Living with Loss*. London: Althea Press.

Warnock, M. and Macdonald, E. (2008). *Easeful Death: Is There a Case for Assisted Dying?* Oxford: Oxford University Press.

Ware, B. (2012). *Top Five Regrets of the Dying.* Carlsbad, CA: Hay House.

Waytt-Brown, A. (2019). *The Big Move: Life Between the Turning Points.* Bloomington, IN: Indiana University Press.

Webb, E. (2020). 'Coronavirus Risk for Older People: The Updated Picture', *Age UK,* <https://www.ageuk.org.uk/discover/2020/06/coronavirus-risk-for-older-people-updated>, accessed 30 September20202.

Weeks, J. (2020). '"An Operational Tsunami": Preparing for a winter surge of COVID-19', *The Guardian*, 30 October,<https://www.theguardian.com/world/2020/oct/30/tsunami-preparing-winter-surge-of-covid-19-university-hospital-coventry>, accessed 30 October 2020.

Welby, J. and Cottrell, S. (2021). 'Letter to the Nation', <https://mcusercontent.com/50eac70851c7245ce1ce00c45/files/c04ce5c3-bbc7-459b-ac6e63aef1f1f31d/20210126_Letter_to_the_nation.pdf?mc_cid=5d6c6a5473&mc_eid=a6fd5d539>, accessed 5 February 2021.

Wicks, E. (2017). 'The Legal Definition of Death and the Right to Life'. In S. McCorristine (ed.), *Interdisciplinary Perspectives on Mortality and Its Timings,* pp. 119–31. London: Palgrave.

Wielnik van, J., Wilhelm, L. and Geelen-Merks, D. (2020). *Loss, Grief, and Attachment in Life Transitions*. London: Routledge.

Wilkinson, I. (2005). *Suffering. Sociological Introduction*. Cambridge: Polity Press.

Willetts, D. (2011). *The Pinch: How the Baby Boomers Took Their Children's Future.* New York: Atlantic Books.

Wittenberg, R., Hu, B. and Hancock, R. (2018). *Projections of Demand and Expenditure on Adult Social Care 2015 to 2040*. London: Personal Social Services Research Unit, London School of Economics, <https://www.pssru.ac.uk/pub/5421.pdf>, accessed 20 January 2022.

Wolfelt, A. D. (2011). *Creating Meaningful Funeral Experiences: A Guide for Caregivers.* Fort Collins, CO: Companion.

Wolpert, L. (2011). *You're Looking Very Well.* London: Faber and Faber.

Wood, A. (2021). *Caritas: Neighbourly Love and the Early Modern Self.* Oxford: Oxford University Press.

Woodhead, L. (2016). 'The Rise of "No Religion" in Britain: The Emergence of a New Cultural Majority', The British Academy Lecture, <https://www.thebritishacademy.ac.uk/documents/1043/11_Woodhead_1825.pdf>, accessed 23 October 2021.

Woolhouse, M. (2022). *The Year the World Went Mad: Scientific Memoir*. Edinburgh: Sandstone Press.

Wootton, S. (2020). *Last Rights: The Case for Assisted Dying (Provocations).* London: Biteback.

World Health Organization (WHO). (2022). 'Dementia', <https://www.who.int/news-room/fact-sheets/detail/dementia>, accessed 20 June 2022.

Wright, L. (2020). 'How Pandemics Wreak Havoc – and Open Minds', *The New Yorker*, 13 June, p. 13.

Xiang, X., Lu, X., Halavanu, A., Xue, J., Sun, Y., Ho, P., Xue, J., Sun, L. and Wu, Z. (2020). 'Pandemic: An Examination of Public Discourse and Sentiment About Older Adults and COVID-19 Using Machine Learning', *The Journals*

of Gerontology: Series B, 76(4) <https://doi.org/10.1093/geronb/gbaa128>, accessed 27 October 2020.
Yong, E. (2022). 'The Final Pandemic Betrayal', *The Atlantic,* 13 April, <https://www.theatlantic.com/author/ed-yong>, accessed 1 June 2022
Zimmermann, C. (2012). 'Acceptance of Dying: A Discourse Analysis of Palliative Care Literature', *Social Science & Medicine*, 75, 217–24.
Zizek, S. (2020). *Pandemic! COVID-19 Shakes the World.* Cambridge: Polity Press.
Zuckerman, P. (2008). *Society Without God: What the Least Religious Nation Can Tell Us About*. New York: New York University Press.

Index

www.ingramcontent.com/pod-product-compliance
Ingram Content Group UK Ltd.
Pitfield, Milton Keynes, MK11 3LW, UK
UKHW021845100926
8556IPUK00019B/1064

9 781800 790025